DATE DUE

3-22-99	11-7		
FEB 2 5	NOV 0 6 2005		
4-20	6-30		
MAR 2 4 2000			
11-28	MAR 2 8 2006		
NOV 3 2000	10-23		
4-23	DEC 1 2 2006		
APR 2 8 2002	4/9		
12/20	APR 2 2 2007		
JAN 1 6 2003	SEP 1 7 2014		
12/19			
DEC 1 0 2004			
5-5			
APR 1 9 2005			PRINTED IN U.S.A.

Alzheimer's Disease
A Handbook for Caregivers

Third Edition

Alzheimer's Disease
A Handbook for Caregivers

Third Edition

Editors

Ronald C Hamdy, MD, FACP, FRCP
Professor of Medicine
Cecile Cox Quillen Professor of Geriatric Medicine and Gerontology
James H Quillen College of Medicine
East Tennessee State University;
Associate Chief of Staff, Extended Care and Geriatrics
James H Quillen Veterans Affairs Medical Center
Johnson City, Tennessee

James M Turnbull, MD, FRCP (C)
Medical Director, Outpatient Service, Frontier Health, Inc
Kingsport, Tennessee;
Clinical Professor of Family Practice and Psychiatry
East Tennessee State University
Johnson City, Tennessee

Joellen Edwards, PhD, RN
Interim Vice President for Health Affairs
Dean and Professor, College of Nursing
East Tennessee State University
Johnson City, Tennessee

Mary M Lancaster, RNC, MSN
Consultant, Center for Geriatrics and Gerontology;
Adjunct Clinical Instructor, College of Nursing
East Tennessee State University;
Clinical Nurse Specialist, Gerontology
James H Quillen Veterans Affairs Medical Center
Johnson City, Tennessee

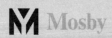 Mosby

St. Louis Baltimore Boston Carlsbad Chicago Minneapolis New York Philadelphia Portland
London Milan Sydney Tokyo Toronto

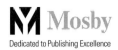

Dedicated to Publishing Excellence

A Times Mirror
Company

Vice President and Publisher: Nancy L. Coon
Editor: Jeff Burnham
Developmental Editor: Jeff Downing
Project Manager: John Rogers
Designer: Yael Kats
Manufacturing Manager: Don Carlisle
Original Illustrations: © Steve Braund, 1997

Printed in the United States of America
Composition by Graphic World, Inc.
Printing/binding by R. R. Donnelley & Sons Company

Mosby–Year Book, Inc.
11830 Westline Industrial Drive
St. Louis, Missouri 63146

Library of Congress Cataloging in Publication Data
Alzheimer's disease: a handbook for caregivers / Ronald C. Hamdy . . .
   [et al.].—3rd ed.
      p.   cm.
   Includes bibliographical references and index.
   ISBN 0-8151-2606-9
   1. Alzheimer's disease.   2. Alzheimer's disease—Nursing.
3. Alzheimer's disease—Social aspects.   I. Hamdy, R. C.
RC523.A386   1997
616.8'31—dc21   97-14558
                                                           CIP

97 98 99 00 01 / 9 8 7 6 5 4 3 2 1

Contributors

Lynda C Abusamra, PhD, RN, SC
Department of Adult Nursing
College of Nursing
East Tennessee State University
Johnson City, Tennessee

Judge Lynn W Brown
Criminal Court
1st Judicial District
Johnson City, Tennessee

Curtis B Clark, MD
Department of Family Practice
University of Tennessee, Health
   Service Center
Jackson, Tennessee

Warren G Clark, BSN, MS
Clinical Nurse Specialist
Catawba Hospital
Catawba, Virginia

JoAnn Cox, LCSW
Coordinator, Outpatient Services
Fairview Associates
Kingsport, Tennessee

Nancy Erickson, MBA
Educational Consultant to Healthcare
   Associations
Chicago, Illinois

Kevin F Gray, MD
Departments of Psychiatry and
   Neurology
University of Texas Southwestern
   Medical Center
Dallas Veterans Affairs Medical
   Center
Dallas, Texas

Ronald C Hamdy, MD, FACP, FRCP
Professor of Medicine
Cecile Cox Quillen Professor of
   Geriatric Medicine and
   Gerontology

James H Quillen College of Medicine
East Tennessee State University;
Associate Chief of Staff, Extended
   Care and Geriatrics
James H Quillen Veterans Affairs
   Medical Center
Johnson City, Tennessee

Larry B Hudgins, MD, FACP
Professor of Medicine
James H Quillen College of Medicine
East Tennessee State University;
Associate Chief of Staff, Ambulatory
   Care
James H Quillen Veterans Affairs
   Medical Center
Johnson City, Tennessee

Lissy F Jarvik, MD, PhD
Distinguished Physician (Emer)
Director, Upbeat and Get Smart
   Programs
West Los Angeles Veterans Affairs
   Medical Center and
Research Professor
Department of Psychiatry and
   Behavioral Sciences
Neuropsychiatric Institute and
   Hospital
University of California
Los Angeles, California

Marcia M Johnson, RNC, BSN, MEd
Nurse Manager, Extended Care &
   Geriatrics
James H Quillen Veterans Affairs
   Medical Center
Johnson City, Tennessee

Linda J Kerley, PhD, RN, CS
Department of Adult Nursing
College of Nursing
East Tennessee State University
Johnson City, Tennessee

Mary M Lancaster, RNC, MSN
Consultant, Center for Geriatrics and
  Gerontology;
Adjunct Clinical Instructor, College of
  Nursing
East Tennessee State University;
Clinical Nurse Specialist, Gerontology
James H Quillen Veterans Affairs
  Medical Center
Johnson City, Tennessee

Eleanor P Lavretsky, MD, PhD
Research Psychopharmacologist
West Los Angeles Veterans Affairs
  Medical Center and Neuro-
  psychiatric Institute and Hospital
University of California
Los Angeles, California

Fredda L Leiter, MD
Clinical Instructor
Neuropsychiatric Institute and
  Hospital
University of California
Los Angeles, California

Sharon Wyatt Moore, MD, MBA
Assistant Professor in Geriatric
  Medicine
Clinical Professor of Family Medicine
James H Quillen College of Medicine
East Tennessee State University;
Staff Physician, Extended Care
James H Quillen Veterans Affairs
  Medical Center
Johnson City, Tennessee

Jorge G Ruiz, MD
Assistant Professor in Geriatric
  Medicine
Clinical Professor of Family Medicine
James H Quillen College of Medicine
East Tennessee State University;
Medical Director, Nursing Home
  Care Unit and Geriatric Evaluation
  and Management Unit
James H Quillen Veterans Affairs
  Medical Center
Johnson City, Tennessee

Lorraine Sambat, RN
Nurse, Medical Ethicist
Johnson City, Tennessee

Patrick Sloan, PhD
Clinical Associate Professor
Department of Psychiatry and
  Behavioral Sciences
Department of Internal Medicine
James H Quillen College of Medicine
East Tennessee State University;
Chief, Department of Psychology
James H Quillen Veterans Affairs
  Medical Center
Johnson City, Tennessee

Vicente Taasan, MD
Chief, Nuclear Medicine Service
James H Quillen Veterans Affairs
  Medical Center
Johnson City, Tennessee

Elizabeth A Turnbull, BA
Research Assistant, J&S Turnbull
  Consulting
Johnson City, Tennessee

James M Turnbull, MD, FRCP (C)
Staff Psychiatrist, Central Appalachia
  Services, Inc
Kingsport, Tennessee;
Clinical Professor of Family Practice
  and Psychiatry
East Tennessee State University
Johnson City, Tennessee

Sharon Turnbull, BS (N), MPH, PhD
Director, Student Health Services
Clinical Associate Professor of Family
  Practice, Psychiatry and Nursing
East Tennessee State University
Johnson City, Tennessee

Lynda Weatherly RN, MSN, C-ANP
Assistant Professor of Nursing
Jackson State Community College;
Facilitator, Alzheimer's Family
  Support Group,

Jackson-Madison County General
    Hospital
Jackson, Tennessee

Sheryl Williams, BS
Educational Consultant to Healthcare
    Associations
Chicago, Illinois

Reviewers

Joan Fritsch Needham, MSEd, RNC
Director of Education
DeKalb City Nursing Home
DeKalb, Illinois

Geraldine Strachan, RN, MSNEd
Nursing Education Supervisor
The George G Glenner Alzheimer's
    Family Centers, Inc
San Diego, California

To
our patients with Alzheimer's disease

and to
their relatives and caregivers,
from whom we have learned
and continue to learn so much

Foreword from First Edition ————————————————•

The full tragedy of Alzheimer's disease, which affects one out of every ten Americans over the age of 65, was impressed upon me during a series of Congressional hearings I chaired in 1984. At a hearing in Tennessee, a woman whose husband suffers from Alzheimer's offered testimony I will never forget. "A few months ago," she began, "my husband asked me to go into the bedroom—we needed to talk privately," he said. I went to the room and closed the door. Turning to me with tears in his eyes he asked, 'Am I losing my mind, honey? Am I going crazy?'" She went on: "My life can be described as a funeral that never ends . . . I want my husband back."

That woman is not alone. Two to three million "never-ending funerals" are sapping the strength of both victims and their families across America. A concerted effort is long overdue to defeat this disease, which erodes the mental and physical health of the patient before his or her time. Part of the solution lies in research to uncover the causes of the disease and develop treatments for it. Just as crucial, however, is ensuring that those who take care of patients with Alzheimer's know as much about the problem as possible.

That is one reason I am so pleased with *Alzheimer's Disease: A Handbook for Caregivers,* which contains a wealth of practical information about the effects of Alzheimer's on the patient's day-to-day life. The book offers detailed descriptions of the stages of the disease, the options for treatment, and the effects of other mental and physical characteristics upon the expression of Alzheimer's. It also offers valuable suggestions for approaching issues such as nutrition, sleep habits, and therapy. The book is a perfect bridge between those who know most about the disease—and those who know most about the patient.

Congress, by establishing regional centers devoted to the research and treatment of Alzheimer's, has taken one step in the right direction. The medical faculty at East Tennessee State University, by creating this fine book, has taken another. Perhaps, through more efforts like these, we can begin to lift some of the fear and uncertainty that surround this national tragedy.

Albert Gore, Jr.
Vice President of the United States

Preface

Alzheimer's disease is often referred to as the "disease of the century." It afflicts approximately 4 million Americans, mostly those over the age of 65. It is the harshest of all incurable diseases because it hits its victim twice. First, the mind dies, slowly and irrevocably, until even the simplest tasks become insurmountable. Then, after many years, the body dies.

Alzheimer's disease is even more devastating for the families and caregivers of its victims. The caregivers often drive themselves to physical and emotional exhaustion while rendering continuous care and experiencing the anguish of seeing a loved one turn into a person who no longer remembers who he or she is.

This is the third edition of a book that was first published in 1990 in response to requests from caregivers in our community following courses and a series of lectures developed in our area. The attendance at these lectures was staggering. Many caregivers braved inclement weather to attend them. We were impressed by the eagerness of caregivers to better understand the disease and how it affects its victims. The time allotted to questions at the end of each lecture had to be greatly expanded. Caregivers wanted to know how best to help and continue helping loved ones or patients under their care.

We recognized the need for a comprehensive book that addresses many of the issues faced by caregivers, which we will define as follows: individuals who care for victims of Alzheimer's disease at home and health care professionals who care for patients in nursing homes. Although a great deal of information is available for professionals and the lay public, we felt there was a need for this particular book. We were very pleased by the reception it received and the opportunity we were given to revise it in the next two editions.

Most of the authors we have selected to write the chapters are actively involved in the care of patients with Alzheimer's disease and are also involved in various local, regional, and national organizations that serve patients and families of patients with Alzheimer's disease. As in the previous two editions, we are emphasizing the need to keep the information on a down-to-earth, practical level.

While preparing the third edition of our book we have taken into account various comments and suggestions made by our readers. We feel these have increased the practical usefulness of the book. We made the following changes in the third edition in content, organization, and features based on our readers' and reviewers' comments in an effort to make the information more accessible to all professionals, laypersons, and family caregivers:

- Chapter 1, "Alzheimer's Disease: An Overview," is a new chapter that sets the stage for the rest of the book and provides a broad overview of the disease and related issues.
- Chapter 20, "Terminal Care of the Patient," is a new chapter designed to provide an understanding of the special issues involved in caring for patients in the end stage of the disease.
- Chapter 23, "Stress in Caregivers," combines two separate chapters on stress for caregivers and stress in nursing care from the second edition to identify the

common stress factors that affect anyone caring for or living with a person with Alzheimer's and to discuss strategies for managing the stress.
- Two new appendixes provide addresses, phone numbers, and Internet addresses of Alzheimer's organizations and additional references as resources for caregivers and families interested in learning more about the disease.
- Key points highlighted throughout the text provide rapid access to key information.
- Coverage of newly released medications such as Aricept that are being used to manage the symptoms of Alzheimer's disease is provided.
- Many new illustrations are included throughout the text to make the presentation of the material more interesting and accessible.

As in the past two editions, the contents of the book should be valuable to nursing assistants, health care professionals, and the lay public. We have retained the glossary, located at the end of the book, which explains most of the technical terms used. Similarly, although the authors have attempted to be as accurate as possible with regard to drug dosages, readers are advised to consult the *Physicians' Desk Reference* for the dosages, indications, and contraindications of various medications that have been referred to.

We believe we are living through historical times; major advances have been made in the diagnosis and treatment of Alzheimer's disease. Very significant progress also has been made in defining the causes of the disease. In the relatively short period since writing the first edition, two medications have been approved by the Food and Drug Administration for the treatment of Alzheimer's disease.

Our dearest wish is that there will be no need for a fourth edition of the book because an effective and safe therapy will be available.

We hope that as we move toward the next century the "disease of the century" will soon become the "disease of the PAST century" and will soon be in the same category as most other readily treatable diseases.

Ronald C Hamdy
James M Turnbull
Joellen Edwards
Mary M Lancaster

Acknowledgments

We thank all our colleagues who have referred to us patients with dementing illnesses, including Alzheimer's disease, thus allowing us to gain a wider experience in this field. We also thank the patients' relatives and caregivers, who have given us so much information and insight on the illness and its impact on their lives. We thank the staff at Mosby, in particular Jeff Burnham, for their work on this book. Finally, we thank Kathy Whalen and Janice Lyons for their painstaking secretarial work and efficient help in producing this manuscript.

Contents ━━━━━━━━━━━━━━━━━━━━━━━━━━━━━━━━━●

1   **Alzheimer's Disease: an Overview, 1**
Ronald C Hamdy
James M Turnbull

Unit One
The Normal Brain

  2   **Higher Brain Functions, 11**
Patrick Sloan

  3   **Neuropsychological Assessment of Dementia, 27**
Patrick Sloan

  4   **Imaging the Brain in Alzheimer's Disease, 41**
Vicente Taasan

Unit Two
Alzheimer's Disease

  5   **Historical Perspectives, 51**
Lorraine Sambat

  6   **Etiology and Pathogenesis: Current Concepts, 60**
Eleanor P Lavretsky
Fredda L Leiter
Lissy F Jarvik

  7   **Clinical Presentation, 74**
Ronald C Hamdy

  8   **Clinical Diagnosis, 87**
James M Turnbull

  9   **Factors that Aggravate the Symptoms, 104**
Ronald C Hamdy
Larry B Hudgins

  10   **Other Dementias, 117**
Jorge G Ruiz

Unit Three
Management

11   General Principles of Management, 143
Lynda C Abusamra

12   Management of Difficult Behaviors, 150
Mary M Lancaster
Lynda C Abusamra
Warren G Clark

13   Psychopharmacology in Dementia, 171
James M Turnbull

14   Specific Drug Therapy, 183
Sharon Wyatt Moore

15   Urinary and Fecal Incontinence, 199
Ronald C Hamdy
Larry B Hudgins

16   Management of Urinary Incontinence, 213
Mary M Lancaster

17   Safety and Accident Prevention, 227
Mary M Lancaster

18   Daily Care and Management, 243
Mary M Lancaster

19   Developing a Day's Activity, 259
James M Turnbull
Elizabeth A Turnbull

20   Terminal Care of the Patient, 276
Marcia M Johnson
Mary M Lancaster

Unit Four
Special Issues

21   Ethical Issues, 293
Sharon Turnbull

22   Legal Issues for Caregivers, 306
Lynn W Brown

23   **Stress in Caregivers, 316**
     Linda J Kerley
     James M Turnbull

24   **Elder Abuse, 328**
     Curtis B Clark
     Lynda Weatherly

Unit Five
Community Support

25   **Caregiver Education and Support, 341**
     Mary M Lancaster

26   **Social Services, 354**
     JoAnn Cox

27   **The Alzheimer's Association, 367**
     Nancy Erickson
     Sheryl Williams

28   **Dementia Care Units, 377**
     Larry B Hudgins

Unit Six
Future Prospects

29   **Promising Areas of Research, 393**
     Robert A Kuwik
     Judith A Martin

Appendix A
     Some Useful Addresses and Phone Numbers, 399

Appendix B
     Additional References, 415

     Glossary, 423

Alzheimer's Disease
A Handbook for Caregivers

Third Edition

Alzheimer's Disease: an Overview

Ronald C Hamdy
James M Turnbull

*Science tells us what we can know, but what we
can know is little, and if we forget how much
we cannot know, we become insensitive to
many things of great importance.*

—Bertrand Russell

The announcement by Ronald Reagan that he had Alzheimer's disease galvanized the American public into recognizing their own vulnerability in a way no other public figure has done. Norman Rockwell and Rita Hayworth, both victims of Alzheimer's disease, were beloved and admired, but they were not former presidents of the United States and did not have the aura of the former president. As a direct result of this announcement, President Reagan challenged politicians and lawmakers to properly fund research into the cause and treatment of this disease.

—• Alzheimer's disease is often referred to as the "disease of the century."

In addition to affecting the patient and caregivers, Alzheimer's disease has very significant social and economic implications. It is identified as "dementia of the Alzheimer's type" in the fourth edition of the *Diagnostic and Statistical Manual of Mental Disorders* (DSM-IV). Alzheimer's disease illustrates and emphasizes the concept of the global village: when a person is afflicted by Alzheimer's disease, it is not only that person who suffers, but also the family, neighbors, friends, relatives, and society by and large. As John Donne said, no man is an island.

Alzheimer's disease is the most common cause of dementia. It now afflicts nearly 4 million Americans. These numbers are expected to increase dramatically as the U.S. population ages. By the year 2050 approximately 14.5 million people will suffer from Alzheimer's disease.

Alzheimer's disease is not part of the normal aging process, although it affects predominantly elderly people. Whereas only 10% of those 65 years of age and older are affected by this disease, the percentage may be as high as 48% in those 85 years of age and older.

ECONOMIC IMPLICATIONS

▬▬● The annual cost of Alzheimer's disease exceeds $100 billion.

The annual cost of nursing care, social services, caregivers' time, and medical care for Alzheimer's disease is estimated at over $100 billion a year. These figures make Alzheimer's disease the third most expensive disease in the U.S., after heart disease and cancer. In 1991 the total Medicaid cost for Alzheimer's disease was $5.7 billion, exceeding the $4.2 billion total cost for acquired immunodeficiency syndrome (AIDS) during that year.

In 1991 the lifetime costs for the patient and caregivers were estimated to total $47,500 for direct costs such as physician visits, diagnostic tests, hospital care, nursing home care, medication, day care, respite care, and transportation services. The costs went up to $174,000 when unpaid informal caregiver services provided by family and friends and the value of time lost by the patient and caregivers from productive activities were taken into account.

The expected increase in the prevalence of this disease will have significant implications on the health care system in the U.S., especially with the present tendency to change from a fee-for-service health insurance plan to a managed care model of health care–delivery system.

The number of Medicare recipients who are enrolled in managed care plans has steadily increased from approximately 800,000 in 1985 to 1.5 million in 1990, 3.1 million in 1995, and 5 million in 1996. By the turn of the century, as many as 12.6 million are expected to be enrolled in this program.

Patients with Alzheimer's disease consistently use more health care resources than the rest of the population in the following areas: trips to the emergency room, physicians visits, and hospitalizations. The median length of stay in nursing homes for patients with Alzheimer's disease is over 10 times the national average for all other diagnoses, including strokes and hip fractures. It is also not uncommon for patients with severe dementia to receive more intensive care than those with mild-to-moderate dementia. Patients with Alzheimer's disease use hospital facilities nearly twice as frequently as controls over the age of 45 years. The financial implications of Alzheimer's disease are therefore staggering.

Nearly half of all caregivers share a residence with the patient, making caregiving a full-time, 24-hour–a–day job. Although most caregivers describe their task as a "labor of love," the majority admit that this task is frustrating, draining, depressing, and painful, and it leads to family stress. Many admit not getting enough sleep. Caregivers whose loved one is in a nursing home or other institution report being depressed more often than those whose loved one is at home. The psychological, physical, social, and economic impacts on family caregivers cannot be overlooked. Family caregivers are often called the "hidden victims" of Alzheimer's disease.

ETIOLOGY

The exact cause of Alzheimer's disease remains obscure, but several hypotheses have been put forward. Some forms of the disease are probably inherited. Genetic defects have been identified in three chromosomes involved in Alzheimer's disease, and some apolipoprotein E genotypes may have a protective effect on the development of Alzheimer's disease.

Several factors increase the likelihood that Alzheimer's disease will develop in an individual. These include head injuries and age. A family history of Alzheimer's disease or Down syndrome is a significant risk factor. Women have a higher incidence than men. Moderate coffee and alcohol consumption and exposure to medications have not been shown to be risk factors, and the jury is still out on smoking.

CLINICAL MANIFESTATIONS

Alzheimer's disease, a slowly progressive degenerative disease of the brain, impairs the victim's mental abilities. Initially the only manifestation may be a tendency to forget recent events or to repeat oneself.

Even in the early stages, the victim is mentally impaired in areas other than memory, and judgment may also be affected.

Afflicted individuals find it increasingly difficult to concentrate on tasks, learn information, or acquire skills. Their work performance may deteriorate. They may become anxious or depressed. Personality changes are often also present in the very early stages.

As the disease progresses, victims tend to lose track of current events. The personality changes become more obvious, judgment is impaired, and patients are no longer able to balance their checkbooks or perform complex tasks. As the disease progresses still further, victims are no longer able to care for themselves and may inadvertently expose themselves (and others) to a number of physical hazards. Sleep patterns are often disrupted.

Eventually a stage is reached when caregivers can no longer care for their loved ones at home and institutionalization in a health care facility becomes necessary. Many patients spend their last five years in a nursing home or need 24-hour home care.

DIAGNOSIS

At present the only way a firm diagnosis of Alzheimer's disease can be established is by examining parts of the brain under the microscope and noting the characteristic decrease in the number of brain cells and the presence of typical senile plaques, and neurofibrillary tangles in between the surviving brain cells. It is reassuring to see that brain biopsies have not become as popular as gastrointestinal, liver, or kidney biopsies. The confirmation of the diagnosis can therefore be done only on postmortem examination.

Clinicians can make an accurate diagnosis of Alzheimer's disease without relying on the microscopic examination of the brain in at least 80% of the cases. In some instances it could be as high as 90%.

The diagnosis is based on not only a thorough review of the patient's memory impairment, but also a meticulous assessment of the mental functions, a clinical examination, and a few laboratory tests and brain-imaging procedures such as the computerized tomography (CT) scan and the single photon emission computed tomographic (SPECT) scan. A number of guidelines have been developed to assist clinicians in their task. The latest guidelines, issued in September 1996, are those of the Agency on Health Care Policy Research (AHCPR).

Even though no cure is available yet, it is very important for a diagnosis to be established in the earliest possible stage for several reasons:

1. Many diseases manifest themselves with memory loss and impaired mental functions. In these instances establishing the correct diagnosis will not only alleviate a lot of anxiety and apprehension for the patient and caregivers, but often a diagnosis may also lead to an improved prognosis if a reversible cause is detected. Even if no such cause can be found, further deterioration can sometimes be stopped.

2. Time to plan finances and future health care. Establishing a diagnosis as early as possible will give time to the victim and family to make arrangements concerning their finances and plans for future health care.

3. Availability of medication that may alter the course of Alzheimer's disease. Two available medications—donezepil (Aricept) and tacrine hydrochloride (Cognex)—may at least slow down the rate of deterioration. There is also some evidence that the administration of these medications may improve the patient's mental functions. It is obviously advantageous to start these medications as early as possible in the course of the disease to maintain the individual at the highest possible level of functioning and postpone the time when institutionalization is necessary. We have no doubt that many other medications will become available in the near future.

MANAGEMENT

Since no single identifiable cause has been established for Alzheimer's disease, it is not going to be cured or prevented by controlling only one factor. People responsible for the management of patients with Alzheimer's disease should have four goals:

1. Treat Other Diseases that may Worsen Mental Functions.

Clinicians should ensure that any other concomitant disease that may further impair the patient's mental functions is adequately treated. Since most patients with Alzheimer's disease are elderly, a number of other medical diseases may interfere with their mental functions if they are not adequately treated. These include heart failure, obstructive airways disease, and pneumonia; loss of blood through the gastrointestinal tract may also be a factor. The patient's compliance with the prescribed medication is very important.

2. Review the Patient's Medication.

Clinicians should review the patient's medications to ensure that they are indeed needed by the patient and that they are administered in the correct dosage. Elderly patients are often very sensitive to medication, especially sleeping tablets, tranquilizers, and sedatives. A dosage that is appropriate for a 48-year-old person may be excessive for an 84-year-old person. Patients should not be given any medication without consulting with a health care professional. Even some cold remedies that can be purchased over the counter could detrimentally affect patients with Alzheimer's disease.

3. Manage the Patient's Abnormal Behavior.

A number of behavioral problems can be managed by the judicious use of psychotropic medication. A variety of behavioral techniques are also available to control some of these symptoms, such as agitation, depression, sleep disturbances, psychotic thinking, and wandering.

4. Slow the Rate of Deterioration.

Although the treatment of the underlying cognitive symptoms is still in its infancy, the presently available medications may maintain the victim at a reasonable level of functioning and may therefore postpone the need for admission to a nursing home or other institution. The majority of caregivers agree that any improvement in the patient's condition is important and consider a lack of deterioration as an improvement.

ETHICAL ISSUES

The possibility of early diagnosis, linked with the possible genetic predisposition to develop the disease, raises very significant ethical issues. Should, for instance, the relatives of patients with Alzheimer's disease be screened for genetic defects and apolipoprotein genotypes, or even undergo brain imaging studies such as positron emission tomography (PET) scans or single photon emission computed tomography (SPECT)? At least one study has shown that brain imaging is abnormal even in the absence of symptoms!

The authors of this manuscript do not recommend these tests for individuals whose memory and mental functions are intact, even if one of their close relatives is afflicted by Alzheimer's disease. The reasons for this are twofold. First, having abnormal genes, or the alleles for apolipoprotein E4, or an abnormal brain imaging test, does not necessarily mean these people will develop Alzheimer's disease. Second, at present nothing can be offered to these potential victims. Telling them they are likely to develop Alzheimer's disease and not being able to offer any steps to avert it is sadistic!

A number of other ethical issues arise when managing patients with Alzheimer's disease. For instance, should they be told of the diagnosis? Should their families be told of the diagnosis? What if the patients demand that their families not be told of the diagnosis? When should a power of attorney be recommended? Should it be as soon as the diagnosis is made or should it be left until later stages are reached, which would risk the patient's making serious judgmental errors, with potential disastrous financial implications for the entire family? Should the power of attorney be a *durable power of attorney?*

Should the patient be allowed to continue driving? What if the spouse is so physically disabled that the patient's continued driving is the only means of transportation the couple has, and without it they would be completely isolated?

Other ethical questions include: when should a patient be admitted to a nursing home or other institution? Should the spouse or relatives be bound by a promise made many years ago not to send the patient to a nursing home? Often this promise has been made and reinforced by "under any circumstances"! Should the well-being of the spouse and the family be sacrificed for the sake of a promise that was made under entirely different circumstances?

Should advance directives be made for the patient? Should a patient be resuscitated if a cardiac arrest develops? Should the patient be hospitalized when pneumonia or another life-threatening condition develops? Should pneumonia be treated in the very late stages of Alzheimer's disease, or should it be viewed as Osler, often referred to as the father of contemporary medicine, did many years ago as "the old person's best friend"?

There are clearly no right or wrong answers to any of these questions. Each question should be addressed in the very specific context of the patient, spouse, and relatives. Open discussions with all interested parties are extremely important if guilt and anxiety are to be avoided at later stages. A number of professionals and professional organizations are available to discuss these issues and help the spouse and relatives reach the proper decision.

SUMMARY

The past few years have witnessed a tremendous increase in the number and quality of research projects on the cause, diagnosis, and management of Alzheimer's disease. There is no doubt that in the near future it will be possible to make a definite diagnosis of Alzheimer's disease without examining the brain microscopically. More important still, an effective and safe treatment will be made available, and early in the 21st century Alzheimer's disease will be relegated to being the *disease of the past century.*

BIBLIOGRAPHY

Alzheimer's Association: *Alzheimer's disease: statistics,* New York, 1994, The Association.

Becker JT, Boller F, Lopez OL et al: The natural history of Alzheimer's disease: description of study cohort and accuracy of diagnosis, *Arch Neurol* 51:585-594, 1994.

Blass JP: Pathophysiology of the Alzheimer's syndrome, *Neurology* 36:922-931, 1985.

Costa PT, Williams TF, Sommerfield M et al: *Early identification of Alzheimer's disease and related dementias: clinical practice guideline—quick reference guide for clinicians,* US Public Health Service, AHCPR Publication no. 97-0703, November 1996.

American Psychiatric Association: *Diagnostic and statistical manual of mental disorders,* ed 4, Washington, DC, 1994, The Association.

Ernst RL, Hay JW: The US economic and social costs of Alzheimer's disease revisited, *Am J Public Health* 84:1261-1264, 1994.

Evans DA, Funkenstein HH, Albert MS et al: Prevalence of Alzheimer's disease in a community population of older persons: higher than previously reported, *JAMA* 262:2551-2556, 1989.

Evans DA, Scherr PA, Cook NR et al: Estimated prevalence of Alzheimer's disease in the United States, *Milbank Quarterly* 68 (2):267-289, 1990.

Gottfries CG: Therapy options in Alzheimer's disease, *Br J Clin Psychiatry* 48:327-330, 1994.

Knopman D, Schneider L, Davis K et al: Long-term tacrine (Cognex) treatment: effects on nursing home placement and mortality, *Neurology* 47:166-177, 1996.

Lubeck DP, Mazonson PD, Bowe T: Potential effect of tacrine on expenditures for Alzheimer's disease, *Medical Interface* p 132-138, Oct 1994.

Max W: The cost of Alzheimer's disease: will drug treatment ease the burden? *Pharmacoeconomics* 1:5-10, 1996.

Max W: The economic impact of Alzheimer's disease, *Neurology* 43 (suppl 4):S6-10, 1993.

National Foundation for Brain Research: *The cost of disorders of the brain,* Washington, DC, 26, 1992.

Rice DP, Fox PJ, Max W et al: The economic burden of Alzheimer's disease care, *Health Aff* Summer 1993:164-176.

Snow C: Medicare HMOs develop plan for future of Alzheimer's programming, *Modern Healthcare* Sept 23, 1996:66-70.

Stern RG, Mohs RC, Davidson M et al: A longitudinal study of Alzheimer's disease: measurement, rate, and predictors of cognitive deterioration, *Am J Psychiatry* 151:390-396, 1994.

Tariot PN: Neurobiology and treatment of dementia. In Salzman C, editor: *Clinical geriatric psychopharmacology,* ed 2, Baltimore, 1992, Williams & Wilkins.

Welch HG, Walsh JS, Larson EB: The cost of institutional care in Alzheimer's disease: nursing home and hospital use in a prospective cohort, *J Am Geriatr Soc* 40:221-224, 1992.

Unit One

I use not only all the brains I have, but all I can borrow.

—Woodrow Wilson

The Normal Brain

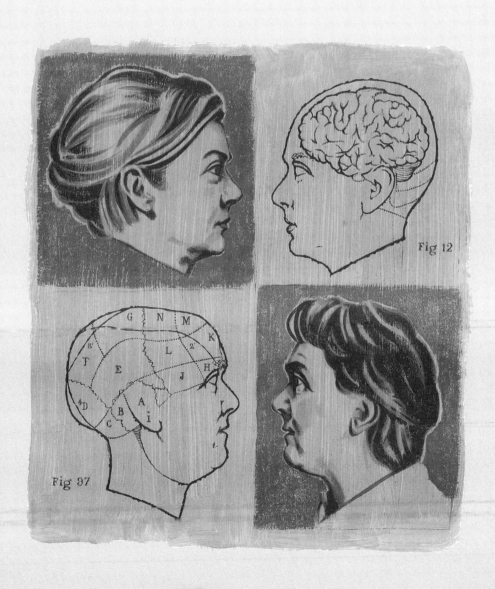

Fig 12

Fig 97

Higher Brain Functions

Patrick Sloan

. . . . Last scene of all,
That ends this strange eventful history,
Is second childishness, and mere oblivion,
Sans teeth, sans eyes, sans taste, sans everything.

—Shakespeare

This chapter presents an overview of normal brain functions with emphasis on higher brain (cortical) functions. It will describe in general terms how brain systems function and how Alzheimer's disease impairs these systems. This basic description should help prepare the reader for subsequent chapters on the effects and management of Alzheimer's disease.

People have known for centuries that the human brain is the primary organ of thought (cognition) and emotion. The brain grows to weigh approximately 3 pounds by the time a person reaches age 30, and then it slowly begins to lose tissue. By using the brain's capacity for complex planning, problem solving, and communicating, humans have been able to travel to the moon, solve medical mysteries, and build elaborate computer networks, but much still needs to be learned about how the brain actually works. A great deal of what people have already learned about the brain has come through the study of brain lesions caused by injuries or diseases such as Alzheimer's disease, Parkinson's disease, and others that affect the nervous system.

CENTRAL NERVOUS SYSTEM

The central nervous system is composed of the spinal cord and the brain. The brain is structurally divided into two cerebral hemispheres that correspond to the left and right sides of the body. The hemispheres are connected by a large bundle of white matter called the corpus callosum. The two halves are essentially symmetrical in appearance but certainly not in function.

Each hemisphere specializes in different cognitive functions, but both typically work with one another. Whether we consider the brain as a whole or two halves, it can be further divided into four basic divisions, or lobes. These lobes are essentially structural divisions at the deepest fissures and are visible to the naked eye. The frontal lobe constitutes the anterior half of the brain, the temporal lobe rests behind each temple, and the occipital lobe sits at the very posterior pole above the cerebellum. Between the front and the extreme back of the brain is the parietal lobe. The parietal lobe occupies most of the posterior portion of the brain. The frontal, temporal, occipital, and parietal lobes are evident on the outside, or lateral, surface, and each overlaps into the middle, or medial, surface of the cortex (Figure 2-1).

———• The neocortex distinguishes humans from lower animals.

The neocortex is that portion of the cerebral cortex that is most complex in structure and considered phylogenetically most recent. It is 6-layered and covers the lateral cerebral hemispheres. All other cortical areas contain fewer layers and are located medially. Its specialized abilities such as language separate humans from lower animals. The brain is folded and wrinkled so the entire surface area fits nicely into the human skull. The brain has many ridges (gyri), deep grooves (fissures), and shallow grooves (sulci) that make up the cerebral cortex and give it its wrinkled appearance.

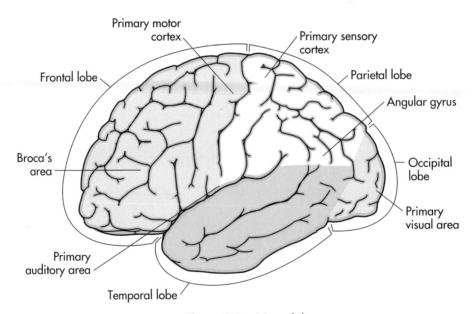

Figure 2-1. Map of the cortex.

HIGHER BRAIN (CORTICAL) FUNCTIONS

Describing the anatomy of the brain is much simpler than describing its functions, because the brain operates in a complex, integrated fashion.

> An analogy can be made between the functions of various parts of the brain and those of individual musical instruments in an orchestra.

When comparing the various functional parts of the brain to instruments in an orchestra, a piece of music is immediately seen not as a function of the individual instruments but as a composition of the whole. Likewise all parts of the brain must be functional for it to perform properly.

In general these functions have been recognized for the following areas:

The Frontal Lobe

The front part of the brain, the frontal lobe, is primarily involved with the programming and execution of motor functions. It comprises much of the neocortex. Since the functions of the frontal neocortex are complex, they are the least understood and measured of all the brain's functions. We know the frontal lobe is responsible for the initiation and execution of motor behavior. It is also instrumental in the normal functioning of higher thought processes, such as planning, abstract reasoning, trial-and-error learning, decision making, complex thinking, and problem solving. The frontal lobe is involved with intellectual insight, judgment, and the expression of emotions.

A.R. Luria, the famous Russian neuropsychologist, described a farmer with frontal lobe damage. The farmer was in danger of starvation, not because he would fail to eat from the cupboard when he had food, but because he had lost his ability to plan ahead to initiate the planting of next year's crops, and eventually he would fail to replenish the cupboard and therefore starve.

The Parietal Lobe

The posterior part of the brain, the parietal lobe, is involved with sensory perception, or the taking in of information from the environment. The parietal lobe is responsible for the monitoring and organizing of all sensory input: visual, auditory, and tactile-kinesthetic. This makes sense geographically, because the parietal lobe lies between the temporal and occipital lobes. The parietal lobe is the hub of sensory information and association.

The inferior, or lower, portion of the left parietal lobe is believed to be the "association area of association areas." This brain region in the dominant cerebral hemisphere must be working normally for one to speak and understand language, to read, and to write. The corresponding parietal lobe in the right cerebral hemisphere must be functioning normally for a person to accurately follow directions on a map, read a clock, and construct objects such as those used in sewing a dress, building a bird house, or even dressing. The parietal lobe is also involved in organizing information and communicating it to the frontal lobe.

The Temporal Lobe is Primarily Responsible for Audition
The Occipital Lobe is Primarily Involved with Vision

The four basic lobes and their respective functions are as follows:
frontal lobe—motor
parietal lobe—sensory
temporal lobe—audition
occipital lobe—vision

MAPPING BRAIN FUNCTIONS

One way of mapping brain functions is by stimulating the brain with tiny electrodes and recording what happens when certain parts of the brain are touched. This method has shown that the brain's primary motor and sensory functions work largely in a contralateral fashion. This means that the side of the body that moves (motor function) or brings in information (sensory function) is on the opposite side of the half of the brain in which this information is processed.

➤ The left half of the brain *controls* the right side of the body, and vice versa.

Specialization of the Left Cerebral Hemisphere

Most people are right-handed. Since the brain tends to function contralaterally, language in most people is predominantly controlled by, or located in, the left cerebral hemisphere. Research has shown that 99% of all right-handed people have language functions represented in the left cerebral hemisphere. That is why after a large stroke on the left side of the brain, patients are paralyzed on the right side of the body and tend to lose speech and language functions such as speaking, reading, spelling, and writing.

The left hemisphere specializes in language and other related abilities such as reading, listening, comprehending and remembering verbal material, and using logical thought processes.

Broca's area, which is responsible for expressive language, is situated between the left temporal lobe and the motor strip. Verbal memories are generated and stored in the left temporal lobe, and the motor cortex controls the verbal mechanisms for output of speech.

In the majority of left-handed people language is also *located* in the left cerebral hemisphere. Cases have been reported in which language was controlled by both cerebral hemispheres or predominantly managed by the right hemisphere. These cases usually resulted from familial, or genetic, left-handedness or early developmental brain injury.

Specialization of the Right Cerebral Hemisphere

The right cerebral hemisphere specializes in visuospatial configurations such as:
• Recognizing the parts of a puzzle
• Following directions on a map
• Building a house from a blueprint

The right hemisphere specializes in holistic, musical, and other nonverbal activities, such as recognizing and appreciating emotions and solving problems or puzzles.

The right hemisphere also contributes to the synthesis, pacing, or organization of language functions. This again emphasizes the integrative capacities and functions of the two hemispheres as a whole. The right hemisphere functions have been described generally as more "creative" or "artistic" and the left hemisphere functions as more "logical" or "analytical." The right hemisphere is also involved in the recognition and expression of emotional responses or behaviors, such as facial expressions.

Integration of Both Cerebral Hemispheres

Although the two hemispheres and other more specific brain areas are specialized for certain functions, the entire cerebral cortex governs cognition, or thinking.

The cerebral cortex includes the frontal, parietal, temporal, and occipital lobes and other brain areas, such as the cingulate gyrus and hippocampus of the limbic system, which are not directly involved in primary, sensory, and motor abilities.

While different areas of the brain have specialized tasks, some functions are distributed throughout the brain. Memory is a prime example. It depends on not only the cortex, but also on the nucleus basalis of Meynert (basal nucleus of Meynert), the subcortical (below the cortex) region of the basal forebrain. Figure 2-2 illustrates the projected lines of communication from the basal nucleus of Meynert to the distant areas of the cortex. Patients with Alzheimer's disease often have an unusually high number of neurofibrillary tangles and senile plaques in the basal nucleus of Meynert, which interferes with the transmission of information into the higher levels of the brain. Neurofibrillary tangles are abnormal bundles of filaments in a nerve cell. Senile plaques are patches of degenerating axon terminals and dendrites.

NERVE CELLS

The brain is made up of approximately 140 billion nerve cells, 20 billion of which are directly involved in information processing. Each of those cells has up to 15,000 direct physical connections to other brain cells. Information is acquired and stored in the brain by processes involving chemical and structural changes at the sites of the connections of these nerve cells, or synapses (Figure 2-3, A).

> The vast number of synaptic interconnections and the complexity of the processes involved in the acquisition and transfer of information help us understand why the brain is far more complex and sophisticated than a main frame computer.

Each nerve cell, or neuron, has a cell body, a stem (axon), and connecting branches (dendrites) (See Figure 2-3, B). Neurons within the brain are interconnected and operate primarily on the basis of electrical and chemical activity. The combination of the electrical and chemical activity enables a great amount of information to be communicated among cells, both within certain areas and to distant parts of the brain. Neurons do not simply relay information; they actually collect, transform, and send signals to many other nerve cells.

In Alzheimer's disease, neurofibrillary tangles and senile plaques interfere with the function of neurons, and some of the normal cells degenerate and die. The number of senile plaques found in postmortem brain tissue of patients with Alzheimer's disease relates directly to the degree of cognitive impairment demonstrated on neuropsychological testing by these patients when they were still able to be tested.

This positive correlation between the number of senile plaques and the degree of cognitive impairment has been shown to be particularly high in regard to the number of plaques found in the frontal and temporoparietal cortices and in the hippocampus and related limbic system structures. These brain areas and structures are described later in this chapter.

A great loss of neurons also occurs in the basal nucleus of Meynert. Axons from the nucleus of Meynert extend far into cortical regions (see Figure 2-2). These cells contain acetylcholine, a neurotransmitter. Deficiencies in acetylcholine and other neurotransmitters positively correlate with cognitive impairment in Alzheimer's disease patients, as described in the next section.

Gray and White Matter

The cell bodies give the brain a gray appearance on visual inspection of a brain specimen. The term *gray matter* is often used to describe the brain or its thinking

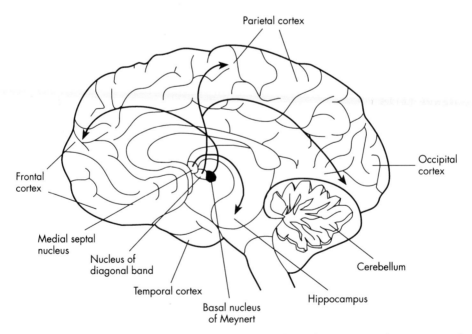

Figure 2-2.   Projections of pathways from basal nucleus of Meynert to distant areas of cortex.

or problem solving functions. The outer layer of the brain, the cortex or neocortex, is made up of mostly gray matter (cell bodies) and is primarily involved in higher cognitive operations.

The connecting nerve tissues are composed of glia cells. Because the axons of nerve cells bind easily to lipids, or fats, these axons have a white appearance; hence the term *white matter* is often used in describing the connecting tracks between areas of gray matter. The white sheaths around the axons, which are made of myelin (See Figure 2-3), help speed conduction of nerve impulses that carry information along the nerve cells. White tracks run from the outer layer of the cortex throughout the brain, spinal cord, and peripheral nerves.

How Nerve Cells Work

When a neuron is stimulated, an electrical impulse is generated and moves along the nerve cell. When the impulse reaches the end of the neuron, it stimulates the production and release of chemical compounds called neurotransmitters. These neurotransmitters then move across the synapse. When they reach the dendrite of an adjacent cell, they transmit the stimulus that caused them to be released to that neighboring cell. The stimulus then migrates along the axon until the synapse is reached, and the process is repeated.

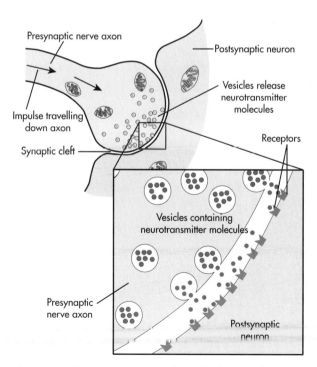

Figure 2-3, A.   A synapse. (From Lewis SM et al: *Medical-surgical nursing: assessment and management of clinical problems,* ed 4, St Louis, 1996, Mosby.)

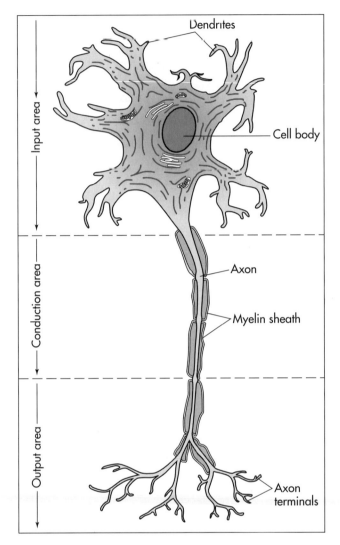

Figure 2-3, B.   Structural features of neurons: dendrites, cell body, and axons. (From Lewis SM et al: *Medical-surgical nursing: assessment and management of clinical problems,* ed 4, St Louis, 1996, Mosby.)

> Acetylcholine is one of the neurotransmitters that has been studied extensively in regard to Alzheimer's disease.

A deficiency in the number and function of nerve cells sensitive to this neurotransmitter has been found in patients with Alzheimer's disease, particularly in certain areas of the brain where these neurons are normally plentiful, such as in the hippocampus and basal nucleus of Meynert. These areas, deep in the brain's limbic system, play an important role in registering memories in the cortex. Thus when this neurochemical system is affected by Alzheimer's disease, memory functions are often the earliest and most prominently impaired of all affected brain functions.

Other neurotransmitters that have received much attention in the past couple decades include dopamine, noradrenaline, serotonin, and enkephalins, or endorphins. Neurons containing these neurotransmitters appear to be organized in systems, and researchers try to relate these systems to particular brain functions or behaviors. The chemicals in some drugs used for medicinal or recreational purposes can either increase or decrease the activity of these neurotransmitters.

Drugs that affect cognitive activity, or *psychoactive* drugs, act on neurotransmitters in different ways, depending on the neurotransmitter system affected. Researchers continue to report on the effectiveness of certain drugs in improving cognition in groups of dementia patients. For example, selegiline hydrochloride has improved attention and episodic memory in Parkinson's and early Alzheimer's disease patients.

Stimulant drugs, such as amphetamines, release noradrenaline and block its reabsorption, or reuptake, in the nerve cells. These drugs cause a general increase in arousal. Conversely, tricyclic antidepressants, such as desipramine and imipramine, block the reuptake of noradrenaline and serotonin, respectively, causing an antidepressant effect.

Antipsychotic drugs, such as chlorpromazine (Thorazine), block the transmission of dopamine, creating a tranquilizing effect. Sedative-hypnotic drugs, such as alcohol, benzodiazepines (Valium), and barbiturates, reduce anxiety at low doses but produce sedation or coma at high doses. These drugs decrease the activity of the neurotransmitter systems that produce arousal, such as noradrenaline.

The neurotransmitter systems in nondisabled elderly people are usually more vulnerable to the effect of psychoactive drugs than the systems in younger people. This vulnerability increases if Alzheimer's disease or other dementing illnesses have altered the normal numbers or activity of brain cells. Drug and neurotransmitter interactions can also cause a variety of complex reactions such as oversedation, which is why physicians should use great care in prescribing psychoactive drugs for persons with suspected dementia. In clinical practice very low doses of antipsychotic medications such as haloperidol (Haldol) are often effective when prescribed for agitation in patients with Alzheimer's disease, whereas higher doses are needed in individuals with no dementia.

The brain and spinal cord are nourished by cerebrospinal fluid (CSF), which flows around the spinal cord and into the brain in a system of cavities called ventricles. In the normal brain after the CSF is produced and circulated it is reabsorbed freely. The ventricles can be viewed on a CT scan, which is a computer—generated X-ray picture of the brain. If there is a decrease in brain tissue—a loss of neurons—then the ventricles may become enlarged to fill the space left by the loss of nerve cells. This shrinking of cortical matter is called cortical atrophy. Cortical atrophy and the resulting enlarged ventricles sometimes can be clues in diagnosing dementia but are not an unequivocal indication of it because many nondisabled elderly people show signs of cortical atrophy as a function of normal aging. However, cortical atrophy in certain brain areas such as the hippocampus occurs frequently in persons with Alzheimer's disease. Cortical atrophy and ventricular enlargement can be seen in nondisabled elderly people in the absence of dementia.

PICTURING BRAIN STRUCTURE AND FUNCTION

Much of what was learned about the brain in the past century was acquired through clinical and anatomical research. With the advent in recent years of sophisticated radiological techniques, we have been able to study brain functions in other ways. Brain imaging techniques are discussed in Chapter 4.

Another way brain functions can be studied relatively inexpensively is through the systematic study of cognitive and emotional behavior by use of the neuropsychological evaluation.

With the neuropsychological evaluation we can study indirectly what the brain actually does by examining what a person can and cannot do on various behavioral tasks. Sensory, motor, and higher cortical functions are tested, including those of attention, concentration, memory, cognition, problem-solving skills, and expression of emotions.

A.R. Luria studied thousands of brain-damaged people and compared their brain functions to those of people without brain damage. He divided levels of brain activity into functional units. These units are related to both areas, or zones, within the brain and to theoretical levels of functioning. Luria labeled these levels primary, secondary, and tertiary.

1. The primary level refers to immediate sensory and motor input and output.
2. The secondary level relates to the association among or between the primary areas or zones.
3. The tertiary level involves the zones that are overlapping and higher levels of integration and organization of brain functions. Luria's model helps explain brain functions from the most simple to the most complex.

The Integration of Brain Functions

Figure 2-4 illustrates the integration of various levels of brain functions in the speaking of a heard word from the perspective of a lateral (side) view of the left cerebral hemisphere. First, one must be awake at the basic level of arousal, a precursor to the activation of the primary projection areas of the brain. Projection refers to the actual recording or reception of sensory information. Once aroused, the temporal lobe is the primary projection area for audition. Second, in order to repeat a word that has been heard, there has to be normal functioning of the auditory cortex in the left temporal lobe.

Third, after the sound is sensed, the signal is then carried to Wernicke's area in the temporal-parietal area, where it is translated or decoded from a sound into a recognizable word. The passage of this signal and its translation involve the secondary area, or level of association. Fourth, in turn, the message is carried forward by the white matter tracks, the arcuate fasciculus, to Broca's area in the frontal lobe. Fifth, Broca's area translates or encodes the signal into its spoken form. Sixth, Broca's area is directly adjacent to the motor strip, which controls the

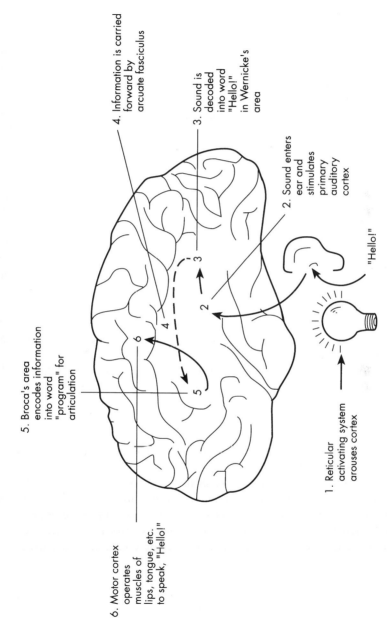

5. Broca's area encodes information into word "program" for articulation

4. Information is carried forward by arcuate fasciculus

3. Sound is decoded into word "Hello!" in Wernicke's area

2. Sound enters ear and stimulates primary auditory cortex

6. Motor cortex operates muscles of lips, tongue, etc. to speak, "Hello!"

"Hello!"

1. Reticular activating system arouses cortex

Figure 2-4. Speaking a heard word. Process is depicted in order of sequence (counter-clockwise). (Modified from Geschwind N: *Sci Am* 241: 180-199, 1979.)

lips, tongue, vocal cords, and palate so the word can be verbalized. This communication between primary and secondary levels of the brain involves the tertiary level of complex brain functioning—our actually thinking and recognizing what we are doing as we do it.

The tertiary level also includes forethought and conscious appreciation of this process. These processes also require intact "working memory," which is composed of the temporary processes that allow the acquisition, retention, and retrieval of memories and information necessary to orchestrate such complex higher cortical functions.

Because Alzheimer's disease often affects, selectively and prominently, the temporoparietal areas of the brain, working memory, language, and visuo-constructive functions are usually disrupted in various combinations and degrees. This is described further in Chapter 3.

In order for a person to say a written word or name an object, the image is projected into the visual cortex of the occipital lobe. Next, it is carried into the association area of the parietal lobe, and then into the motor speech area, which results in a verbal response.

Naturally, any disruption in the structures or processes that govern these functions will likely result in conditions such as visual agnosia, in which people are unable to recognize familiar objects or symbols. People are also likely to encounter difficulties in confrontation naming. Both of these are common symptoms in Alzheimer's disease.

At first glance, this seems to be a fairly simple, straightforward process. It is not difficult to relate a functional-anatomical correlate to these particular higher cortical functions once one understands some of the anatomical structures and their basic functions.

These examples show that there is a relatively well-understood neurology for vision and audition. However, the neurology for cognition, or complex thinking, is not yet as thoroughly understood.

In order to better understand some of these higher cognitive processes, a few other brain structures and their basic functions will be described and related to some of the more complex brain activities called higher cortical functions. For instance, what processes are involved when someone not only sees and hears an activity, but also thinks and takes appropriate actions? This processing includes understanding various perceptions and ideas congruently, and then planning one's next action or some future action. For all of the motor, sensory, and associative processes to respond and go smoothly, the various brain functions must be working both independently and in concert. This has sometimes been referred to as the "executive" function of the cortex. Some researchers have described the breakdown in multiple brain areas as a result of Alzheimer's disease as the "dysexecutive syndrome"—when these higher integrative powers are impaired due to multiple brain lesions throughout the cortex.

BASAL GANGLIA

The basal ganglia, which are made up of cell bodies, are closely involved with motor functions. They are symmetrically arranged and lie under the frontal cortex, with many connections to both the cortex above and midbrain structures below. Loss of brain cells or neurochemicals in the basal ganglia and their connections can cause severe motor problems, and to a lesser extent, cognitive problems. Parkinson's disease, for example, affects nerve cells and neurochemicals in the basal ganglia, specifically the substantia nigra, which results in difficulties with the following: posture; gait; and initiation and speed of motor activity.

The basal ganglia are also involved in the learning and programming of behavior. Activities that are well learned and rehearsed over the course of one's life become somewhat "automatic." For example, the complex motor skills involved in walking, eating, or driving become so ingrained that one does not have to think consciously to perform them. Some of these complex but well-programmed activities apparently are relegated to the basal ganglia. This may help explain why some of these complex behaviors are retained in people with dementia sometimes long after severe loss of memory or language has occurred.

LIMBIC SYSTEM

Needs, instincts, drives, and emotions are considered part of the functions of the deeper structures of the brain—the limbic system or limbic lobe. It is referred to as a system because its functions are thought to be related and working together. Part of the limbic system, the amygdala, is instrumental in emotional functioning and is sometimes removed surgically in people with epilepsy, whose seizures are refractory to anticonvulsant medication.

The hypothalamus is another part of the limbic system that rests deep within the brain and generates physical drives such as hunger and sex. It also helps regulate other basic functions such as sleep, body temperature, and, like the amygdala, emotions; it is also responsible for endocrine functions. The pituitary gland, which is very important to endocrine functions, is located close to the hypothalamus.

Besides emotional and instinctual activities, the limbic system is involved in cognitive activities. As we will see in the discussion of the hippocampus, the limbic system is extremely important in both the recording and generating of memories.

Hippocampus

The hippocampus, which is located in the inside fold of each temporal lobe, is one of the major gray-matter areas that comprise the limbic system due to its connections with the functions of memory and emotions. It has direct connections with other limbic structures such as the hypothalamus and amygdala, which are strongly involved in emotionality. The hippocampus is the site of intersection between the storage of memories and their reproduction with emotional coloring. It helps store information, temporarily sequences memories, and aids in their recall. Loss of neurons in the left hippocampus impairs verbal memory, whereas right hippocampal impairment causes a defect in the recognition and recall of complex visual information.

———• The hippocampus plays a direct role in the formation of declarative memory.

Declarative memory is directly accessible to recollection, whereas nondeclarative memory, or procedural memory, is shown by performance on a task. Experiments have shown that the hippocampus plays a major role in the encoding, consolidation, and retrieval of memories. Damage to the hippocampus from diseases such as Alzheimer's affects short-term memory and learning ability more than long-term memory.

Several areas of the brain are involved in working memory, or the ability to hold information temporarily for more than 30 seconds so it can be stored into long-term memory or retrieved for use in the present. For example, the prefrontal cortex and inferior temporal cortex are involved in recognizing specific forms such as faces. The encoding of this information involves the hippocampus, medial temporal regions, and left prefrontal cortex. The network for recognition involves the right prefrontal cortex, right parietal cortex, and bilateral ventral occipital cortices, whereas the network for encoding the information involves the left prefrontal cortex and the right hippocampus.

The hippocampus, septohippocampal pathway, and basal nucleus of Meynert are strongly involved in the neuropathology of Alzheimer's disease. The age-related decline in memory functions has been correlated with shrinkage of the hippocampus. Formation of short-term memories involves neurochemical changes at existing synapses, whereas formation of long-term memories involves structural changes in existing synapses and in the number of synapses. Formation of long-term memories requires protein synthesis. Loss of synapses correlates strongly with severity of symptoms in Alzheimer's disease. Researchers have infused growth hormone into the brains of Alzheimer's disease patients to help alleviate or prevent the deterioration of hippocampal neurons and preserve memory functions. Other researchers have found that hypothalamic activity is associated with the degeneration in dementia. They believe a disconnection between the hippocampus and the hypothalamic areas may explain uncontrolled activity in the hypothalamic-pituitary-adrenal axis in Alzheimer's disease patients.

In summary, the hippocampus plays a key role in memory functioning. Thus it is understandable that early and severe loss of neurons in that part of the brain correlates strongly with early and prominent symptoms of memory disturbance in Alzheimer's disease patients.

Integration and Specialization of Higher Cortical Functions

In moving from the deep brain structures and their functions to the cortex, we encounter complex cognitive functions referred to as higher cortical functions. One may wonder what processes are involved in logical thinking, associating, remembering, and problem solving, which are examples of higher cortical functions. Many interconnections exist between the limbic system and the cortex and within the cortex itself, and all of these connections contribute to the network of higher cortical functions. As was described above, separate yet complex networks are responsible for encoding and recognizing complex visual stimuli such as faces. Like the instruments in an orchestra, all of the deeper and higher brain structures have to be operational and working in concert for the tune (thought, behavior) to evolve as effective and synthesized.

With this description of normal brain functions, it is easier to understand why patients with Alzheimer's disease have difficulty with cognitive functions. In an early stage of Alzheimer's disease, a larger distribution of neurofibrillary tangles and senile plaques can be found in the hippocampus and the temporal and parietal lobes than in other brain areas. This disruption of normal brain functions in an early stage results in predominant impairment in memory, language, and constructional abilities.

As the disease progresses, the frontal lobes and their connections may be affected. This can result in behavioral changes that result from the loss of initiative, spontaneity, and the ability to plan and organize behavior. Other personality changes also occur. For example, the person may become less inhibited due to disconnection or loss of neurons in the frontal lobes, leading to impulsive or agitated behavior.

Perhaps this overview of normal brain functions will allow us to arrive at a definition of normal brain functioning and behavior. We could define normal brain functioning as follows: when all of these structures and their functions are working properly, both independently and in concert. This is, of course, relative to the individuals and their cultural surroundings. This definition is analogous to how we attempt to define normal intelligent behavior using such methods as intelligence tests and other neuropsychological instruments.

David Wechsler, who developed the cognitive tasks and intelligence tests often used in assessing patients with suspected dementia, said the tests do not measure intelligence per se. Instead, he said, the tests simply correlate with other more widely accepted criteria of intelligent behavior. Thus the normal brain and its functions are defined in the context of the individual's given abilities, peer group, and culture. In Chapter 3, we review the neuropsychological assessment of higher brain functions as part of an evaluation of suspected dementia in an individual.

BIBLIOGRAPHY

Balldin J, Blennow K, Brane G et al: Relationship between mental impairment and HPA axis activity in dementia disorders, *Dementia* 5 (5):252-256, 1994.

Bannister R: Brain's clinical neurology, New York, 1985, Oxford University Press.

Becker JT, Bajulaiye O, Smith C: Longitudinal analysis of a two-component model of the memory deficit in Alzheimer's disease, *Psychol Med* 22:437-445, 1992.

Begley S, Carey J, Sawhill R: How the brain works, *Newsweek*, Feb 7, 1983: pp 40-47.

Chusid, JG: *Correlative neuroanatomy and functional neurology*, Los Altos, Calif, 1976, Lange Medical Publications.

Galomb J, de-Leon MJ, George AE et al: Hippocampal atrophy correlates with severe cognitive impairment in elderly patients with suspected normal pressure hydrocephalus, *J Neurol Neurosurg Psychiatry* 57(5):590-593, 1994.

Gazzaniga MS: *The bisected brain*, New York, 1970, Appleton-Century-Crofts.

Geschwind N: Disconnection syndromes in animals and man, *Brain* 88:237-294, 1965.

Geschwind N: Specializations of the human brain, *Sci Am* 241:180-199, 1979.

Heilman KM, Bowers D, Velenstein E: Emotional disorders associated with neurological diseases. In Heilman KM, Valenstein E, editors: *Clinical neuropsychology,* New York, 1985, Oxford University Press.

Huerta PT, Lisman JE: Heightened synaptic plasticity of hippocampal CA1 neurons during a cholinergically induced rhythmic state, *Nature* 364(6439):723-725, 1993.

Hyman BT, West HL, Rebeck GW et al: Neuropathological changes in Down's syndrome hippocampal formations, *Arch Neurol* 52(4):373-378, 1995.

Katzman RD: Alzheimer's disease, *N Engl J Med* 314:964-973, 1986.

Kolb B, Whishaw IQ: *Fundamentals of human neuropsychology,* San Francisco, 1980, WH Freeman.

Lees AJ: Selegiline hydrochloride and cognition, *Acta Neurol Scand* 84:91-94, 1991.

Lezak MD: *Neuropsychological assessment,* New York, 1995, Oxford University Press.

Luria AR: *Higher cortical functions in man,* New York, 1966, Basic Books.

Luria AR: *The working brain,* New York, 1973, Basic Books.

McKhann G et al: Clinical diagnosis of Alzheimer's disease, *Neurology* 34:939-944, 1984.

Mitchell AJ: HPA axis function in depression and dementia; review, *Int J Geriatric Psychiatry* 9(4):331-334, 1994.

O'Brien JT, Ames D, Schweitzer I: HPA axis function in depression and dementia: a review: *Int J of Geriatric Psychiatry* 8(11):887-898, 1993.

Rosenzweig M, Leiman A, Breedlove SM: *Biological psychology,* Sunderland, Mass, 1996, Sinauer Associates Inc.

Samuel WA, Henderson VW, Miller CA: Severity of dementia in Alzheimer disease and neurofibrillary tangles in multiple brain regions, *Alzheimer Dis Assoc Disord* 5(1):1-11, 1991.

Samuel W, Masliah E, Hill LR et al: Hippocampal connectivity and Alzheimer's dementia: effects of synapse loss and tangle frequency in a two-component model, *Neurology* 44(11):2081-2088, 1994.

Snyder SH: Basic science of psychopharmacology. In Kaplon HI, Sadock BJ, editors: *Comprehensive textbook of psychiatry,* vol 4, Baltimore, 1985, Williams & Wilkins.

Wechsler D: *The measurement and appraisal of adult intelligence,* Baltimore, 1958, Williams & Wilkins.

Zandi T: Changes in memory processes of dementia patients. In Zandi T, Ham RJ, editors: *New directions in understanding dementia and Alzheimer's disease,* New York, 1990, Plenum Press.

Neuropsychological Assessment of Dementia

Patrick Sloan

Be careful about reading health books.
You might die of a misprint.

—Mark Twain

Neuropsychological evaluation of dementia employs measurement and qualitative observation to describe brain dysfunction as it is expressed in motor, sensory, emotional, and cognitive performance. The goal of the evaluation is to measure and describe what the patient can and cannot do on various tasks that are part of the activities of daily living.

The typical neuropsychological evaluation attempts to address the following questions:

1. Is there evidence of brain dysfunction?
2. If there is dysfunction, is the degree of impairment mild, moderate, or severe?
3. Is there a particular pattern of impairment?
4. Are the degree and pattern of impairment consistent with a specific type of dementia?

Neuropsychologists use a combination of standardized tests and observations to address these questions, with results that can be replicated by various practitioners. For example, the Consortium to Establish a Registry for Alzheimer's Disease (CERAD) used a multi-center, controlled study of a large sample of patients to develop a brief battery of neuropsychological tests for the assessment and follow-up evaluation of patients with probable Alzheimer's disease. The greatest strengths of neuropsychological tests are in their ability to distinguish between groups of patients with and without early brain impairment, and their usefulness in tracking the progression of the illness over time.

For example, the CERAD battery, which measures the primary cognitive manifestations of Alzheimer's disease at different levels of severity, is able to discriminate between nondisabled subjects and those with mild and moderate dementia. In addition, the battery is able to detect deterioration of language, memory, praxis, and intellectual functions on reassessment 1 year later. Such testing allows assessment of subtle cognitive and behavioral changes that may not be readily identifiable or quantifiable in a typical bedside neurological or psychiatrical examination. Because the tests record subtle or specific changes in mentation, they are well suited for measuring such changes over time. Patterns of performance on neuropsychological tests can be used to differentiate between various dementing illnesses.

CLINICAL NEUROPSYCHOLOGICAL EVALUATION PROCEDURES

Neuropsychological assessments attempt to "map" the brain in terms of its various integrated, functional systems. A typical battery, comprised of a number of tests, may require up to 3 hours of testing. The cost of evaluation depends upon the amount of time required, but is typically less expensive than a magnetic resonance imaging (MRI) head scan.

Except for patients in the very early stages of dementia, most patients suspected of having dementia are unable, due to cognitive impairment and fatigue, to undergo several consecutive hours of testing. For those reasons and others, patients are often available for only a single testing session of limited duration. Thus the neuropsychologist must make good use of a selected number of measures that have been shown empirically to reveal dementia, distinguishing it from other causes of brain dysfunction.

Special Considerations

Pressures from managed care and governmental agencies for cost containment, with the attendant reduction in length of hospital stays, have led to an increasing reliance on outpatient evaluation and on the use of technicians and psychometricians to administer and score test batteries. The neuropsychologist's role is increasingly devoted to interpretation, diagnostic consultation, teaching, and research.

However, the test administrator needs to be well trained to handle demented patients with comfort. These patients are often apprehensive, cognitively slow, distractible, fatigable, and vulnerable to emotional distress. The testing environment should be quiet, pleasant, and free from distractions.

Special consideration must also be given to cultural, ethnic, and language differences between patients and evaluators. Several investigators have noted that age, gender, education, and social class influence test results. Cultural and racial differences are also found, with results favoring English-speaking patients. Wilder and co-workers reviewed the use of brief screening measures for dementia in a multicultural population and found large numbers of false positive diagnoses in nonwhites with low levels of education. The authors noted that most studies have shown these commonly used scales report increased rates of cognitive impairment among minority groups or persons with less than a high school education and that these scales typically include items that are racially or ethnically biased. Thus the careful use and interpretation of various measures, with appropriate allowances, and modifications such as the use of functional measures are indicated.

The ideal neuropsychological evaluation incorporates information from the medical and social histories, combined with the clinical psychological examination and various psychometric and functional measures. Functional behaviors, such as kitchen tasks, have been shown to correlate with neuropsychological tests and may assess global dysfunction in Alzheimer's disease.

Most neuropsychologists use a group of tests designed to measure brain impairment. A neuropsychological evaluation includes interviews with the patient and caregivers, behavioral observations, and mental status examinations. Depending upon the referral question concerning the patient's clinical condition, other psychometric procedures may be added to these routine procedures. The specific procedures required may include an individually administered intelligence test and other standardized tests, including measures of attention, concentration, verbal and nonverbal memory, language, motor and somatosensory functions, and specific higher order cognitive functions, such as complex reasoning, learning, and problem-solving skills. Table 3-1 lists a brief battery of tests included in the CERAD battery.

A number of brief cognitive screening instruments such as the Blessed Dementia Scale and the Mini-Mental State Examination (MMSE) are reliable in differentiating demential from nondemential persons. The Modified Blessed, for example, has been correlated with neuropathological findings indicative of Alzheimer's disease dementia. Another brief checklist, the Hachinski Ischemic Scale, has been shown to help differentiate Alzheimer's disease from multiinfarct dementia (MID). The use of these brief scales is an example of the basic quantitative measurement of cognitive impairment and the empirical correlation of such impairment with different types of dementia.

The MMSE assesses orientation, attention, concentration, memory, and basic dominant and nondominant hemisphere functions, but not to the extent of formal neuropsychological assessment. Screening tests can also provide helpful measures

---

Table 3-1

Example of Brief Cognitive Screening Battery of Neuro-psychological Tests Developed by the Consortium to Establish a Registry for Alzheimer's Disease (CERAD)

Blessed Dementia Scale
Short Blessed Test
Verbal Fluency
Boston Naming Test
Mini-Mental State
Constructional Praxis
Word List Memory
Word List Recall
Word List Recongition

From Morris JC et al: the Consortium to Establish a Registry for Alzheimer's Disease (CERAD): part 1—clinical and neuropsychological assessment of Alzheimer's disease, *Neurology* 39: 1159-1165, 1989.

of the rate of deterioration in patients with Alzheimer's disease. Cognitive screening instruments, however, are limited in the following way: even though they may measure cognitive decline from 1 year to the next, they may not be able to predict the disease progression beyond the second year.

Tests such as the MMSE have been used successfully in differentiating dementia from depression. The Mattis Dementia Rating Scale as described by Shay and co-workers, which has been validated in determining the stages of dementia, correlates well with clinical ratings of dementia on the Instrumental Activities of Daily Living scale and may be useful in making level-of-care decisions.

Linn and co-workers suggest that cognitive deficits in verbal learning, memory, and immediate auditory attention span may be detected up to 7 years before the clinical diagnosis of Alzheimer's disease is made. Thorough and accurate neuro-psychological assessment early in the course of suspected dementia is clearly useful.

Great attention has been paid to memory and language impairment because these are commonly the earliest and most prominent clinical symptoms of dementia, particularly in Alzheimer's disease. The memory processes include the following: the acquisition, retention, and retrieval of information.

After Hodges, Salmon, and Butters used a battery of tests to assess semantic knowledge—permanent representation of facts, objects, words, concepts, and meanings—in patients with Alzheimer's disease and age-matched controls, they found that impairment in semantic memory is due to storage degradation rather than a sensory input or acquisition problem.

> Patients with Alzheimer's disease, who are susceptible to distractions, have impaired working memory and problems with learning and retrieval.

Patients with Alzheimer's disease suffer a breakdown in the understanding of semantic relationships. They lose the connection between words and what they represent; however, syntax remains intact. They have difficulty recognizing the emotional tones in speech and emotionally laden facial expressions. Alzheimer's disease patients produce a decreased quantity of words when asked to write, and they experience a general loss of verbal spontaneity.

Even when given cues, patients with Alzheimer's disease perform more poorly than nondisabled people, especially when distracted. Their responses often include intrusions of previous responses; they do not seem able to activate storage of information in memory and do not benefit from repetition. Patients with Alzheimer's disease seem to benefit somewhat from conceptual cues, such as categories in which they are to name or remember objects; however, they display rapid forgetting. Their ability to learn simple motor tasks, however, is relatively preserved until late in the disease. Table 3-2 summarizes disruption and cognitive features of Alzheimer's disease.

CLINICAL DIFFERENTIATION

Neuropsychological tests prove useful in identifying the specific cause of dementia. Patients with Alzheimer's disease perform more poorly on standardized tests than those with MID, who in turn perform more poorly than nondisabled people.

Table 3-2

Sequence of Disruption and Most Distinguishing Cognitive Features for Alzheimer's Disease

Sequence of Disruption in Alzheimer's Disease:

Memory functions
Attention
Mental quickness and reasoning
Impairment of language and visuospatial abilities (may occur at any point)

Most Distinguishing Cognitive Features for Alzheimer's Disease

Severe verbal memory disorder
Impaired verbal expression
Impaired verbal comprehension
Deficits in: Attention
            Orientation
            Psychomotor performance
            Reasoning

From LeZak, M: *Neuropsychological assessment*, ed 3, New York, 1995, Oxford University Press.

Although individual patients with Alzheimer's disease may perform somewhat differently from one another on the tests, their relative strengths and weaknesses typically remain consistent from initial diagnosis through the end-stages of the disease.

In addition to having a greater degree of general cognitive impairment, patients with Alzheimer's disease differ from patients with MID in other characteristic ways. Patients with Alzheimer's disease who have an impairment in nonverbal memory but relatively good verbal skills will show these characteristics over the course of the illness, regardless of how severe the impairment becomes.

Patients with MID show more variation in their test patterns from patient to patient and within the same patient over a period of time than those with Alzheimer's disease. This finding is presumably due to the more multifocal nature and "stuttering" course of MID.

The Wechsler Adult Intelligence Scale (WAIS), a commonly used and well-known intelligence quotient (IQ) test, is both a content- and age-appropriate test for elderly persons and is a thorough yet nonthreatening test for most patients.

In a series of studies, Fuld used some subtests of the WAIS to identify characteristic patterns of performance among various groups of demented and nondemented persons. Based on previous studies showing the cholinergic deficiency in patients with Alzheimer's disease, she found that a particular pattern of test results correlated highly with the diagnosis of Alzheimer's disease.

The "Fuld profile" based on the WAIS is highly specific for Alzheimer's disease since it produces few false positives (patients characterized as having Alzheimer's disease who do not), but the profile is only moderately sensitive since it identified

Table 3-3
Example of the Use of Fuld's Profile (Formula) in Assessment in Case 1, a 69-Year-Old Man with Probable Dementia of the Alzheimer's Type

Wechsler Adult Intelligence Scale (WAIS)

WAIS subtests used for the Fuld Profile and scores for Case 1:

Information	= 12
Similarities	= 5
Digit Span	= 9
Vocabulary	= 12
Digit Symbol	= 7
Block Design	= 6
Object Assembly =	8

Fuld's Profile formula using *age-corrected* scaled scores:

A = Information + Vocabulary /2   = 12.0
B = Digit Span   + Similarities /2   =   7.0
C = Digit Symbol + Block Design /2=   6.5
D = Object Assembly   =   8.0

Fuld profile is suggestive of Dementia of Alzheimer's Type if:
  $A > B > C \leq D$; $A > D$

In Case 1, A = 12 + 12/2   = 12.0
          B = 5 + 9/2   =   7.0
          C = 7 + 6/2   =   6.5
          D = 8   =   8.0

Thus, in Case 1: A (12.0) > B (7.0) > C (6.5) ≤ D (8.0)
                A (12.0) > D (8.)

The Fuld profile is positive in Case 1 and suggests the probability of Dementia of the Alzheimer's Type, if other causes of dementia have been excluded and the clinical history and other data are consistent with this clinical diagnosis.

---

only about 50% of all testable patients with Alzheimer's disease (Table 3-3). In addition, later studies using the Fuld formula showed high specificity but lower sensitivity than that found by Fuld, suggesting the possibility of a high number of false positive diagnoses of Alzheimer's disease. My clinical experience suggests that, although the accuracy of the profile is somewhat limited, particularly in patients who are culturally or educationally deprived, the procedure is particularly useful as a measure of deterioration over time in a population of patients with dementia.

The following case illustrates the use of the Fuld formula and profile. Additional case examples describe some frequently encountered diagnostic issues and other clinical considerations in the neuropsychological assessment of dementia syndromes. Table 3-4 gives examples of a battery of tests used in these cases.

| Table 3-4

Example of a Battery of Tests Used in the Assessment of Dementia and the Neuropsychological Functions Measured

Wechsler Adult Intelligence Scale (WAIS) (Intelligence)

Information   (fund of information, remote memory)
Similarities   (verbal abstracting ability)
Digit Span   (attention, concentration, immediate memory)
Vocabulary   (language usage, remote memory)
Digit Symbol   (psychomotor speed, immediate memory)
Block Design   (novel visuospatial perception and construction)
Object Assembly (cued visuospatial perception and construction)

Wechsler Memory Scale Russell Revision

Russell's Semantic Memory (verbal memory encoding, retrieval, recognition)
Russell's Figural Memory   (visual memory encoding, retrieval, recognition)

Rey Auditory Verbal Learning Test (new verbal learning, encoding, retrieval, recognition)

Mini-Mental State Examination (brief screen of orientation, basic attention, concentration, memory, verbal and constructive cognitive functions)

Tests from the Halstead-Reitan Neuropsychological Test Battery

Aphasia Screening Examination (expressive and receptive language, including reading, writing, spelling, naming, recognition; calculation, right/left orientation, praxis, drawing)

Finger Oscillation (Tapping) Test (Coordination, Motor Speed)

Grip Strength (Motor Strength)

Sensory-Perceptual Examination

A. Bilateral Simultaneous Sensory Perception (attention, tactile sensation)
B. Tactile Finger Recognition Test (tactile sensation, spatial awareness, naming)
C. Finger-tip Number Writing Perception Test (graphaesthesia)
D. Tactile Form Recognition Test (stereognosis)

Trail Making Test (higher order cognition, visual tracking, spatial attention, trial and error learning, working memory, visuomotor coordination, and speed)

Beck Depression Inventory (brief screen for depressed mood)

Selected neuropsychological and personality tests as indicated.

• Case Study—Dementia of the Alzheimer's Type (DAT)

A 69-year-old college-educated, retired professional man with an 18-month history of cognitive decline was referred as an outpatient for neuropsychological evaluation of dementia after an unremarkable extensive medical evaluation. No history or symptoms of cerebrovascular disease were found. Although his attention and concentration were adequate, the patient showed prominent memory loss for both recent and well-learned, (or remote), information. His WAIS scores revealed global intellectual decline (verbal IQ = 94, performance IQ = 82, full scale IQ = 88) compared with his estimated premorbid level of above-average–to–superior intellect based on his educational and occupational history (average IQ = 90 to 110).

Age-corrected scores on each of the selected WAIS subtests were consistent with the Fuld profile (i.e., (A) Vocabulary + Information/2 > (B) Digit Span + Similarities/2 > (C) Digit Symbol + Block Design/2 < (D) Object Assembly; (A) Vocabulary + Information/2 > (D) Object Assembly). Table 3-4 shows how to calculate the Fuld formula. (See Figure 3-1 of the WAIS profile.)

The interpretation of these data revealed that this man's vocabulary and general fund of information were relatively well preserved, though still lower than expected for his educational and vocational experience. This was expected, since these well-learned areas of knowledge are well retained—they are the last to deteriorate in either normal aging or dementing illness. His ability to recite strings of digits forward and backward in the Digit Span portion of the WAIS and his analysis or verbal similarity skills—for example, how oranges and bananas are alike—were more impaired than his abilities that were tested on the Vocabulary and Information subtests. The WAIS Digit Span and Similarities subtests, which reflect auditory processing, immediate memory, abstract reasoning, and more complex cognitive functions, are likely to deteriorate early in Alzheimer's disease. This man's performance on the WAIS timed tasks requiring visuospatial organization and visuomotor coordination and speed, the Digit Symbol substitution task and the visuoconstructive Block Design subtest, was even more impaired, suggesting dysfunction in temporoparietal areas of both cerebral hemispheres.

Finally, his ability to construct puzzles of familiar objects, which was tested in the Object Assembly, was less impaired than the last two pairs of subtests but more impaired than the first pair. These results are consistent with empirical data from Fuld's studies of patients with Alzheimer's disease. With the respective pairs of tests each represented by a letter, this man's age-corrected scores for the seven WAIS subtests corresponded to Fuld's profile—(A > B > C < D; A > D)—which is suggestive of probable Alzheimer's disease.

This man also made one or more intrusive-type perseverative errors, which have been found frequently among patients with dementia and are suspected to be characteristic of Alzheimer's disease in particular. These are errors wherein the patient gives an inappropriate response to a question by carrying forward a response to a previous question despite other responses occurring in between. For example, having given correctly the name of the current president earlier in the test, when later asked the name of a character in a brief story that had been read to him (after several intervening questions), the man answered again with the name of the president.

The remainder of the neuropsychological tests given to the patient revealed no particular pattern of sensorimotor or cognitive asymmetries suggestive of localized or lateralized brain dysfunction. That is, there were no findings suggestive of focal brain disease such as those found in patients with a brain tumor or stroke. Memory and other global intellectual impairments were prominent in this man, and there were no significant motor findings suggestive of "subcortical" disease. His wife described personality changes of decreased spontaneity and initiative.

The history and neuropsychological findings in this case were consistent with those of patients with Alzheimer's disease, which is the most definitive statement that can be made on the basis of the clinical neuropsychological evaluation. Periodic reevaluation, referral to the local Alzheimer's support group, and consultation with the family were recommended.

Case Study—Multiinfarct Dementia (MID)

A 53-year-old right-handed, disabled laborer with an eighth-grade education was referred for neuropsychological evaluation of dementia upon admission to an inpatient psychiatry service. The patient was brought to the hospital by police, who reported he was confused and had been rummaging through a large trash dumpster. His history included treatment for chronic hypertension and several episodes of suspected transient ischemic attacks (TIA). On testing several days after admission, his orientation, attention, concentration, and verbal memory (immediate, recent, and remote) were all commensurate with his education, despite his disorientation and confusion on admission. Recall for figures and visuoconstructive drawings was extremely impaired. The WAIS profile did not correspond to Fuld's profile for Alzheimer's disease and suggested instead mild intellectual decline and specific impairment in functions served by the right cerebral hemisphere. Asymmetries were found on the sensorimotor examination, such as decreased index finger tapping speed on the left hand and impaired ability to recognize numbers written on the left fingertips (i.e., agraphesthesia).

The Hachinski Ischemic Score was elevated and was positive for several markers suggestive of cerebrovascular disease such as abrupt onset, history of hypertension, stuttering course, and focal neurological signs and symptoms. The clinical neuropsychological evaluation was strongly suggestive of right cerebral hemisphere dysfunction and MID, and thorough neurological evaluation for suspected stroke was recommended. Concurrent neurological examination, EEG, CT scan, and noninvasive blood flow studies suggested an infarct in the distribution of the right middle cerebral artery and bilateral carotid artery disease. Following appropriate treatment the patient improved, and eventually reached a plateau in cognitive functions.

Multiple infarctions, either clearly identifiable or subtle, often appear in a "patchy" distribution of deficits on the neuropsychological examination and tend to plateau after each event, each episode causing more dysfunction than the previous one. Typically, however, the course is one of a less severely progressive and rapid decline than in the typical patient with Alzheimer's disease unless a larger stroke occurs in the process. Yet, even when large strokes occur, unaffected areas of the brain often will be relatively functional. This picture is somewhat contrary to the global diminution in cortical function seen in Alzheimer's disease, particularly in the middle to late stages of the disease. In "mixed" cases with evidence of both Alzheimer's disease and MID this distinction is more difficult to determine.

Case Study—Depression and Other Pseudodementias

A 66-year-old retired administrative assistant with a college education was referred as a psychiatric inpatient where he was being treated for depression. He had a family history of affective disorder, and had become clinically depressed after his recent retirement and the death of his wife. On interview, he showed psychomotor slowing, was generally oriented (with close questioning), and appeared sad and despondent. His response to formal testing was generally cooperative but slowed. He frequently stated, "I don't know" to questions and could not be motivated to respond. No sensorimotor asymmetries were noted and constructional drawings were adequate though sparse. Attention and concentration were severely impaired. Verbal recall was adequate for recent news events though he did poorly on formal memory tests. Abstract reasoning and topographical direction finding were intact. The history, clinical behavior, and cognitive test data strongly suggested depression rather than dementia, although the latter could not be ruled out due to the patient's inability and the unavailability of family to provide adequate history. It is sometimes difficult to determine whether depression is the cause of cognitive decline or whether it represents a reaction to the patient's recognition of increasing cognitive impairment. Personality testing suggested depressed mood rather than confusion or disorientation. Vigorous treatment of depression was recommended to the referring psychiatrist.

Following a positive response to a few weeks of antidepressant pharmacotherapy, the patient's cognitive performance, psychomotor speed, and mood improved measurably.

Virtually any medical illness can masquerade as dementia. A thorough history and complete medical evaluation are precursors to good diagnosis and treatment, as it is possible to reverse many treatable causes of dementia (i.e., pseudodementia) such as thyroid disease, pernicious anemia, and other conditions.

Neuropsychological testing is useful because it can help distinguish between cognitive impairment and emotional paralysis, as in depression, and can document improvement or diminishing cognitive functioning over time. Memory complaints, for example, are very common among depressed elderly adults, and neuropsychological testing has been demonstrated to differentiate among patients with Alzheimer's disease, depression, and normal control subjects on such factors as rates of forgetting, WAIS Digit Symbol performance, and other cognitive tasks.

Contrary to anecdotal reports that patients with dementia do not appear depressed, patients in the early stages of dementia are frequently depressed to at least a mild degree. In addition, many patients in chronic medical and/or psychiatric populations also have varying degrees of dementia (particularly milder forms). The former group includes, but is not limited to, cancer patients and those with vascular, lung, systemic, or neurologic disease. Psychiatric illnesses that may accompany mild dementias include chronic schizophrenia, affective disorders, and substance abuse disorders.

EMOTIONAL FACTORS

In the typical neuropsychological evaluation of dementia, much of the focus is on assessment of cognitive factors. Yet, the importance of evaluating emotional variables should not be underestimated. Not only is this important when emotional variables are involved in the primary differential diagnosis, but the patient's and family/caretaker's reaction to the condition is always of critical importance.

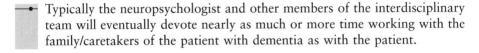

Typically the neuropsychologist and other members of the interdisciplinary team will eventually devote nearly as much or more time working with the family/caretakers of the patient with dementia as with the patient.

Assessment of emotional factors can take two forms: an evaluation of the patient and also of the family system. The evaluation of the patient's objective mental status may include formal testing of emotional variables as well as observations of emotionality during interviewing and cognitive testing. In early stages of dementia, the patient may be able to complete self-report inventories of feelings/personality, such as the Minnesota Multiphasic Personality Inventory (MMPI-2). More typically, the patient is too impaired to complete long questionnaires. Thus, projective tests such as the Rorschach may be useful. Although the Rorschach test is not primarily intended to be a test of brain dysfunction per se, it can be helpful in eliciting and documenting empirically how a person with dementia is perceiving his or her environment, mood states, and the likelihood of acting out. It may help to individualize the treatment plan, particularly in regard to psychotherapeutic interventions for the individual and/or family. The following example illustrates this point:

● **Case Study—Stroke Victims with Dementia and Compulsive Personality Traits**
The neuropsychological and personality evaluation of a 57-year-old man with mild multiinfarct dementia and a right cerebral hemisphere stroke revealed his having significant difficulty with maintaining sustained attention and emotional control. He quickly changed topics of conversation, was highly impatient, and laughed or cried disinhibitedly with the slightest stimulation. His emotionality during the cognitive testing provided ample data that were used in later efforts to teach him and his wife how to cope with his poststroke problems.
   Personality testing of the patient and the conjoint interviews with him and his wife helped elucidate emotional strengths, weaknesses, and communication patterns within the family. Testing revealed this patient's paternalistic relationship with his wife, his compulsive need to organize his environment, and the painful emotion he experienced when he felt emotionally "out of control." This information was most helpful in constructing his individual treatment plan and planning the psychotherapeutic strategies to be used with the couple.

SUMMARY

Neuropsychological assessment is designed to provide detailed information concerning the specific cognitive skills and deficits that characterize an individual patient's dementia. This information confirms the diagnosis of Alzheimer's disease, making it possible at times to identify other treatable diseases that may confuse the diagnosis. Additionally, neuropsychological evaluation can be used to measure the extent of disease progression. Most importantly, it can aid in the development of treatment plans that capitalize on the patient's and family's strengths and, as much as possible, bypass the specific cognitive deficits that impair optimal function. An important contributor to the understanding of dementing illness, neuropsychology also plays a vital role in the clinical management of the patient with Alzheimer's disease.

BIBLIOGRAPHY

Bau C, Edwards D, Yonan C et al: The relation of neuropsychological test performance to performance of functional tasks in dementia of the Alzheimer type, *Arch Clin Psychol* 11(1):69-75, 1996.

Blessed G, Tomlinson BE, Roth M: The association between quantitative measures of dementia and of change in the cerebral grey matter of elderly subjects, *Br J Psychiatry* 114:787-81, 1968.

Bowler JV, Hachinski V: Vascular cognitive impairment: A new approach to vascular dementia, *Baillieres Clin Neurol* 4(2):357-376, 1995.

Braekhus A, Laake K, Engedal KA: Low "normal" score on the Mini-Mental State Examination predicts development of dementia after three years, *J Am Geriatrics Soc* 43(6):656-661, 1995.

Butters N, Delis DC, Lucas JA: Clinical assessment of memory disorders in amnesia and dementia, *Annu Rev Psychol* 46:493-523, 1995.

Claman DL, Radebaugh TZ: Neuropsychological assessment in clinical trials of Alzheimer Disease, *Alzheimer's Dis Assoc Disord* 5(Suppl. 1):S49-S56, 1991.

Fillenbaum GG, Heyman A, Wilkinson WD et al: Comparison of two screening tests in Alzheimer's disease, *Arch Neurol* 44:924-927, 1987.

Fuld PA: Psychometric differentiation of the dementias: an overview. In Reisberg B, editor: *Alzheimer's disease,* New York, 1983, MacMillan, Inc.

Furey-Kurkjian ML, Pietrini P, Graff-Radford NR et al: Visual variant of Alzheimer's disease: distinctive neuropsychological features, *Neuropsychology* 10(2):294-300, 1996.

Gainotti G, Parlato V, Montelcone D et al: Neuropsychological markers of dementia on visual-spatial tasks: a comparison between Alzheimer's type and vascular forms of dementia, *J Clin Exp Neuropsychol* 14:239-252, 1992.

Galasko D, Corey-Bloom J, Thal LJ: Monitoring progression in Alzheimer's disease, *J Am Geriatr Soc* 39:932-941, 1991.

Golden CJ: A standardized version of Luria's neuropsychological tests. In Filskov S and Boll TJ, editors: *Handbook of clinical neuropsychology,* New York, 1981, Wiley-Interscience.

Grasel E, Cameron S, Lehri S: What contribution can the Hachinski Ischemic Scale make to the differential diagnosis between multiinfarct dementia and primary degenerative dementia? *Arch Gerontol Geriatr* 11(1):63-75, 1990.

Green RC, Woodward JL, Green J: Validity of the Mattis Dementia Rating Scale for detection of cognitive impairment in the elderly, *J Neuropsychiatry Clin Neurosci* 7(3):357-360, 1995.

Hart RP, Kwentus A, Taylor JR et al: Rate of forgetting in dementia and depression, *J Consult Clin Psychol* 55:101-105, 1987.

Hart RP, Kwentus JA, Wade JB et al: Digit Symbol performance in mild dementia and depression, *J Consult Clin Psychol* 55:236-238, 1987.

Hodges JR, Berrios G: The neuropsychological differentiation of patients with very mild Alzheimer's disease and/or major depression, *J Am Geriatr Soc* 43(11):1256-1263, 1995.

Hodges JR, Salmon DP, Butters N: Semantic memory impairment in Alzheimer's disease: failure of access or degraded knowledge? *Neuropsychologia* 30:301-314, 1992.

Horton AM, Alana S: Validation of the Mini-Mental State Examination, *Int J Neurosci* 53(24):209-212, 1990.

Kawas C, Karagiozis H, Resau L et al: Reliability of the Blessed Telephone Information-Memory-Concentration test, *J Geriatr Psychiatry Neurol* 8(4):238-242, 1995.

Kolanowski A: Everyday functioning in Alzheimer's disease: contribution of neuropsychological testing, *Clin Nurse Spec* 10(1):7-11, 1996.

Lesher EL, Whelihan WM: Reliability of mental status instruments administered to nursing home residents, *J Consult Clin Psychol* 54:726-727, 1987.

Linn RT, Wolf PA, Bachman DL et al: The "preclinical phase" of probable Alzheimer's disease: A 13-year prospective study of the Framingham Cohort, *Arch Neurol* 52(5):485-490, 1995.

Lowenstein DA, Arguelles T, Arguelles S et al: Potential cultural bias in the neuropsychological assessment of the older adult, *J Clin Exp Neuropsychol* 16(4):623-629, 1994.

Luria AR: *Higher cortical functions in man,* New York, 1966, Basic Books.

Madsen J, Kesner RP: The temporal-distance effect in subjects with dementia of the Alzheimer type, *Alzheimer Dis Assoc Disord* 9(2):94-100, 1995.

Mahler ME, High WM et al: Assessment of cognitive, psychiatric, and behavioral disturbances in patients with dementia: The Neurobehavioral Rating Scale, *J Am Geriatr Soc* 40(6):549-555, 1992.

Mayeaux R, Stern Y, Rosen J et al: Is "subcortical dementia" a recognizable clinical entity? *Ann Neurol* 1(4):278-283, 1983.

McFadden L, Sampson M, Mohr E: Screening for cognitive dysfunction in neurodegenerative illness, *J Neurol* 57(10):1282, 1994.

Nadler JD, Relkin NR, Cohen MS et al: Mental status testing in the elderly nursing home population, *J Geriatr Psychiatric Neurol* 8(3):177-183, 1995.

Nebes RD, Brady CB: Generalized cognitive slowing and severity of dementia in Alzheimer's disease: implications for the interpretation of response-time data, *J Clin Exp Neuropsychol* 14:317-326, 1992.

Pantoni L, Inzitari D: Hachinski's ischemic score and the diagnosis of vascular dementia: a review, *Ital J Neurol Sci* 14(7):539-546, 1993.

Paolo AM, Troster AI, Glatt SL et al: Differentiation of the dementias of Alzheimer's and Parkinson's disease with the Dementia Rating Scale, *J Geriatr Psychiatry Neurol* 8(3):184-188, 1995.

Pearsall TS, O'Neill D, Wilcock GK: Use of the Mini-Mental State Examination to determine the usefulness of subsequent cognitive assessment in moderately to severely demented subjects, *Int J Geriat Psychiatry* 10(11):975-980, 1995.

Reitan RM, Wolfson D: *The Halstead-Reitan neuropsychological test battery: theory and clinical interpretation,* Tucson, 1985, Neuropsychological Press.

Rosen WG, Terry RD, Fuld PA et al: Pathological verification of ischemic score in differentiation of dementias, *Ann Neurol* 7:486-488, 1980.

Schmand B, Lindeboom J, Hooijer C et al: Relation between education and dementia: The role of test bias revisited, *J Neurol Neurosurg Psychiatry* 59(2):170-174, 1995.

Shay KA, Duke LW, Conboy T et al: The clinical validity of the Mattis Dementia Rating Scale in staging Alzheimer's dementia, *J Geriatr Psychiatry Neurol* 4:18-25, 1991.

Skelton WP, Skelton NK: Alzheimer's disease: recognizing and treating a frustrating condition, *Postgrad Med* 90:33-41, 1991.

Sloan P: Clinical neuropsychology in evaluating and treating brain dysfunction, *South Med J* 77:4-6, 1984.

Solomon DP, Thal LJ, Butters N: Longitudinal evaluation of dementia of the Alzheimer type: A comparison of three standardized mental status examinations, *Neurology* 40:1225-1230, 1991.

Stoudemire A, Hill C, Gulley LR et al: Neuropsychological and biomedical assessment of depression-dementia syndromes, *J Neuropsychiatry Clin Neurosci* 1(4):347-361, 1989.

Tierney MC, Snow WG, Szalai JP et al: A brief neuropsychological battery for the differential diagnosis of probable Alzheimer's disease, *Clin Neuropsychologist* 10(1):96-103, 1996.

Welsh KA, Fillenbaum G, Wilkinson W et al: Neuropsychological test performance in African-American and white patients with Alzheimer's disease, *Neurology* 45(12):2207-2211, 1995.

Wilder D, Cross P, Chen J et al: Operating characteristics of brief screens for dementia in a multicultural population, *Am J Geriat Psychiatry* 3(2):96-107, 1995.

Imaging the Brain in Alzheimer's Disease

Vicente Taasan

A picture is worth a thousand words.

—Author Unknown

The development of imaging techniques within the last 15 years has dramatically altered the field of neurosciences. A variety of techniques capable of imaging the brain became available in the late 1980s. Brain anatomy now can be mapped in exquisite detail.

Changes in brain metabolic activity due to emotional, motor, and cognitive aberrations can be documented by new imaging techniques. It is now possible to identify the anatomic, metabolic, and neurochemical bases of numerous mental illnesses. The techniques that permit observation of the brain can be divided into two broad groups:

1. Techniques measuring structure (anatomic imaging)
2. Techniques that measure function (functional imaging)

Anatomic imaging techniques include Computerized Tomography (CT) and Magnetic Resonance Imaging (MRI). In both, brain anatomy and alterations in brain structure are depicted by anatomic techniques.

Functional imaging techniques include Single-Photon Emission Computed Tomography (SPECT) and Positron Emission Tomography (PET), which measure metabolic and neurotransmitter functions. In Alzheimer's disease, anatomic imaging alone is often inadequate.

As a general rule, structural changes in the brain are late findings in Alzheimer's disease; in some mental illnesses, no structural changes are discernible at all. Functional imaging in Alzheimer's disease is clearly beneficial for this reason.

ANATOMIC IMAGING

Computed Tomography (CT)

The earliest of these techniques is Computerized Tomography (CT). Abnormalities in CT scans are not specific to any type of mental illness and, therefore, do not serve as a specific test for any such illness. Nonspecific abnormalities in

41

CT scans of patients with schizophrenia, bipolar disorder, depression, alcoholism, multiinfarct dementia, and Alzheimer's disease have been reported. CT is widely used because of its availability, low cost, and capability of identifying structural changes. Areas of atrophy, infarction (strokes), hemorrhage, and space-occupying lesions can be easily identified. Its disadvantages include lack of sensitivity, underestimation of brain atrophy, and the inability to take images in the sagittal and coronal views.

Patient preparation includes removal of metallic objects on the head. Items such as eyeglasses, earrings, and hair clasps produce artifacts that scatter x-rays and degrade CT images. And, as with all brain imaging techniques, the patient must be thoroughly instructed in the importance of keeping the head still to prevent motion artifacts.

It is the consensus of opinion that CT has a limited role in the diagnosis of Alzheimer's disease; however, it is useful in documenting organic causes of dementia such as brain neoplasms, atrophy, or infarcts. These issues are discussed further in Chapter 8.

Magnetic Resonance Imaging (MRI)

MRI provides better detail of the brain than CT and the information is in three planes (transverse, sagittal, and coronal), whereas CT provides information in the transverse plane only. Another attractive feature of MRI is that it does not use radiation. MRI can differentiate water, iron, fat, and blood using physical and biochemical properties of tissues.

MRI is unaffected by bone, and unlike CT, brain structures close to the skull such as the posterior fossa, orbits, and the skull base are imaged in good detail. MRI technology is readily available in most hospitals. MRI scanners are enclosed in a copper-lined windowless room. Prior to scanning, all metallic objects are removed from a patient. To prevent motion artifacts, a head holder is used during the scanning procedure. The procedure takes 35 to 45 minutes, and motion during this period will cause blurring and loss of structural detail. The procedure is painless. Those with back abnormalities, however, may experience discomfort. Postural hypotension may follow prolonged recumbency. Patients should be routinely advised against abruptly standing up after an MRI procedure.

Patients are often unprepared for the close quarters during the procedure. Also, a significant number find machine noise disturbing. Spatial limitation causes anxiety and sometimes claustrophobia in patients.

● MRI Cannot be Performed in the Following Patient Groups:

- Individuals with pacemakers
- Individuals with metallic objects such as screws, prostheses, orthopedic devices, shrapnel, etc.
- Patients on life-support systems
- Individuals with claustrophobia, who are often unable to complete the study

Patients with Alzheimer's disease usually show the following MRI findings: atrophy of the parahippocampal gyrus and temporal cortex, enlargement of the temporal horn, and atrophy of the hippocampal formation. Quantitation MRI has shown that patients with Alzheimer's disease have smaller brain volume, and in the temporal lobe, atrophy and loss of gray matter is often observed.

Other causes of dementia should be excluded before the diagnosis of Alzheimer's disease is made. This is best accomplished by CT or MRI.

Patients with dementia who will most likely benefit from CT or MRI include the following:

- Age less than 70 years
- Those with incontinence, gait changes, and a past history of head injury
- Those with focal neurologic signs to exclude "organic" causes of dementia

FUNCTIONAL IMAGING

From 1965 to 1975 nuclear medicine progressed from the research laboratory to standard hospital practice. Brain imaging was one of the earliest procedures offered by nuclear medicine, and the first nuclear medicine tomograms preceded CT scans. In the late 1970s, introduction of photo-multiplier tubes and 99mTechnetium agents simplified nuclear medicine procedures, and the acquisition of nuclear medicine images became relatively easy.

Information about blood flow to the brain is used as the basis of diagnosis in PET and SPECT scanning. PET uses radiopharmaceuticals that readily cross the intact blood-brain barrier to provide functional mapping. In the last decade, significant progress has been made in the availability and clinical application of single photon radiopharmaceuticals that cross the intact blood-brain barrier and are readily imaged by commercial (SPECT) systems. Unlike SPECT, PET remains in the forefront of neurochemistry research but its cost has prevented its introduction into standard hospital practice.

Currently, functional imaging offers the most information in the diagnosis of Alzheimer's disease. More importantly, because functional imaging is independent of changes in brain structure, early Alzheimer's disease may be diagnosed by functional (PET or SPECT) imaging. Low-metabolic activity in the brain cortex may be seen in PET scanning long before brain atrophy can be seen in CT or MRI.

Functional imaging is especially useful in differentiating Alzheimer's disease from depression and other dementing disorders such as multiinfarct dementia, Pick's disease, and Parkinson's disease.

This differentiation is important clinically since depression is an illness that can be treated with medications.

Positron Emission Tomography (PET)

PET was the first functional imaging procedure introduced and remains as the "gold standard" to which SPECT and other functional imaging techniques are compared. Despite its elegance and utility, PET has not gained the widespread use it deserves because of the expense and expertise required.

PET relies on "coincidence scanning." Images of the brain are produced when a positron-emitting radionuclide interacts with an electron. Both particles cease to exist and they are converted into two photons, which travel in opposite directions. The event (annihilation) is detected and an image can be obtained by recording the location, intensity, and direction of these photons using coincidence circuitry.

Positron-emitting radionuclides can only be produced by a cyclotron and a support team of physicists, chemists, and computer experts is required to run a PET facility. Functional imaging of the brain with PET is usually done with intravenous injection of Fluorine-18 Fluorodeoxyglucose (^{18}FDG) or compounds labeled with carbon-11 (^{11}C). Glucose is ideal since it is the basic nutrient of brain metabolism. PET scans show neuronal patterns of glucose metabolism. Areas of decreased photon activity reflect dysfunctional neurons.

The patient is imaged 4 to 6 hours after fasting. Fasting is necessary to control the amount of glucose in the brain during the imaging procedure. An arterial line may be necessary if quantitation procedures are added to the usual imaging process. The radionuclide is injected via an intravenous line. Because the procedure is lengthy, patients are asked to void prior to it. During the procedure, motion and conversation are not allowed. The patient remains supine throughout the procedure with only the head inside the scanner.

Despite its general clinical usefulness, the value of the PET in the diagnosis of Alzheimer's disease remains controversial. Additionally the expense makes it a toll beyond the financial means of most health care plans and patients.

Single Photon Emission Computer Tomography (SPECT)

Recent improvements in instrumentation and radiopharmaceuticals point to an increasing role of SPECT in the diagnosis of a number of neurologic disorders. Evaluation of patients with certain neurologic and psychiatric diseases now routinely involves SPECT scanning, attesting to the power of this procedure as a window to peer into the functions of the brain. Even the most sophisticated SPECT technique is more widely available and less expensive than PET.

The radiopharmaceutical model for SPECT imaging is the microsphere model. This model assumes that the tracer is freely diffusible from the blood. From the blood, the tracer is completely extracted into the brain, where it remains fixed in one location. Intravenous injection of brain radiopharmaceuticals result in brain distribution following the above-mentioned model. Brain SPECT tracers cross the blood-brain barrier, distribute proportionally to regional blood flow, and remain in the brain to permit SPECT imaging.

The most widely used agent in brain SPECT imaging is HMPAO (hexamethylpropyleneamineoxime [Ceretec]). It is labeled with 99mTechnetium, a radionuclide that has optimal physical characteristics for imaging. HMPAO can be labeled on-site, has an ideal half-life of 6 hours, and has a 140 keV single energy peak—a characteristic that makes it ideal for imaging. Additionally, a variety of commercial systems are capable of imaging with high resolution.

Modern imaging systems have overcome drawbacks of the older systems such as poor head alignment, inadequate uniformity and linearity, and magnetic field limitations. Resolution with the modern systems is fairly good as compared to older systems—state-of-the-art systems provide a resolution ranging from 6 to 9 mm. Multidetector systems are capable of resolving 6-mm structures in the cortex and 7 mm at the brain center.

Clinical studies comparing patients with Alzheimer's disease and normal controls or those with multiinfarct dementia have shown that SPECT has an acceptable accuracy. The sensitivity of SPECT in mildly demented patients is 80% to 87%. In severe dementia, sensitivity as high as 95% has been reported. Bilateral posterior temporal and parietal perfusion defect are predictive of Alzheimer's disease.

The reduction in tracer uptake in the posterior association cortex in patients with Alzheimer's disease is due to multiple factors, including reduced blood flow, cortical thinning of the temporal area, and a corresponding decrease in the number of neurons in these areas. Most of the abnormality, though, is due to reduced blood flow, and in conjunction with reduced brain size (atrophy) in these areas, the characteristic scan appearance is produced.

Other scan patterns may be present in patients with dementia and even Alzheimer's disease. In frontal dementia, considered by some as a subset of Alzheimer's disease, bilateral frontal or frontal and temporal abnormalities are noted. These abnormal patterns occur in Alzheimer's disease, schizophrenia, depression, Pick's disease, and other diseases, and by themselves are not characteristic of Alzheimer's disease. On the other hand, the probability of Alzheimer's disease is relatively low with normal perfusion or if defects are noted in areas other than in the temporal or parietal lobes.

Holman and others, in a controlled study to determine the value of brain SPECT studies with HMPAO in the diagnosis of Alzheimer's disease, have estimated the predictive value of different SPECT imaging patterns. These authors have shown that the probability of Alzheimer's disease is 82% when the scan shows bilateral temporal abnormalities. When additional defects are noted in conjunction with bilateral temporal defects, the probability is 77%. Unilateral defects and frontal defects have a probability of 57% and 43%, respectively, for Alzheimer's disease. The probability of the disease is 0% when multiple small defects were noted. These authors concluded that unilateral or frontal defects are not predictive of Alzheimer's disease, while bilateral perfusion defects have a high predictive value for the disease. An example of bilateral perfusion defects is shown in Figure 4-1.

SUMMARY

Most clinicians believe that an anatomic scan (CT or MRI) is useful in some patients with dementia to exclude diseases other than Alzheimer's disease. Table 4-1 shows the duration, preparation, cost, and the entities best identified by CT, MRI, PET, and SPECT. Since SPECT is readily available and considerably less expensive than PET, it is the scan of choice in the diagnostic work-up of Alzheimer's disease.

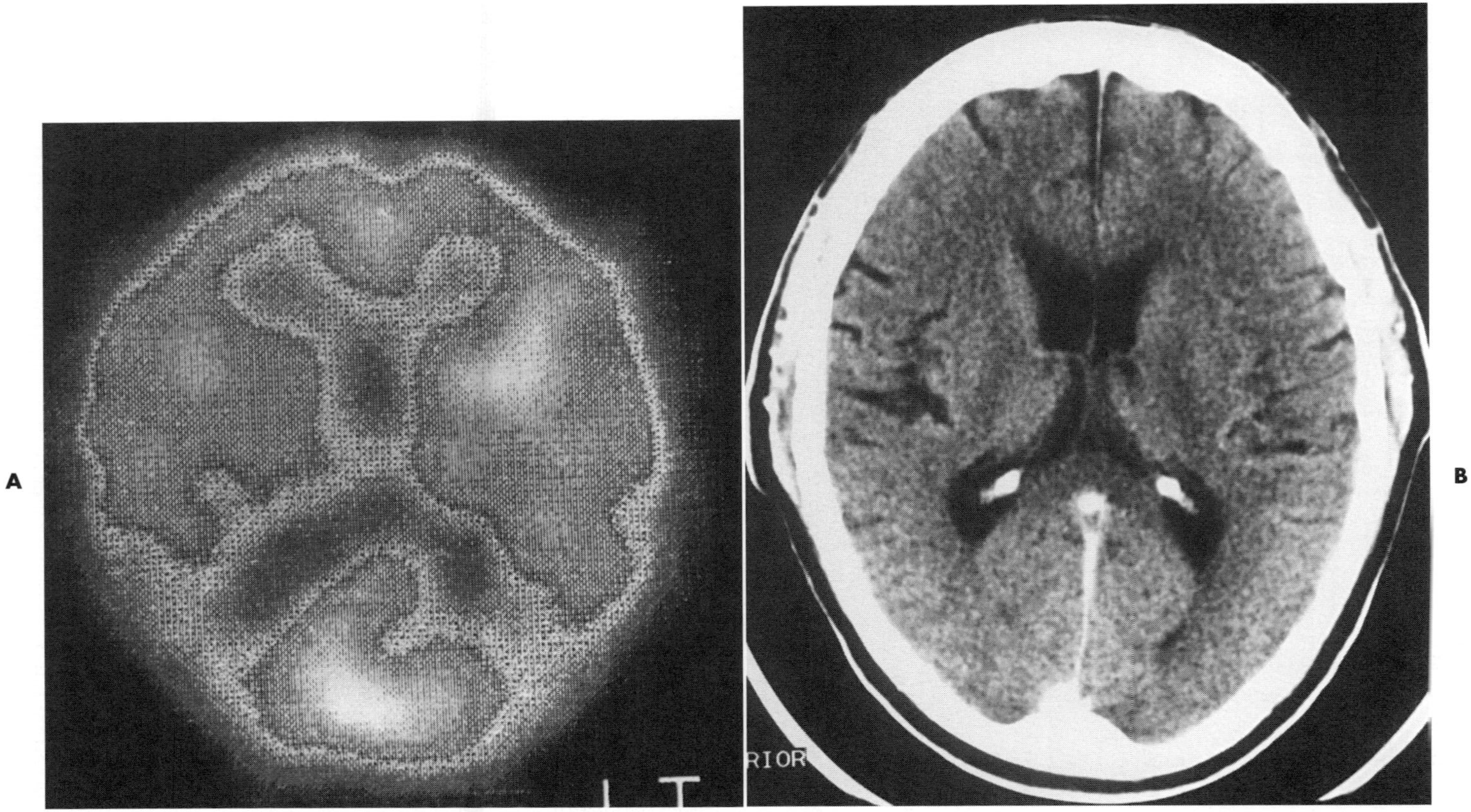

Figure 4-1 Fifty-eight-year-old male with dementia. **A,** The SPECT scan of the brain shows absent activity in both temporal lobes. Absence of activity indicates reduced perfusion in the temporal lobes. **B,** Note that the CT scan shows normal findings. The SPECT scan findings in this patient are typical of Alzheimer's disease.

Table 4-1

Comparison of Imaging Time, Cost, Preparation, and Utility of CT, MRI, PET, and SPECT in the Diagnosis of Alzheimer's Disease

Test	Time	Prep	Cost	Utility
CT	20 minutes	Remove objects on head	$700–900	Tumors, hemorrhages, infarct atrophy
MRI	35–45 minutes	Remove metallic objects	$1,100–1,300	More sensitive than CT for above indications
PET	2–3 hours	4–6 hour-fast	$1,500–2,000	Not readily available, expensive
SPECT	45 minutes–1 hour	Instruct patient not to move	$700–800	Generally available, picture quality very good with modern scanners, ideal for AD

BIBLIOGRAPHY

Andreasen, NC: Brain Imaging: Applications in Psychiatry, *Science* 239:1381-1388, 1988.

Bonte FJ, Horn J, Tiortner R et al: Single photon tomography in Alzheimer's disease and the dementias, *Semin Nucl Med* 20:342-352, 1990.

Clarfield AM, Larson EB: An opposing view, *J Fam Pract* 31:405-409, 1990.

Davis PC, Mirra SS, Alazraki N: The brain in older persons with and without dementia: findings on MR, PET and SPECT images, *American J Radiology* 162:1267-1278, 1994.

Herholz K, Adams R, Kessler J et al: Criteria for diagnosis of Alzheimer's disease with Positron Emission Tomography, *Dementia* 1:156-164, 1990.

Holman BL, Devons MD: Functional brain SPECT: the emergence of a powerful clinical method, *J Nucl Med* 33:1888-1904, 1992.

Holman BL, Johnson KA, Gerada B et al: The scintigraphic appearance of Alzheimer's disease: a prospective study using Technetium-99m-HMPAO SPECT, *J Nucl Med* 33:181-185, 1992.

Jaqust WJ, Budinger TF, Reed BR: The diagnosis of dementia with Single Photon Emission Computed Tomography, *Arch Neurol* 44:258-262, 1987.

Powers WJ, Perlmutter JS, Videen TD et al: Blinded chemical evaluation of Positron Emission Tomography for the diagnosis of probable Alzheimer's disease, *Neurology* 42:765-770, 1992.

Souder E, Alavi A: Á comparison of neuroimaging modalities for diagnosing dementia, *Nurse Pract* 20:66-74, 1995.

Tanna NK, Kohn MI, Horwich DN et al: Analysis of brain and cerebrospinal fluid volumes with MR Imaging: impact on PET data correction for atrophy; Part II. Aging and Alzheimer's dementia, *Radiology* 178:123-130, 1991.

Unit 2

When health is absent,
wisdom cannot reveal itself,
art cannot become manifest,
strength cannot fight,
wealth becomes useless,
and intelligence cannot be applied.

—Herophilus

Alzheimer's Disease

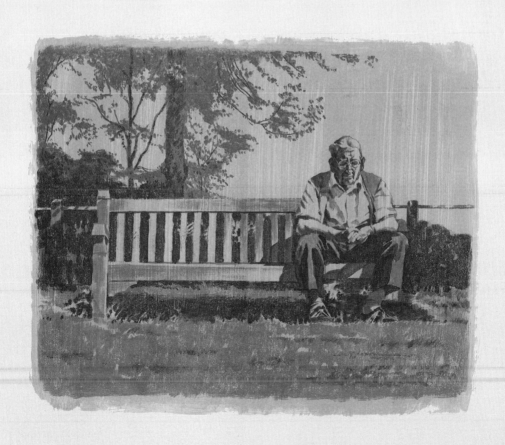

Historical Perspectives

Lorraine Sambat

One of the most remarkable and beneficial re-
forms of the nineteenth century has been in
the attitude of the profession and the public to
the subject of insanity, and the gradual formation
of a body of men in the profession who labour
to find out the cause and the means of relief of
this most distressing of all human maladies.

—William Osler

The history of Alzheimer's disease began in 1906 with Dr. Alois Alzheimer's presentation of the clinical case of a 55-year-old woman suffering from progressive dementia. Dementia, however, has been recognized since early antiquity, and has often been associated with old age.

EARLY HISTORY OF SENILE DEMENTIA

References to senile dementia were first recorded around 600 B.C. Solon, an Athenian lawgiver known as one of the seven wise men of Greece, acknowledged the fact that judgment may be impaired in old age and revised the usual practice of dividing an inheritance within the family, taking into account that judgment while making a will may be affected by old age.

Plato also recognized senile dementia in his *Republic,* and stated that the commission of certain crimes (sacrilege, treachery, treason) is excusable in a state of madness, when under the influence of drugs or alcohol, in extreme old age, or in a fit of childish wantonness.

It is interesting to note that although dementia was often associated with old age, the ancient Greeks recognized that it was not part of the normal aging process. In fact, in that era of history, the government was usually run by the elderly because of their greater experience, loyalty, and wisdom. This was in line with the ancient Greek tradition of placing emphasis on philosophical arguments and the prowess of the mind, rather than on the body.

Hippocrates, on the other hand, whose major contribution to medicine was to free it from the hold of the supernatural by attributing diseases to natural rather than supernatural forces, did not include senile dementia among the mental disorders, giving the impression that he may have felt senile dementia was part of the normal aging process. One of the leading thoughts at that time was that human life went through stages governed by two numbers: 3 and 7. At 3 the child started to talk and was able to express himself. At 7 he was able to understand abstract concepts, at 21 (3×7) he reached the peak of his physical abilities and was legally responsible for his actions, at 49 (7×7) he reached the peak of his mental abilities, at 63 ($3 \times 3 \times 7$) he should retire from active work, and at 81 ($3 \times 3 \times 3 \times 3$) he should contemplate the end of life. At no stage was the individual expected to be mentally incompetent.

In ancient Rome where more emphasis was placed on youth, vigor, health, and physical fitness, the elderly tended to be somewhat denigrated. In 40 B.C. Horace expressed in a letter the characteristics of old men as, *"desire for gain, miserliness, lack of energy, quarrelsomeness, praise of the good old days, and a condemnation of the younger generation."*

Cicero, however, answered this accusation by stating, *"As wantonness and licentiousness are faults of the young rather than of the old, yet not of all young men but only of the depraved, so the senile folly called dotage is characteristic not of all old men but only of the frivolous."*

It was not until about 200 years later that the general opinion of the elderly improved in Rome under the philosopher-emperors Trajan, Hadrian, and Marcus Aurelius. It was at this time in history that Galen, who had achieved the pinnacle of Greek medicine, added "morosis" (dementia) to the list of mental diseases, and included old age as one of the stages in which it occurred.

In the ensuing centuries dementia was thought to be simply a result of old age. In 1599, Du Laurens, a physician to the court of Henry IV of France, wrote a discourse on old age in which he noted, *"All the action of the bodie and minde are weakened and grown feeble, the senses are dull, the memorie lost and the judgement failing so that they become as they were in their infancie."*

Salmon, a London practitioner, issued a remarkable evaluation in a case report of senile dementia, *"For Sir John was not mad, or distracted like a man in Bedlam, yet he was so depraved in his intellect that he was become not only a perfect child in understanding but also foolish withall."*

Even as late as the nineteenth century, senile dementia was considered by many to be an inevitable accompaniment of aging. It was generally accepted that as individuals grew older, their mental faculties declined. Older persons became unable to remember or to communicate, and they often developed eccentric habits, such as talking to themselves or hoarding useless possessions.

Unfortunately, the diseases of the aged were considered relatively unimportant until the second half of the nineteenth century, when interest in geriatric medicine began to grow.

This interest was initiated by the French, who introduced more humane treatment of the impoverished sick, elderly, and insane patients housed in their asylums. Until the end of the eighteenth century, conditions at these asylums had been decidedly inhumane.

At Bethlehem Hospital in London, commonly referred to as Bedlam (which became a synonym for chaos), the conditions were appalling. Patients were subjected to filthy living conditions, poor food, isolation, darkness, and brutal guards. Common treatments for these patients and others throughout western Europe included the use of emetics and purgatives (substances used to induce vomiting and evacuation of the bowels, respectively), bloodletting, and other procedures such as dousing the patient with ice cold water or putting him in a gyrating chair (a spinning chair that left the patient unconscious) in order to cause a shock to his system.

King George III of England may even have been subjected to some of these treatments. In 1788, in addition to arguing over whether he was insane or physically ill, physicians disagreed about whether he should *"have his skull blistered, his intestines purged, be bled, be made to vomit, or be walked around the gardens of the royal castle while he listened to soothing music."*

PATIENT CARE REFORM MOVEMENT AND ORIGINS OF CONTEMPORARY VIEWS ON DEMENTIA

The evolution of the clinical recognition of senile dementia as a disease entity, and not part of the normal aging process, occurred in the latter half of the 18th century. Cullen, a professor of medicine in Scotland (1710 to 1770), made the following observations: *"Imbecility of judgement, by which men either do not perceive the relation of things or forget them due to diminished perception and memory when oppressed with age [senile dementia]."*

The leader of the movement to reform the asylums in France was Philippe Pinel, a French physician who was greatly influenced by the science of psychology, which was then a new field. Pinel became physician-in-chief at the Bicetre asylum in Paris in 1793. Before he took charge, conditions at the Bicetre asylum, where patients were kept in chains, had been as appalling as those at Bedlam.

Pinel instituted radical changes in the treatment of those deterred in Bicetre. Shackles were removed, patients were allowed freedom to sunshine and air, and healthy nutritional food was served. Kindness and understanding were made mandatory by Pinel's policy. He insisted that the staff physicians live with the insane patients in order to study their habits and personalities and to follow the progression of their illnesses. Pinel believed that if a physician had no understanding of human behavior, he was not qualified to work with the mentally ill.

During his tenure at Bicetre, Pinel studied his patients carefully, systematically described their symptoms, and determined whether those symptoms were linked to difficulties with memory, attention, or judgment. Unlike most of his predecessors, Pinel believed that mental illness was not inflicted on victims by evil spirits or other sources. Instead, he thought it was caused by adversities in their lives or by heredity.

Esquirol, who worked with Pinel, wrote a chapter on dementia in his book, *A Treatise on Insanity,* published in 1845. He said, *"Senile dementia is established slowly. It commences with enfeeblement of memory, particularly the memory of recent impressions. The sensations are feeble; the attention, at first fatiguing, at length becomes impossible; the will is uncertain and without impulsion; the movements are slow and impractical."*

Since many elderly people were placed in asylums because of their poverty or eccentric behavior, a large population of elderly patients was available for physicians to study. As a result, French physicians began to build up a large body of work on geriatrics, and they called for more attention to be given to the problems of the elderly. The French were soon followed by the Germans and the English. Together, physicians from the three countries developed the founding principles of modern geriatrics.

Soon the rest of society began to accept these new attitudes concerning the treatment of the elderly. However, there were a few notable exceptions. In 1874 George M. Beard, an American neurologist, concluded that the sharpness of the mind diminished as one aged. He estimated that 70% of a person's work was accomplished before age 45 and that 90% was done before age 50. In 1905 Sir William Osler repeated Beard's conclusions in a speech and joked that men should be put to sleep when they reach age 60. Beard was severely criticized by his peers, among them Sir James Chricton-Browne, who believed that, although there was no way to avoid the aging process, many of the ailments that accompany old age could be prevented. Like many of his contemporaries, Chricton-Browne was a proponent of more humane treatment of the elderly.

Alois Alzheimer

It was in this milieu in 1906 that Alois Alzheimer presented his findings on what was first called presenile dementia. Alois Alzheimer, a German neuroscientist, was born in Marktbreit-am-Main, Bavaria, in 1864. He was the son of a government officer in Marktbreit, Bavaria. He studied medicine at the universities of Würzburg, Tübingen, and Berlin, and received his medical degree in 1887 from the University of Würzburg after completing a thesis on the wax-producing glands of the ear.

Alzheimer next served as an assistant at Irrenanstalt in Frankfurt am Main, where he met Franz Nissl in 1889. It was Nissl who inspired Alzheimer to study neuropathology and stimulated his interest in brain pathology research. As a young medical student, Nissl had demonstrated his flair for experimentation by winning a competition on the "Pathological Changes of Nerve Cells in the Cerebral Cortex." The resulting method of staining neuronal cell bodies, now called Nissl's stain, was considered a scientific breakthrough in 1892 and a major advance in neuroanatomy and neuropathology.

Nissl's research captivated the attention of Alzheimer and through their shared interest, their lives intertwined with yet another giant in the history of psychiatry, Emil Kraepelin, one of the founders of biologically based psychiatry. In 1895 Nissl joined Emil Kraepelin in Heidelburg to study the framework of psychiatric disease. Alzheimer followed in 1902 and then moved to Munich with Kraepelin in 1903.

In Munich, Alzheimer and Kraepelin devoted themselves to presenting the exact clinical-anatomical relationships in psychiatric diseases. Alzheimer acquired a reputation for being a great teacher and is remembered for training and encouraging his protégés, who would become the next generation of neuropathologists.

Alzheimer and Nissl complemented each other perfectly. Alzheimer had meticulous research practices and strong reasoning ability, and Nissl had imagination and original ideas. For seven years the two men worked together at the psychiatric hospital in Frankfurt. During this time they introduced new laboratory techniques, new methods of microscopically examining brain cells, and new ways of handling the brain during autopsy.

The First Patient with Alzheimer's Disease

In 1906 Dr. Alois Alzheimer presented a case before the meeting of South-West Germany Psychiatrists in Tübingen. This was the first case of the disease that would later bear his name. The patient was a 55-year-old woman suffering from dementia who had been admitted to the psychiatric hospital in Frankfurt. Her symptoms had begun at the age of 51 with an unreasonable jealousy of her husband. As her illness progressed, the woman endured a rapid decline in memory, paranoid delusions, auditory hallucinations, and, finally, complete dementia. Within four and a half years of the onset of symptoms, the woman died.

Other cases of dementia had been noted previously, but Alzheimer is credited for his extraordinary clinical observations in this specific case of a disease that later came to bear his name. This patient's illness also was unique because of her age, the speed of the disease's progression, and the neuropathological findings. Unlike senile dementia, which begins at age 65 or older and progresses slowly, this woman's illness began at a relatively young age and progressed very rapidly.

At autopsy, using the techniques developed by Nissl, Alzheimer noted the presence of multiple foci known as plaques, which had been described by Emil Redlich in 1898 as the distinctive feature of senile dementia. In addition, however, Alzheimer noted the presence of neurofibrillary tangles, thick, coiled fibers within the cytoplasm of the cerebral cortical neurons. This discovery led Alzheimer to note in his report, *"On the whole, it is evident that we are dealing with a peculiar, little-known disease process."*

Senile dementia had previously been associated with the age group of 65 and older, and was an accepted part of aging.

Alzheimer's discovery of senile plaques in presenile dementia was especially significant. Alzheimer was never certain of the distinction between presenile dementia and senile dementia, but Kraepelin believed presenile dementia with anatomical findings of senile dementia to be an independent disease process. Gaetano Perusini, an Italian physician, also believed that early onset and clinical features of presenile dementia were sufficient symptoms for it to be considered a separate disease process. In 1910 Kraepelin proposed naming the presenile form of dementia after Alzheimer. The name *Alzheimer* is now known worldwide.

During the next 5 years, 12 other cases of this new disease were reported. The condition was already being referred to by many authors as "Alzheimer's disease." This designation was in part the result of its endorsement as a separate disease by Alzheimer's mentor, Emil Kraepelin, who was the leader of the organic school of psychiatry. This school of thought held that psychiatric ailments could be traced to an organic origin. This was in direct contrast with the functional school of psychiatry, which taught that psychological elements, such as an unhappy childhood, could produce mental disease. Alzheimer's discovery effectively established the organic school and Emil Kraepelin as the chief authorities on the causes of mental illness.

The most prolific of the authors who described Alzheimer's disease from 1906 to 1911 was not Alzheimer but Gaetano Perusini, who reported four cases in 1910 alone. Because of Perusini's efforts, many Italian authors still refer to the condition as Alzheimer-Perusini disease. Another Italian physician, Francesco Bonfiglio, reported the second case of Alzheimer's disease in 1908. His paper described in detail the neuropathological findings and included the first drawing of neurofibrillary tangles as seen under a microscope. It was not until 1911, however, that Alzheimer reported his second case of the disease.

Alzheimer did not make his discovery in a vacuum. His research was made possible by the work of other researchers, such as Nissl, and Max Bielschowsky, whose silver-based stain permitted Alzheimer to view neurofibrillary tangles. Senile plaques such as those detected by Alzheimer in the brain of his first patient were initially described by Paul Blocq and Georges Marinesco in 1892, and were later described by Emil Redlich in 1898, to be characteristics of senile dementia.

Alterations in neurofibrils similar to those discovered by Alzheimer had been found in the brains of experimental animals before Alzheimer reported on his findings in humans. In fact, in 1845 Wilhelm Griesinger had been the first researcher to recognize presenile dementia. Even though Griesinger's book was translated into French and English, his report was overlooked. Although the disease bears Alzheimer's name, its discovery can also be credited to many other scientists whose work enabled Alzheimer to make his discovery.

In 1912 Alois Alzheimer accepted a position as a psychiatry professor and director of the Psychiatric Institute at the University of Breslau. Three years later he developed a heart condition and died at the age of 51. Although there were many international contributions, Nissl, Kraepelin, and Alzheimer were credited with making possible early contributions to the investigation of numerous brain disorders. Using Nissl's silver stain, Alzheimer identified the distinctive features of Alzheimer's disease that are now considered the hallmark neuropathological features: neuronal loss, neurofibrillary tangles, and senile plaques.

Presenile vs. Senile Dementia

After Alzheimer's discovery, many questions were still unanswered. It seemed likely that since the first patient reported as having Alzheimer's disease was only 51 years old and the next few cases involved patients under the age of 65 years that Alzheimer's disease predominantly affected younger people. At the turn of the century, it was thought that mental functions tended to deteriorate as an individual aged. Since different terms were needed to distinguish the impairment of mental functions that occurs in old age, known as senile dementia, from that which occurs in younger people, the term *presenile dementia* was introduced. A few cases in which the disease manifested itself in the fourth decade were reported, which reinforced the concept that Alzheimer's disease should be classified as a presenile dementia. In fact, until the 1970s the diagnosis of Alzheimer's disease was restricted to patients less than 65 years of age.

However, as clinical and postmortem findings resulted in more cases being described in patients over 65 years of age, it was acknowledged that Alzheimer's disease was not confined to younger people but also was affecting older patients. Thus another term was introduced, "senile dementia of the Alzheimer's type."

For many years the debate continued in regard to whether Alzheimer's disease affecting younger people, or presenile dementia, was the same condition as senile dementia of the Alzheimer's type. Some experts raised the question of whether the disorder was one disease that could have an early onset (presenile dementia) and a late onset (senile dementia) or whether there were two different diseases that sometimes displayed the same or similar features.

A publication in the *American Journal of Psychiatry* by Charles Wells in 1978 clearly demonstrated that the autopsy findings in patients with Alzheimer's disease and what was then referred to as senile dementia were identical. Citing the 1970 study of Tomlinson, Blessed, and Roth, who did 50 successive autopsies in elderly patients with dementia, Wells concluded that Alzheimer's disease accounted for at least 50% of the cases of dementia.

In the early 1980s a consensus was reached, and it is now generally accepted that the presenile and senile types of Alzheimer's disease are actually the same. The currently accepted position is to refer to Alzheimer's disease and to note that its onset can occur early or late in life.

The Aging Population

The incidence of Alzheimer's disease increases with advancing age.

The aging of the American population is increasing dramatically. Average life expectancy in the United States today is 75.5 years, with some demographer's placing the average at 85 years. The average life expectancy at the turn of the century was 47 years. Since 1950, the 65-and-older group has increased 7%, totaling a startling 34 million people. The 3.8 million seniors 85 years old and older constitute the fastest-growing segment of our population. The U.S. Census Bureau projects that by 2030 this group will number 9 million and increase to 19 million in the following two decades. A research team in Denmark projected that today's newborns will live on average to 100 years.

Dementia affects about 10% of all people over the age of 65, and as many as 50% of those over age 85. Alzheimer's disease is the most common cause of dementia in the elderly—there are currently 4 million recognized cases in the United States alone. By the year 2040, there could be 14 million cases of Alzheimer's disease in the U.S. Alzheimer's disease is the fourth leading cause of death for the elderly, accounting for more than 100,000 deaths per year. The cost of caring for Alzheimer's patients is estimated at a staggering $125 billion annually. The rising prevalence of dementia is directly related to the aging of the American population.

ALZHEIMER'S DISEASE RESEARCH

Almost 90 years after Alzheimer first reported on the disease, scientists still do not understand the causes of Alzheimer's disease and have yet to discover a cure. Because of our aging population, Alzheimer's disease is a much greater problem now than it was at the beginning of the twentieth century. Therefore, findings about this disease are more important now than they were at the time of their discovery. In 1900 there were only 3 million Americans aged 65 or older, and in 1989 there were more than 27 million. By the year 2050 approximately 67 million Americans will be 65 or older. Unless a cure or method of prevention is found, of those 67 million people, it is estimated that 14 million will have Alzheimer's disease.

Because of the rapidly growing elderly population, the prevalence of the disease, and the high cost of patient care, much more attention is being given to Alzheimer's disease than in the past. This attention resulted in the formation of the Alzheimer's Disease and Related Disorders Association (ADRDA) in 1980. From a handful of dedicated family members and researchers with an initial budget of $85,000, this association has become the largest nonprofit health organization in the U.S., with a budget exceeding $60 million. The ADRDA has encouraged a great deal of media attention for Alzheimer's disease, and it has acted as a source of information for the public. Increasing public awareness of Alzheimer's disease has resulted in the establishment of support groups for families and caregivers of patients with Alzheimer's disease and adult day care for the patients themselves.

Another benefit of public interest in Alzheimer's disease is increased funding for research. The number of articles related to Alzheimer's disease published in medical journals has increased from none in 1966, 49 in 1976, 785 in 1986, and 1560 in 1996. This increase in publication on Alzheimer's disease in the last three decades has been nothing short of phenomenal. A journal exclusively devoted to the subject, *The Journal of Alzheimer Disease and Associated Disorders* began its quarterly publication in 1986.

Although a cure for Alzheimer's disease has not yet been found, researchers have made considerable advances since Alzheimer first identified the disease in 1906. Whereas in the past a diagnosis of Alzheimer's disease could be made only by ruling out all other possibilities and then examining the brain at autopsy, now researchers are on the brink of being able to make a positive diagnosis before death by using laboratory tests or brain imaging studies.

In addition to making advances in diagnostic procedures, researchers are currently experimenting with new treatments for patients with Alzheimer's disease. One reason for optimism in the area of treatment is the similarity of Alzheimer's disease to Parkinson's disease. In Parkinson's disease one neurotransmitter is missing, whereas in Alzheimer's disease five or six neuro-transmitters are lacking. Since researchers have discovered several treatments for Parkinson's disease, they hope to develop similar treatments for replenishing the missing neurotransmitters in the brains of Alzheimer's disease patients.

The dedication and effort of those striving to shed light on Alzheimer's disease can be compared to Dr. Bernard Rieux in Camus' *The Plague*. Dr. Rieux's chronicle, like those aforementioned and many others, "could be only the record of what had to be done and what assuredly would have to be done again in the never-ending fight against terror and its relentless onslaughts, despite their personal afflictions, by all who, while unable to be saints but refusing to bow down to pestilences, strive their utmost to be healers." These advances offer hope that a cure for Alzheimer's disease is on the horizon.

BIBLIOGRAPHY

Alexander FG, Selesnick ST: *The history of psychiatry: an evaluation of psychiatric thought and practice from prehistoric times to the present,* New York, 1966, Harper & Row.

Alois Alzheimer: *JAMA* 208:1017-1018, 1969.

Alzheimer's Disease and Related Disorders Association: *Alzheimer's disease statistics,* Chicago, 1990, The Association.

Beach TG: The history of Alzheimer's disease: three debates, *J Hist Med* 42:327-349, 1987.

Brick K, Amaducci L, Pepeu G: *The early story of Alzheimer's disease,* New York, 1987, Raven Press.

Evans DA et al: Estimated prevalence of Alzheimer's disease, *Milbank Q* 68(2):267-289, 1990.

Kreutzberg GW: 100 years of Nissl staining, *Trends Neurosci* July:236-237, 1984.

Pendleburg WW, Solomon, PR: "Alzheimer's Disease," Clinical Symposium, *Ciba* 48(3):2-32, 1996.

Rocca WA, Amaducci LA: Letter to editor, *Alzheimer Dis Assoc Disord* 2:56-57, 1988.

Tomlinson BE, Blessed G, Roth M: Observations on the brains of demented old people, *J Neurol Sci* 11:205-242, 1970.

Wells CE: Chronic brain disease: an overview, *Am J Psychiatry* 135(1):1-12, 1978.

Wisniewski HM: Milestones in the history of Alzheimer disease research. In Wisniewski HM, Winblad B, editors: *Alzheimer's disease and related disorders,* New York, 1989, Alan R Liss.

Etiology and Pathogenesis: Current Concepts

Chapter 6

Eleanor P Lavretsky
Fredda L Leiter
Lissy F Jarvik

*On the whole, it is evident that we are dealing
with a peculiar, little-known disease process.
In recent years these particular disease-processes
have been detected in great numbers. This fact
should stimulate us to further study and analysis
of this particular disease. We must not be satisfied to force it into the existing group of well-
known disease patterns. It is clear that there exist many more mental diseases than our
textbooks indicate.*

—Alois Alzheimer

Life expectancy has increased dramatically during this century due to many
factors, including the discovery of cures for many infectious diseases, the
development of sophisticated medical and surgical technologies, and the
promotion of healthier lifestyles. Many people now reach an age at which
degenerative diseases of the brain, particularly Alzheimer's disease, become
common. Dementia, the loss of our most human qualities—reasoning, memory,
and language—formerly was accepted as the natural consequence of reaching
advanced old age. A grandparent who became confused and forgetful suffered
from "hardening of the arteries in the brain." In the past, two etiologic factors
were thought to be responsible for initiating the dementing process: advanced
age and arteriosclerosis or atherosclerosis. It is now obvious that they are neither
necessary nor sufficient for the development of dementia.

Old age is an important risk factor for Alzheimer's disease, but epidemiologic
studies have demonstrated that a large proportion of individuals do not have
dementia, no matter how old they are. The number of individuals at a given time
(prevalence) with dementia from all causes ranges from 5% to 10% among
persons age 65 and older, and increases exponentially with age. A recent study
performed in England demonstrated that new cases per year (incidence) doubled

with every five years of age: from 2.3% for persons aged 75-79, to 4.6% for ages 80-84, and 8.5% for ages 85-89 years.

NEURITIC PLAQUES, AMYLOID, AND GENETICS

The etiologic basis of the degenerative changes in Alzheimer's disease is still unknown.

It is becoming clear that understanding the genesis of neuritic (senile) plaques may provide powerful clues to the pathogenesis of the disease.

In 1907 Alois Alzheimer described the following microscopic changes in his first Alzheimer's disease patient: "Scattered through the entire cortex, especially in the upper layers, are found foci that were caused by the deposition of a *peculiar substance* in the cerebral cortex." This "peculiar substance" is now known as the β-amyloid protein (BAP). The neuritic plaque, which contains BAP, is a complex, slowly evolving structure believed to require up to decades to reach maturation. It consists of a central amyloid core surrounded by abnormal neurites, altered glial cells, and cellular debris.

These deposits had been described some 50 years earlier (in 1853) by Rudolf Virchow, the great German pathologist who called them "amyloid," an unfortunate term because it implies that the deposits are made of a starchlike substance. In fact, chemical studies have shown that the principal constituents of the amyloid filament are actually proteins, and that various types of protein characterize the different diseases marked by the deposition of amyloid. The common thread linking these amyloidoses is the extracellular deposition of normal or mutated protein fragments, always folded in a particular three-dimensional pattern called a beta-pleated sheet. This characteristic feature enables researchers to observe apple-green birefringence in polarized light after the tissue has been stained with Congo red dye.

The formation of amyloid deposits in different diseases seems to follow a common chain of events: normal protein-altered protein-amyloid deposition. In Alzheimer's disease the sequence starts within the amyloid precursor protein (APP), a membrane-bound glycoprotein that is present in normal neurons and in nonneuronal cells (Figure 6-1). Its exact role in the adult brain is not known, but it does have a trophic function and is required to maintain both fibroblast and hippocampal cells in tissue culture.

The central portion of senile plaques, β-amyloid protein consists of a 39 to 43 amino acid fragment derived from APP. The normal pathway of APP metabolism produces a long portion of soluble APP rather than BAP. A shift in APP metabolism from the production of soluble APP to the production of insoluble β-amyloid is now believed to be the metabolic abnormality leading to Alzheimer's disease.

The possible causes of this shift are yet to be determined. One hypothesis is that point mutations in the APP gene may alter APP metabolism in some familial cases. Another hypothesis suggests the overproduction of APP may bring on a subsequent shift to the alternative metabolic pathway that leads to the production of β-amyloid. Observations of increased APP synthesis in experimental brain injuries, severe head trauma, and in Down syndrome are in accord with that hypothesis.

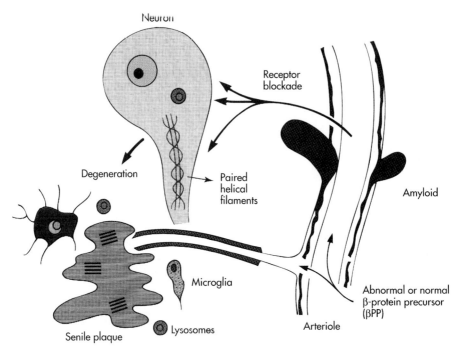

Figure 6-1   Diagram of the theory of brain damage in Alzheimer's disease. An abnormal β protein precursor (βPP) circulates in the blood, forming amyloid fibrils. These fibrils break the blood-brain barrier, causing leakage into brain tissue. There they block receptors necessary for proper metabolism of nerve cells and lead to the formation of paired helical filaments (tangles), which destroy the nerve cell. The βPP also seeps into other brain areas, where it accumulates, forming senile plaques (From Fortinash KM et al: *Psychiatric mental health nursing,* St Louis, 1996, Mosby. Courtesy George G. Glenner.)

It is not clear whether β-amyloid is a cause or a result of Alzheimer's disease.

Several studies have shown that β-amyloid may induce neuronal death or apoptosis (programmed cell death) or stimulate glial cells (that support neurons) to form toxic substances such as tumor necrosis factor. New transgenic technology has made it possible to engineer mice with a mutant human APP gene, with overexpression of a normal APP gene or with neurons overproducing APP. In all these models neuropathologic changes characteristic of Alzheimer's disease were found. These models may be useful in the search for medications to slow amyloid production or prevent its toxic effects on the brain (Figure 6-2).

Inflammatory Process

Inflammatory mechanisms may also stimulate synthesis of APP and influence amyloid formation. In addition to β-amyloid, neuritic plaques contain an acute-phase reactant (APR). Synthesis of APR is positively regulated by Interleukin-6 (IL-6), the primary cytokine mediator of the acute-phase inflammatory response. Involvement

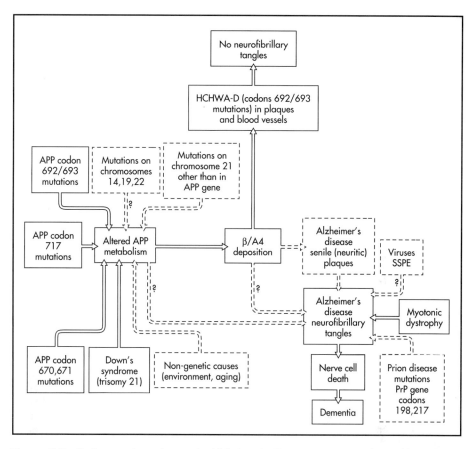

Figure 6-2   Pathogenetic pathways in Alzheimer's disease. Diagram of possible pathogenetic pathways in Alzheimer's disease associated with the "amyloid hypothesis." (From Mann MA: *Color atlas of adult dementias*, St Louis, 1994, Mosby.)

of the immune system and inflammation in the pathophysiology of Alzheimer's disease have been supported by the following findings in patients: the presence of APR in cerebrospinal fluid; elevated levels of various cytokines (including tumor necrosis factor in serum and interleukins 1-beta and 6 in the brain); cellular immune responses (including T4 and T8 lymphocytes and microglia); and the production of complement. This hypothesis is further supported by the low incidence of Alzheimer's disease in patients with rheumatoid arthritis and prolonged exposure to antiinflammatory therapy. Therefore, antiinflammatory medications may be helpful in the treatment of Alzheimer's disease. These are further discussed in Chapter 14.

Genetic Process

A major focus of investigation of the etiology of Alzheimer's disease in the 1990s has been the contribution of genetic factors. Earlier family, twin, and survey studies

Table 6-1

Genes Involved in Alzheimer's Disease (AD)

Gene Location	Gene Pathology	Protein	Effect
Chromosome 21	Several point mutations	APP	Small number of early-onset autosomal dominant AD families
Chromosome 14	Several point mutations	Presenilin 1	Majority of early-onset autosomal dominant AD families
Chromosome 1	Mutation	Presenilin 2	Small number of AD families
Chromosome 19	APOEe-4 genotype confers increased risk	APOE4	Majority of late-onset AD families

yielded strong clinical evidence for a genetic basis of Alzheimer's disease, showing that approximately 50% of adult members in families with AD developed the disease. This ratio is expected for an autosomal dominant trait, but the genetics of Alzheimer's disease turn out to be far more complex than that. Several different genetic changes have already been found to contribute to the etiology of Alzheimer's disease (Table 6-1). The first discoveries were related to point mutations in the APP gene on chromosome 21. However, the frequency of these mutations was very low: all occurred in families with autosomal dominant transmission of early-onset familial AD, and none of the mutations led to changes in the β-amyloid portion of the APP molecule. However, several different point mutations were identified in the first five families examined.

Two other chromosomes have also been involved in the etiology of Alzheimer's disease. Missense mutations in the Presenilin 1 gene, located on chromosome 14, are associated with approximately 70% of early-onset familial Alzheimer's disease (FAD). PS1 has been implicated in alteration of a pathway called the Notch pathway that determines the ultimate function of a cell. This pathway may also affect how cells process APP to create a β-amyloid variant, Beta A42, which may lead to the formation of new plaques. Mutant PS1 genes introduced into mice have been found to increase Beta A42 in the brain. The PS2 gene, located on chromosome 1, may account for some of the nerve cell loss in Alzheimer's disease by coding proteins that induce apoptosis. Research is just beginning to delineate the effects of normal and mutated presenilins and to determine if this mutation is a primary cause of Alzheimer's disease or part of multifactorial etiologies.

Late-onset (age 65 and over) familial AD (not autosomal dominant kindreds) has been linked to apolipoprotein E (APOE) genes on chromosome 19. Apolipoproteins comprise the protein part of lipoproteins that transport cholesterol in the blood stream. APOE binds the low density lipoprotein, the major transporter of cholesterol. Gene pairs, or alleles, determine isoforms of APOE.

These alleles are e-2, e-3, and e-4. At present, the e-4 allele, found more frequently in Alzheimer's disease patients than in the general population, is considered the most significant allele in determining risk for late-onset Alzheimer's disease. Individuals homozygous for the e-4 allele have an eight times greater risk of developing Alzheimer's disease than do non-e-4 carriers. They also have an earlier age at onset of the disease. However, not all e-4 carriers develop Alzheimer's disease, which suggests that other undetermined factors are necessary for manifestation of the disease. Approximately 60% to 70% of North Americans carry two e-3 alleles, and therefore do not carry e-4, the allele linked to increased risk for Alzheimer's disease. The e-2 allele (the gene frequency in the general population is 7%) is associated with decreased risk of developing Alzheimer's disease and lower LDL cholesterol, and may protect individuals from dementia and cardiovascular disease.

The APOE4 protein binds to β-amyloid more tightly than proteins coded by the e-2 and e-3 alleles. It has been hypothesized that the altered binding of APOE4 to the amyloid fragment results in abnormal metabolism of the APP molecule, with accumulation of β-amyloid. Another postulate is that the APOE protein itself produces amyloid fibrils. Discovery of mechanisms of increased (with APOEe-4 allele) and decreased (with APOEe-2 allele) susceptibility may lead to specific therapies for Alzheimer's disease.

NEUROFIBRILLARY TANGLES, MICROTUBULES, TAU, AND LEWY BODIES

Neurofibrillary tangles, like neuritic plaques, are not specific to Alzheimer's disease. They occur in about a dozen other chronic diseases of the human brain and in normal aging brains. However, unlike neuritic plaques, neurofibrillary tangles have only been observed in humans, so there is no animal model available for study. The core structures of the neurofibrillary tangles are paired helical filaments. These filaments contain the proteins tau and ubiquitin, which may be important in the pathogenesis of Alzheimer's disease. Tau protein stabilizes microtubules and promotes their assembly.

Several lines of evidence point to altered phosphorylation as an aspect of Alzheimer's disease pathology. Tau protein can exist in different isoforms, which can be excessively phosphorylated in Alzheimer's disease. Abnormalities of protein kinase C and casein kinase II, enzymes involved in protein phosphorylation, result in excessive phosphorylation of tau. It has been demonstrated that APOE4 binds with less affinity to tau protein when compared with APOE3, and especially APOE2. It has been suggested that the binding of tau to APOE prevents the early phosphorylation that initiates the formation of neurofibrillary tangles. Thus, 8-amyloid accumulation may be secondary to the abnormal phosphorylation of tau.

Microtubules

Microtubules are tiny structural components present in all cells and essential for numerous cellular functions. An impaired microtubule system could account for many of the abnormalities observed in Alzheimer's disease: formation of neurofibrillary tangles, loss of neurons, abnormal function of nerve growth factor, and interference with neurotransmitter activity. Other diminished cell functions in Alzheimer's disease include cell division, goal-directed motion, and axonal transport of neurotransmitters. The effects of these changes accumulate with time and eventually reach threshold levels sufficient for the manifestation of the neuropathologic changes and symptomatic behaviors characteristic of Alzheimer's disease.

New experimental data suggest that protein generated by APOEe-4 allele lacks microtubule-protective properties characteristic of proteins generated by alleles APOEe-2 and APOEe-3. Absence of these alternate alleles may increase risk for Alzheimer's disease in patients with genotype APOE 4/4. On the other hand, agents with APOE2- and APOE3-like microtubule-stabilizing properties may be candidates for treatment agents.

Lewy Bodies

Lewy bodies are round, eosinophilic cytoplasmic inclusions with a diameter of 5–25 µm. When found in the substantia nigra, they are a hallmark of Parkinson's disease. They are also frequently found in the cerebral cortex of autopsy-confirmed Alzheimer's disease patients. Some patients have both Lewy bodies and neuron loss in the substantia nigra and the cortex. These patients have been described as Lewy body variant (LBV) of Alzheimer's disease, which is a different entity than Lewy body dementia. LBV, present in almost one-third of autopsied clinically diagnosed Alzheimer's disease patients, is associated with the development of mild parkinsonian symptoms during the course of Alzheimer's disease which do not respond well to antiparkinsonian agents. Some LBV patients are described as having prominent hallucinations, paranoid ideation, unexplained falls, and loss of consciousness. The prevalence of neurofibrillary tangles in these patients was much lower than in "pure" Alzheimer's disease patients, but neuritic plaque counts were similar. Patients with Lewy body dementia have Lewy bodies throughout the cortex without Alzheimer's disease pathology. This group slowly develops dementia with extrapyramidal features.

NEUROTRANSMITTERS, NEUROTROPHIC FACTORS, AND ESTROGEN

A long-held hypothesis regarding the cause of Alzheimer's disease is that it is a neurotransmitter disease, specifically a cholinergic disorder. Currently, most investigators believe that the cholinergic abnormalities are secondary rather than primary factors in the disease. Nonetheless, the importance of the cholinergic system remains beyond dispute when it comes to memory and the other higher mental functions impaired in patients with Alzheimer's disease.

It has been established that there is decreased cholinergic activity in Alzheimer's disease patients. This observation is supported by a significant loss of neurons in the basal nucleus magnocellularis, which provides cholinergic innervation to the brain. The patient with Alzheimer's disease has a 40% to 70% loss of presynaptic cholinergic neurons in the brain. Moreover, the activity of choline acetyltransferase, the enzyme that synthesizes acetylcholine, is consistently reduced in the cerebral cortex of such patients.

Deficits in the level of cholinergic activity correlate significantly with cognitive impairment, but treatment with cholinomimetic agents and anticholinesterase inhibitors has generally been disappointing. It seems that the regulation of memory and other cognitive functions by the cholinergic system is much more complicated than previously suspected. Electrophysiologic and other studies suggest that the cortical cholinergic system may serve to modulate or amplify other afferent inputs rather than to initiate specific behavioral functions. Treatments with cholinesterase inhibitors and muscarinic agonists may actually disengage the remaining presynaptic cholinergic neurons and increase, rather than alleviate, the deficit. Therefore, it might be appropriate to focus on presynaptic modulation of cholinergic activity with agents increasing acetylcholine release.

The data on neurotransmitters other than the cholinergic ones are less clear, although both noradrenergic and serotonergic denervation have been reported in patients with Alzheimer's disease who die at a relatively early age. Reduction in gamma-aminobutyric acid has also been reported, but is believed to be a result of postmortem changes rather than Alzheimer's disease itself. Attempts to correlate the other neurotransmitter deficits with cholinergic changes and cognitive impairment have been largely unsuccessful.

Researchers have also looked at the possible role of excitatory amino acids in Alzheimer's disease. The excitatory amino acids have been most clearly implicated in the pathogenesis of Huntington's disease and stroke. Their involvement in Alzheimer's disease, however, has not yet been demonstrated.

There is strong evidence for the role of neurotrophic factors in Alzheimer's disease. Neurotrophic factors are endogenous polypeptides apparently essential for the function and survival of neurons. Nerve growth factor (NGF), the best characterized neurotrophic factor, is a II 8-amino acid polypeptide that does not cross the blood-brain barrier. NGF seems vulnerable to degeneration in Alzheimer's disease. It has been hypothesized that a dysfunction in neurotrophic systems is directly responsible for the neurodegeneration observed in certain diseases, including Alzheimer's disease. Nerve growth factor injected into cerebral ventricles has been demonstrated in animal models to improve lesion-induced cholinergic deficits and cognitive impairment.

Human NGF has been produced by recombinant techniques to make it available for clinical trials for Alzheimer's disease. Other substances with neurotrophic activities, including epidermal growth factor, brain-derived neurotrophic factor, gangliosides, and the 6 1 -28 peptide of BAP, might have therapeutic potential as well. New pharmaceutical techniques, such as the use of synthetic liposomes, drug lipidization, the development of lipid-soluble prodrugs, and the use of genetically modified NGF-secreting fibroblasts might provide noninvasive delivery to the central nervous system of such compounds that do not normally cross the blood-brain barrier.

According to some epidemiologic studies, supplementary estrogen protected women from the development of Alzheimer's disease or its clinical manifestations. Estrogen has stimulatory effects on the cholinergic system and neurotrophic effects under some conditions. The mechanisms of estrogen's protective effects are currently under investigation.

ABNORMALITIES OF TISSUES OTHER THAN BRAIN

It is important to understand that Alzheimer's disease affects both peripheral and brain tissues. Abnormalities have been reported in fibroblasts, red and white blood cells, and platelets. Fibroblasts from skin biopsies have shown some differences in the potassium channel profile in Alzheimer's disease patients as compared with control groups. Epidermal growth factor was found in capillaries of skin samples and in cerebral blood vessels in postmortem assessment of patients with Alzheimer's disease and other dementias. Further research is needed to confirm the significance of these changes and their role in the etiology and pathogenesis of the disease.

ENVIRONMENTAL RISK FACTORS

Several environmental risk factors have been reported as having a role in Alzheimer's disease (Box 6-1), but in general, confirmation is lacking. Among the putative environmental risk factors are myocardial infarction; prior malnutrition; alcohol consumption; exposure to solvents, aluminum, and lead; lack of education; and a sedentary lifestyle. Even a history of nose picking has been suggested as a risk factor! Several of these factors deserve more attention.

Head Trauma

One risk factor reported independently by more than one group of investigators is head trauma. The evidence linking head injury and Alzheimer's disease includes epidemiologic studies and β-amyloid deposits, which are found in approximately one-third of individuals who die of severe head trauma.

More recent epidemiologic and genetic studies support a synergistic interaction between head trauma and genetic predisposition in the development of Alzheimer's disease. The frequency of APOEe-4 in brain injury patients with amyloid depositions was significantly increased when compared to similar patients without β-amyloid depositions.

The role of head trauma in the development of Alzheimer's disease is readily accommodated by the following conceptual framework. Since there is some evidence that the degree of dementia in Alzheimer's disease is a function of synaptic loss, any condition that reduces the number of synapses could have a role in the development of Alzheimer's disease. Aside from head trauma, such conditions include normal aging with its concomitant neuronal losses, developmental retardation in early life with an associated reduction in synaptic connections, and deficits in formal education or other sources of intellectual challenge to spur the development of synaptic connections. All these could logically be risk factors for Alzheimer's disease. Conditions such as head trauma and periods of ischemia attended by coronary artery disease could lead not only to the death of neurons but

---

● **Box 6-1**
Possible Risk Factors and Potential Protective Factors for Alzheimer's Disease

Possible Risk Factors

Age
Family history
Apolipoprotein Ee-4
Head trauma
Limited education
Lack of mental activity
Down syndrome
Reduced cerebral blood flow
Vascular disease
Anticholinergic drugs
Toxins
Inorganic compounds (Aluminum, Iron, Silicon)
Electromagnetic fields
Inflammation
Infection
Metabolic (Thyroid Disease, Diabetes Mellitus, Folic Acid/B_{12} deficiency)

Potential Protective Factors

Estrogen
Nicotine
Apolipoprotein Ee-2
Nerve growth factors
Antioxidants
Mental activity
Microtubule stabilizers
Cholesterol lowering agents
Control of hypertension
Control of diabetes mellitus
Control of thyroid disease
Control of vitamin deficiencies
Physical activities
Antiinflammatory drugs

---

also to the deposition of diffuse plaques. Eventually, the accumulated damage would exceed threshold values and result in the manifestation of Alzheimer's disease.

One interesting hypothesis suggests that reduced cerebral blood flow, including all those conditions that cause it (such as head trauma, old age, depression, Parkinson's disease, Down syndrome, underactivity, sleep disturbances, and impaired glucose utilization, may be a major risk factor for Alzheimer's disease. Conversely, conditions with increased cerebral blood flow (arthritis/antiinflammatory drugs, occupational attainment/activity, exercise, smoking, etc.) may be protective against the disease.

Thyroid Disease

There has been some evidence that thyroid disease, especially hypothyroidism, may also be associated with Alzheimer's disease. Recent data support this assumption: thyroid epithelium seems to produce large amounts of APP, which can become a source for amyloid deposition and cause impairment of thyroid hormone production.

Infection

The significance of infection in the development of Alzheimer's disease is not clear. It has been discussed in the literature in connection with human prion diseases (Creutzfeldt-Jakob disease, Gerstmann-Straussler-Scheinker disease, and kuru), which are characterized by the development of dementia and protein brain deposits similar to the β-amyloid deposits of Alzheimer's disease. These disorders can be transmitted to animals by injecting brain extracts from deceased patients. There have also been reports of apparently accidental interhuman transmission. Attempts to induce Alzheimer's disease in animals by injecting brain extracts from deceased patients have not been replicated. Nonetheless, the role of infection in the pathogenesis of the disease cannot be ruled out.

Free Radicals

Normal aging and Alzheimer's disease may be associated with increased free radical production, leading to cell damage. Glutamate and 6-amyloid may also cause excessive free radical production in Alzheimer's disease.

It has been hypothesized that antioxidant agents, such as vitamin E, idebenone, and selegiline, may prevent cell death and slow the progression of cognitive decline in Alzheimer's disease.

These data suggest antioxidants as possible therapeutic agents in the disease, which may reduce free radical production and prevent cell injury.

Inorganic Compounds

Attention has also been given to inorganic compounds in the brains of patients with Alzheimer's disease. Various compounds have been considered as potential risk factors for the disease, most notably aluminum and silicon, which have been found in plaques and tangles.

The relevance of the aluminum accumulation is unclear. It may be secondary to incompetence of neuronal membranes and tangle formation. Once in the cell, aluminum may cause further damage by interfering with intracellular transport and transmission systems, possibly by substituting for magnesium in binding to the microtubule-associated protein tau. In addition, aluminum was found to be toxic to the cholinergic system. These findings led to clinical trials of desferrioxamine mesylate, which has high affinity for aluminum and has been used to treat iron and aluminum toxicity. However, this compound was also found to inhibit radical formation.

SUMMARY

After this brief survey of current concepts of the etiology and pathogenesis of Alzheimer's disease, the following three conclusions can be reached. First, Alzheimer's disease is even more complex than has generally been assumed. Second, a vast array of abnormalities in brain function and structure has been reported, many of which require replication. Third, what is called Alzheimer's disease today is most likely a heterogeneous disorder with manifest symptoms that reflect a common final pathway. Our knowledge concerning the etiology and pathogenesis of Alzheimer's disease is expanding, most notably with regard to risk factors and the availability of animal models. Advances in molecular biology, especially genetics, give promise for the further understanding of this devastating disorder, and for its effective treatment and prevention, possibly soon after we enter the twenty-first century.

BIBLIOGRAPHY

Advisory Panel on Alzheimer's Disease: Third report of the Advisory Panel on Alzheimer's Disease, 1991, DHHS Pub No (ADM) 92-1917, Washington DC, 1992, US Government Printing Office.

Alsen PS, Davis KL: Inflammatory mechanisms in Alzheimer's disease: implications for therapy, *Am J Psychiatry* 151:1105-1113, 1994.

Behl C et al: Vitamin E protects nerve cells from amyloid B protein toxicity, *Biochem Biophys Res Commun* 1986:944-950, 1992.

Breitner JCA et al: Inverse relationship of anti-inflammatory treatments and Alzheimer's disease: initial results of a co-twin control study, *Neurology* 44:227-232, 1994.

Citron M et al: Excessive production of amyloid protein by peripheral cells of symptomatic and presymptomatic patients carrying the Swedish familial Alzheimer disease mutation, *Proc Natl Acad Sci* USA 51:11993-11997, 1994.

Clayton RM et al: A long term effect of aluminum in the fetal mouse brain, *Life Sci* 1921-1928, 1992.

Cordell B: B-Amyloid formation as a potential therapeutic target for Alzheimer's disease, *Annu Rev Pharmacol Toxicol* 34:69-89, 1994.

Corder EH et al: Apolipoprotein E, survival in Alzheimer's disease patients, and the competing risks of death and Alzheimer's disease, *Neurology* 45:1323-1328, 1995.

Corder EH et al: Protective effect of apolipoprotein E type 2 allele for late onset Alzheimer disease, *Nat Genet* 7:180-183, 1994.

Crawford JG: Alzheimer's disease risk factors as related to cerebral blood flow, *Medical Hypotheses* 46:367-377, 1996.

Davies P, Maloney AJF: Selective loss of central cholinergic neurons in Alzheimer's disease, *Lancet* 2:1403, 1976.

DeKosky ST: Advances in the biology of Alzheimer's disease. In Weiner MF, editor: *The dementias: diagnosis, management and research,* ed 2, 1996, pp:313-330.

DeKosky ST, Scheft SW: Synapse loss in frontal cortex biopsies in Alzheimer's disease: correlation with cognitive severity, *Ann Neurol* 27:457-464, 1990.

Duff K et al: Increased amyloid-B42 (43) in brains of mice expressing mutant presenilin 1, *Nature* 383:710-713, 1996.

Farrer LA et al: Segregation analysis reveals evidence of major gene for Alzheimer's disease, *Am J Hum Genet* 48:1026-1033, 1992.

Fisher IJ et al: Selecting signaling via unique M I muscarinic agonists, *Ann NY Acad Sci* 695:300-303, 1993.

Games D et al: Alzheimer-type neuropathology in transgenic mice overexpressing V717F β-amyloid precursor protein, *Nature* 373:523-527, 1995.

Hefti F: Development of effective therapy for Alzheimer's disease based on neurotrophic factors, *Neurobiol Aging* 15:S193-S194, 1994.

Henderson VW et al: Estrogen replacement therapy in older women: comparison between Alzheimer's disease cases and nondemented control subjects, *Arch Neurol* 51:896-900, 1993.

Hyman BT et al: Quantitative neuropathology in Alzheimer disease: neuronal loss in high order association cortex parallels dementia, *Neurobiol Aging* 15:S141, 1994.

Jarvik LF, Lavretsky EP, Neshkes RE: The central nervous system: dementia and delirium in old age. In Brocklehurst JC, editor: *Textbook of geriatric medicine and gerontology,* ed 4, Edinburgh, 1992, Churchill Livingstone.

LaFerla FM et al: The Alzheimer's A peptide induces neurodegeneration and apoptotic cell death in transgenic mice, *Nat Genet* 9:21-29, 1995.

Lapchak PA: Nerve growth factor pharmacology: Application to the treatment of cholinergic neurodegeneration in Alzheimer's disease, *Exp Neurol* 124:16-20, 1993.

Lavretsky E et al: Genetics of geriatric psychopathology. In Sadavoy LW et al, editors: *Comprehensive Review of Geriatric Psychiatry—*II: 43-79, 1996.

Marx J: Dissecting how presenilins function and malfunction, *Science* 274:1838-1840, 1996.

Matsuyama SS, Jarvik LF: Hypothesis: microtubules, a key to Alzheimer disease, *Proc Natl Acad Sci USA* 86:8152-8156, 1989.

McGeer PL, McGeer EC: Complement proteins and complement inhibitors in Alzheimer's disease, *Res Immunol* 143:621-624, 1992.

Neurobiology of Aging: Special issue on amyloid protein and neurotoxicity, Sept 1992.

Nicoll JAR et al: Amyloid B-protein, APOE genotype and head injury, *Ann NY Acad Sci* 777:271-275, 1996.

Olson L: NGF and the treatment of Alzheimer's disease, *Exp Neurol* 124:5-15, 1993.

Paykel ES et al: Incidence of dementia in a population older than 75 years in the United Kingdom, *Arch Gen Psychiatry* 51:325-332, 1994.

Pericak-Vance MA et al: Linkage studies in familial Alzheimer disease: evidence for chromosome 19 linkage, *Am J Hum Genet* 48:1034-1050, 1991.

Perry EK, Irving D, Perry RH: Cholinergic controversies (letter to editor), *TINS* 14:483, 1991.

Plassman BL, Breitner JC: Recent advances in the genetics of Alzheimer's disease and vascular dementia with an emphasis on gene-environment interactions, *JAGS* 44:1242-1250, 1996.

Roses AD et al: Clinical application of apolipoprotein E genotyping to Alzheimer's disease, *Lancet* 343:1564-1565, 1994.

Schellenberg GD et al: Genetic linkage evidence for a familial Alzheimer's disease locus on chromosome 14, *Science* 258:668-671, 1992.

Schmitt TL et al: Thyroid epithelial cells produce 8-amyloid precursor protein (APP) and generate potentially amyloidogenic APP fragments, *J Clin Endocrinol Metab* 80:3513-3519, 1995.

Schork MJ, Weder AB: The use of genetic information in large-scale clinical trials: applications to Alzheimer research, *Alzheimer Dis Assoc Disord* 10: Suppl 1:22-26, 1996.

Selkoe DJ: Deciphering Alzheimer's disease: the amyloid precursor protein yields new clues, *Science* 248:1058-1060, 1990.

St. George-Hyslop PH et al: Genetic linkage studies suggest that Alzheimer disease is not a single homogeneous disorder, *Nature* 347:194-197, 1990.

Strittmatter WJ, Roses AD: Apolipoprotein E and Alzheimer disease, *Proc Natl Acad Sci USA* 92:4725-4727, 1995.

Tanzi RE et al: Assessment of amyloid 6-protein precursor gene mutations in a large set of familial and sporadic Alzheimer disease cases, *Am J Hum Genet* 512:273-282, 1992.

Terry RD et al: Structural basis of the cognitive alterations in Alzheimer disease. In Terry RD et al, editors: *Alzheimer disease*, New York, 1994, Raven, pp. 179-196.

Tomlinson BF et al: Observations on the brains of demented old people, *J Neurol Sci* 11:205-242, 1970.

Clinical Presentation

Chapter 7

Ronald C Hamdy

There is a wicked inclination in most people to suppose an old man decayed in his intellects. If a young or middle-aged man, when leaving a company, does not recollect where he laid his hat, it is nothing; but if the same inattention is discovered in an old man, people will shrug up their shoulders, and say, 'His memory is going.'

—Samuel Johnson

Alzheimer's disease is a dementia characterized by an insidious onset and slow rate of deterioration. In addition to the memory impairment that interferes with the patient's daily activities, there is other evidence of cognitive deficits.

Positive Findings:
1. Amnesia, i.e., memory deficit
2. Evidence of cognitive impairment, including: anomia, agnosia, aphasia, and apraxia
3. Insidious onset

Negative Findings:
1. No other disease responsible for mental impairment
2. No medication responsible for mental impairment
3. No clouding of level of consciousness

CLINICAL SYMPTOMS

Memory Impairment

Memory impairment is the hallmark of Alzheimer's disease. However, it is by no means the only characteristic feature, nor is it the most important. Many conditions apart from Alzheimer's disease can lead to memory impairment.

Memory has three different modalities: immediate memory (remembering for

74

a few seconds), short-term memory (remembering for a few minutes or hours), and long-term memory (remembering for a few years).

> Early in Alzheimer's disease, short-term memory is impaired, but long-term memory is preserved.

Immediate memory is also affected, but this change is probably secondary to a short attention span. The main problem for patients with this disease is the short-term memory impairment, which interferes with their social and professional activities. Learning and recalling new information, both verbal and visuospatial, are gradually reduced.

Alzheimer's disease vs. benign forgetfulness. It is important to differentiate the memory impairment of Alzheimer's disease from that sometimes noted in normal people, which is often called "benign forgetfulness, benign senescent forgetfulness, or age-associated memory impairment."
Memory impairment in Alzheimer's disease:
• Is undiscriminating, that is, affects trivial as well as important matters
• Interferes with the patient's social and professional activities.
Memory impairment in benign forgetfulness:
• Usually is sporadic and limited to trivial matters
• Does not significantly interfere with the patient's life, apart from causing frustration and irritation (e.g., when a person cannot remember where the keys were left)

Unlike memory impairment associated with Alzheimer's disease, that seen in benign forgetfulness usually can be remedied fairly easily, for example, by concentrating and trying to remember, or by keeping written records. In Alzheimer's disease, although patients initially may try to overcome their problem by writing down what they want to remember, sooner or later the memory deficit is such that they may forget to check their written record.

Patients with Alzheimer's disease have difficulties encoding material to be recalled. Unlike patients with benign forgetfulness, they are not helped by including the target material in stories, by providing a semantic connection between words to be remembered, or by cueing.

Obviously, the degree of impairment necessary to interfere with a patient's social and professional life depends a great deal on the person's activities. This situation can be demonstrated best by comparing two patients of the same age, a housewife and a professional.

● **Case Study—Cognitive Impairment Not Noticed Until Late**
The housewife lives with her husband and is dependent on him for most of her activities because she has been crippled with osteoarthritis for many years. She does not need to pay bills or shop. She does some cooking, but her husband makes most of the decisions and does most of the housework. By the time this patient's memory impairment affects her day to day activities, it will be severe.

● **Case Study—Cognitive Impairment Noticed Early**
An accountant who lives on her own is finding it increasingly difficult to continue performing her professional activities because of her 'poor memory.' She has to rely more

and more on her secretary to perform these duties. She is often late for meetings, at times forgetting altogether to attend them, at other times taking the wrong files, and at still other times going to the wrong place for the meeting, in spite of clear instructions from her secretary. She also often mixes up her clients' names, addresses, and accounts.

Any degree of memory deficit experienced by most professionals interferes with their professional life. Physicians, pharmacists, attorneys, or accountants, for instance, may find it very difficult to pursue their professional activities with any memory deficit. Even though the degree of mental impairment may be mild, it is constant and sufficient to interfere with the person's professional life and thus must be considered part of a dementia process rather than benign forgetfulness.

Whether the memory impairment is secondary to Alzheimer's disease or not depends on the rest of the patient's clinical picture and laboratory investigations.

How do patients cope with their impaired memory? Early in the course of Alzheimer's disease, patients usually are aware of their memory deficit and may make notes to remember important things, or may trivialize their problem, blaming it on other factors or on being involved with so many different activities and responsibilities that they cannot remember everything. Later they may become frightened and apprehensive about their memory problems and may feel depressed and discouraged.

Late stages of memory impairment. As the disease progresses, patients lose insight into their memory deficit and are no longer aware of it. At this point patients must be protected from themselves.

For instance, they may try to enter into new business ventures or invest their assets with disastrous results. They may prepare a meal and forget that the stove is on, or they may try to drive, oblivious to the fact that they are becoming lost or are making dangerous errors in judgment.

Inability to Acquire and Process New Information

One of the earliest manifestations of Alzheimer's disease is an inability to acquire and retain new information, and to integrate it with previously acquired knowledge. This problem is partly the result of short-term memory impairment. Patients have difficulties keeping abreast of recent developments in their profession and are not able to discuss current events. These difficulties often lead the patient to withdraw from discussions revolving around these topics and to appear to have lost interest in them.

Often the first indication that something is wrong occurs when the patient needs to develop new skills at work. For instance, when computerization is introduced in the office or the individual's job is reorganized, he may be unable to adapt to these changes. Consequently his colleagues may think that he is getting old and set in his ways. At this stage the patient may elect to take early retirement or may be assigned a more routine, less demanding job.

Changes in Personality

In the early stages of Alzheimer's disease, patients also may appear to have a change in personality.

For instance, the keen bridge player may start declining invitations to play the game and may make excuses for not joining his partners. Similarly a golfer may ask a partner to keep the score, or an avid reader may find books "less interesting." At this stage the patient may stop cooking or knitting because of an inability to integrate and process new information.

A sudden change in a person's environment can trigger an episode of severe confusion. The individual suddenly finds himself in a strange place and is unable to remember how he got there. For instance, during a stay in a hotel or a visit with his children, a man may wake up in the middle of the night and be totally disoriented and confused. As a result, he becomes agitated. In the early stages of Alzheimer's disease, this type of state does not last long. With explanations and reassurance, the patient soon becomes reoriented, alert, and rational.

Language Difficulties

Language difficulties are present at the earliest stages of the disease. Initially they may be so subtle as not to be readily apparent to most observers, even professional ones, and can be detected only by neuropsychological tests (e.g., a word list generation, in which the subject is asked to list words in a specific group, such as animals, plants, or fruits beginning with the same letter). As the disease progresses, these language deficits become more marked and are readily noticed by most observers, even lay people.

Anomia. Anomia, the inability to find the right word, is a characteristic feature of Alzheimer's disease. At first the patient usually is aware of these deficits and may try to make up for them by using sentences to describe the object he cannot name (paraphrasia). Thus in the very early stages of Alzheimer's disease, the patient's speech becomes picturesque and interesting as he attempts to overcome the problems of anomia.

In the early stages of the disease, the anomia is confined to objects that the patient does not come into contact with on a regular basis. As the condition worsens, however, anomia also includes common objects. The patient recognizes these objects but is unable to recall their name. For instance, when shown a key, the patient recognizes it, knows what it is used for and can use it, but cannot think of the word "key." It is interesting that in Dr. Alzheimer's original description his patient was unable to recall the word "jug" and instead said "pourer." Rather than referring to the "milk jug" she said "milk pourer."

Agnosia. As the disease progresses, agnosia sets in. Agnosia is more serious than anomia because, in addition to being unable to name an object, the person cannot identify it. For instance, he may not recognize a key—he may think it is a spoon and try to eat soup with it. Alternatively the patient may think that a knife is a comb and may attempt to comb his hair with it.

Patients may not recognize people they have not seen for a long time. For example, grandparents may confuse their grandchildren with their children or their children with their siblings.

▬▶ As the disease progresses, patients may not recognize their spouse or other close relatives and may accuse them of being intruders.

This development is a traumatic experience for the caregivers. One of my patients thought that her only son was her husband. She regularly made sexual advances to him and demanded that they sleep together. This situation was very distressing to the son, who developed severe depression and even contemplated suicide.

As the agnosia becomes more extensive, the patient cannot use sensory information to recognize objects or people. With time, the anomia also becomes more noticeable, and the paraphrasia becomes less related to the target word and more rambling. At this stage conversation becomes very difficult. This situation is worsened by the patient's inability to concentrate for normal periods. Often words and themes related to previous discussions and unrelated to the present conversation intrude. As a result, the listener is unable to follow any coherent train of thought.

Aphasia. Aphasia develops later. This impairment in language prevents the patient from understanding what he hears, from following instructions, and from communicating needs (e.g., the need to go to the toilet or being in pain). This situation is distressing to the patient and trying to the caregivers, who now must guess what the patient's needs are.

As the disease progresses, spontaneous speech deteriorates. The patient tends to repeat words and questions (echolalia) without making any effort to answer the questions. With further deterioration the patient repeats one word (paralalia) or the first syllable of a word (logoconia) again and again. In the advanced stage of the disease, speech becomes unintelligible, and eventually complete mutism occurs.

Impaired Visuospatial Skills and Apraxia

Apraxia, the inability to carry out purposeful movements and actions despite intact motor and sensory systems, is evident early in the course of Alzheimer's disease, but patients and relatives often do not connect it with the disease. In the early stages, for instance, a patient may be unable to lace his shoes but still be able to put on loafers or boots. He may attribute this inability to tie the laces to "lack of practice." In fact, the impairment represents an early stage of apraxia. The patient may be unable to adjust the controls of the video recorder and the television set simultaneously, although he may still be able to adjust each independently. In other words, the more complex or technical skills, particularly those recently acquired or requiring integration of various stimuli, are lost early in the process.

The "automatic" actions, such as eating, walking, dressing, and undressing, tend to be preserved until the late stages. This discrepancy exists because the complex and technical skills are controlled mainly by the cerebral cortex, whereas the control of automatic actions is relegated to the basal ganglia.

Impaired visuospatial skills may be the reason a patient becomes lost in familiar surroundings or while driving a car.

In the latter instance, however, the inability to integrate new information and to make rational decisions also plays an important part.

Apraxia often becomes a source of frustration: minor tasks that the patient once performed easily become major tasks involving almost insurmountable obstacles.

> The patient does not understand what is happening or how or why he is losing control over his environment.

This situation often leads to discouragement and depression. For instance, when asked to set the table, the patient is faced with so many choices (knives, forks, spoons, plates, glasses) and so many alternative positions for each item that he may not be able to tackle this "complex" task. On the other hand, if given only a knife, a fork, and a plate, he may be able to cope with this limited choice and arrange them adequately on the table.

As the disease progresses, simply getting dressed becomes an impossible task. The patient may see his shirt and recognize the front, back, left, and right sides, but he is unable to translate these stimuli and coordinate his movements accordingly to put his right arm through the right sleeve of his shirt while keeping the top part of the shirt up and its front on his chest.

Poor Judgment

Sooner or later the patient's ability to use correct judgment deteriorates. This development is often the point at which relatives recognize the disease. They no longer consider the person odd or eccentric but realize that something is seriously wrong. This situation occurs when the patient pays the same bill twice, does not pay some bills, or cannot balance his checkbook. Difficulty in managing finances is one of the most common reasons relatives insist that a person seek medical attention and is often the first indication of cognitive deficit.

Poor judgment also may be reflected when the patient makes a large donation to a charity after watching a television commercial or after speaking to unscrupulous entrepreneurs on the phone. Sometimes the patient may start buying unnecessary items or giving extravagant gifts.

Self-Neglect

Another degree of mental impairment is reached when, in addition to impaired memory and impaired judgment, the patient shows evidence of carelessness, particularly self-neglect.

One of the earliest manifestations of Alzheimer's disease is that patients stop taking pride in the impression they make.

This very useful sign can be appreciated by looking at the patient's general appearance. For instance, if a patient makes no attempt to comb her hair and if her dress is stained or torn, in the absence of physical incapacitation, the caregiver can assume that self-neglect is present.

In hospitals and nursing homes this carelessness and self-neglect can be recognized easily by asking the patient to get up from her chair and take a few steps. If after standing up the patient adjusts her clothes before walking or makes sure that her hospital gown is properly closed and that her genital area is not exposed, then she is aware of her body image and cares about the impression she projects in public. A patient with Alzheimer's disease, in contrast, when asked to stand up and walk, may do so without realizing that her hospital gown is wide open at the back. She will probably walk the length of the room without making any effort to cover her back and without showing any signs of embarrassment; in fact, she is not aware of and does not care about the image she projects in public.

Personality Changes

Changes in personality are often seen in patients with Alzheimer's disease, and they can be severe. These changes include self-centeredness, withdrawal, increased passivity, and agitation.

Many patients develop delusions of persecution, including infidelity and fear of theft or harm.

Mood changes also have been described in patients with Alzheimer's disease. These changes are manifested by loss of interest, loss of energy, and depressed mood in the early stages, although insight is retained.

Behavioral Problems

Aberrant behavior is almost always distressing to both caregivers and patients. Such behavior may include stubbornness, resistance to care, suspicion of others, use of abusive language, acting in response to delusions or hallucinations, rummaging through other people's rooms, "stealing," hiding articles, urinating in inappropriate places, and angry outbursts (catastrophic reactions) precipitated by apparently trivial events. These abnormal behavioral patterns often are the reason that caregivers seek institutionalization for the patient.

Ironically, these same behaviors frequently are the reason nursing homes refuse to admit patients with Alzheimer's disease, on the grounds that such behavior would disrupt the harmony of the institution, could be offensive and dangerous to other residents, and could lead to litigation. Because of this aberrant behavior, patients with Alzheimer's disease often are prescribed potent sedatives and tranquilizers, and are physically restrained.

Restlessness, aimless wandering, and reversal of the sleep/wake cycle are often seen in patients with Alzheimer's disease and frequently put the patient at risk for self-injury.

Patients with this condition sometimes engage in asocial sexual behavior, such as masturbating in front of others. Although this is distressing to caregivers, especially the patient's children, there is no evidence that patients with dementia pose a sexual threat to others.

Physical Deterioration

Most patients with Alzheimer's disease remain physically well until the late stages of the disease. They gradually become more unsteady, may experience repeated falls, and tend to spend more time sitting in a chair or lying in bed. As time goes by, they develop generalized muscle rigidity. Later they become bedridden, assume the fetal position, and often become incontinent of urine and feces. Grasping and sucking reflexes are often seen in the late stages of the disease. Seizures and myoclonus may affect up to about 10% of the patients in late-stage disease. The three most common causes of death in these patients are pneumonia, urinary tract infection, and infected decubitus ulcers.

Insidious Onset

Alzheimer's disease has a very insidious onset and a slow, relentless progress. One of the best indicators of these two aspects of the disease is the inability of the patient's relatives to agree on a specific date when the symptoms started to manifest themselves. For instance, the patient's daughter may think it was last Christmas, whereas his wife may believe that his condition started to deteriorate much earlier. In contrast to strokes of multiinfarct dementia, no one can pinpoint an exact date or time when the disease manifested itself or the patient's condition suddenly deteriorated.

CLINICAL STAGES

At present, Alzheimer's disease is an irreversible, gradually progressive condition associated with relentless deterioration. In the earliest stage the patient may exhibit only minimal memory impairment and cognitive deficit. In the last stage the patient is commonly bedridden in the fetal position, doubly incontinent, and mute.

Staging the Disease

Several classifications have been developed for categorizing patients according to stage. Although these classifications are useful for determining the level of care a patient needs and for comparing groups of patients with one another, they are not truly useful as prognostic indicators because of the great variability in the rate of deterioration exhibited by different patients.

Table 7-1

Stages of Alzheimer's Disease

	Duration (yr)	Characteristics
Stage 1	1-3	Poor memory
		Impaired acquisition of new information
		Mild anomia
		Minimal visuospatial impairment
		Personality change
Stage 2	2-10	Profound memory loss
		Significant impairment of other cognitive parameters
		Severe impairment of judgment
Stage 3	8-12	Severe impairment of all cognitive functions
		Physical impairment: unsteadiness, repeated falls, reduced mobility
		Loss of ability to care for oneself

Usually, the younger the patient is when the disease manifests itself, the faster will be its rate of progression.

Similarly, when there is a strong family history of Alzheimer's disease, the rate of progress tends to be more rapid than if no such history exists.

The two classifications most widely used involve three or seven stages. It is important to realize that both classifications are arbitrary and that there is a great deal of overlap among the various stages. Furthermore, not all patients go through all these stages. It also must be emphasized that a rapid rate of deterioration is often caused by other diseases or factors (see Chapter 9).

For practical purposes, the three-stage classification is preferred because the characteristic features of each stage are easier to recognize and the needs of the patient in each stage are so different (Table 7-1).

Stage 1. Stage 1, which lasts between 1 and 3 years, is characterized by the following signs:
- Poor recent memory
- Impaired acquisition of new information
- Mild anomia
- Minimal visuospatial impairment
- Personality change
- Lack of initiative
- Poor judgment
- Mood changes

The patient may appear "normal" to people who do not know him. However, his immediate contacts know that there has been a change in his behavior, personality, and intellectual functioning. This stage is difficult because the patient still has some insight into his condition and yet cannot understand or cope with the complexity of his situation. At times the patient may rebel and refuse to accept the implications of his condition; at other times he may realize that he is fighting a losing battle and become depressed and irritable or withdraw into apathy.

This stage can be particularly taxing for the patient's family. On one hand, they understand and appreciate the patient's actions; on the other, they question the validity of his judgment and yet do not want to appear to question or doubt his integrity, intentions, and ability to look after his family. Such a situation may require professional intervention to safeguard the family's financial assets.

> A particularly difficult problem concerns the patient's ability to drive a motor vehicle.

Driving is a symbol of independence and may be the person's only means of transportation. However, while driving, the patient may make serious mistakes that could endanger himself or others. In addition to having poor judgment, many patients with Alzheimer's disease have a slow reaction time and may be easily distracted, both of which make driving hazardous.

Toward the end of stage 1, memory impairment and impaired ability to make rational decisions often cause the patient to become lost even in familiar surroundings. This development is another traumatic and stressful experience for the patient's relatives. For example, a man goes to a store one block away to buy something, and two hours later he has not returned. Five hours later the police call his wife to tell her that they have found her husband a few miles away. It is understandable that a patient's relatives may be reluctant to take away his sense of initiative and independence by confining him indoors. Yet, whenever he leaves home, they worry that he may become lost, be mugged, or be involved in an accident. Often the relatives resort to writing their address and phone number on a card and leaving it in one of the patient's pockets.

Patients with Alzheimer's disease can become lost because they may not recognize familiar signs. Since they do not know where they are, they start to panic. When they panic, their judgment becomes even more impaired and they may not be able to retrace their steps. Although stress may sharpen a normal person's mental abilities, in a patient with dementia, it can lead to severe confusion.

In the first stage of Alzheimer's disease, the clinical examination is essentially within normal limits, although some patients have a reduced sense of smell. While the computed tomography (CT) scan, the magnetic resonance imaging (MRI) scan, and the electroencephalogram (EEG) are usually essentially normal, single photon emission tomography (SPECT) is often abnormal (see Chapter 4).

Stage 2. Stage 2 lasts between 2 and 10 years and is characterized by the following signs:
- Profound memory loss, both remote and recent
- Short attention span
- Problems recognizing people
- Significant impairment of other cognitive parameters, as evidenced by two or more of these symptoms: anomia, agnosia, apraxia, and aphasia

- Severe impairment of judgment
- Restlessness

In stage 2 the anomia and agnosia become much more pronounced and interfere with the patient's daily activities. These signs can be recognized even by people who are meeting the patient for the first time.

Later in this stage the patient may develop significant apraxia, which leaves him unable to perform simple tasks such as feeding or washing himself, even though he has no muscle weakness or coordination difficulties. At this stage patients with Alzheimer's disease tend to become very restless. They often are seen pacing the room or walking outside as if constantly searching for something. They do not like to stay in one place and want to keep moving.

The patient's personality, which in the first stage was variable, now is mostly apathetic.

> The individual has no insight into his condition and does not seem bothered by his relatives' distress over it.

This lack of insight is exemplified by the patient's denial of problems with his memory despite evidence of profound memory loss. If confronted with the fact that his memory is poor, the patient usually makes some excuse, such as that he was not really paying attention, that he is getting old, or that he has other things to remember and cannot be bothered with such details.

The patient may make "near misses." For instance, when asked which day of the week it is, he may say that the day is Monday (rather than Tuesday). When corrected, he may question the relevance of today being Tuesday rather than Monday. If an examiner asks him to remember three or four objects, he may question the importance of being able to do so. In contrast, patients suffering from depression readily acknowledge problems with their memory; rather than making near misses, they refuse to cooperate with the examiner.

In stage 2, a CT scan usually shows evidence of brain atrophy and ventricular dilation. The EEG also may be abnormal and may show generalized slowing of the waves.

Stage 3. Stage 3, which lasts between 8 and 12 years, is notable for the following features:
- Severe impairment of all cognitive functions
- Physical impairment involving unsteadiness, repeated falls, reduced mobility
- Total loss of ability to care for oneself

Gross intellectual impairment is obvious at this stage. For example, a patient may not recognize his wife and children, and may confuse them with his parents. Complete disorientation of time and place, and with other individuals is evident, and the patient cannot cope with his basic needs. As the condition progresses, complete mutism may occur and motor deficits may become apparent. The patient may develop generalized muscular rigidity, and his mobility may be grossly reduced. In contrast to stage 2, in which the patient wandered constantly, he now spends most of the time sitting in a chair or lying in bed. An attitude of generalized flexion gradually is adopted, with the patient lying curled up in bed. Eventually the patient assumes the fetal position. At this stage urinary (and sometimes fecal) incontinence may develop. The CT scan shows gross atrophy and ventricular dilation, and the EEG shows slow waves.

Staging of Patients

In general, stages proceed according to a pattern. In the first stage memory is impaired, but other cognitive deficits are minimal and easily overlooked. In the second stage there is also evidence of gross deficits in other cognitive fields. In the third stage, besides the severe intellectual deterioration, physical deficits become apparent.

Cause of Death

The usual cause of death is not Alzheimer's disease itself. Instead, it is septicemia, which is a complication of pneumonia, urinary tract infection, or infected decubitus ulcers. Decubitus ulcers are very likely to develop unless pressure areas are given special care.

Although Alzheimer's disease is characteristically irreversible and slowly progressive, it often is punctuated by sudden bouts of reversible deterioration caused by other diseases or factors apart from Alzheimer's disease (see Chapter 9).

BIBLIOGRAPHY

Bennett DA, Evans DA: Alzheimer's disease, *Dis Mon* 38:1-64, 1992.

Brooks JO: A comment on age at onset as a subtype of Alzheimer disease, *Alzheimer Dis Assoc Disord* 9 Suppl 1:S28-29, 1995.

Brooks JO, Yesavage JA: Identification of fast and slow decliners in Alzheimer disease: a different approach, *Alzheimer Dis Assoc Disord* 9 Suppl 1:S19-25, 1995.

Donnelly RE, Karlinsky H: The impact of Alzheimer's disease on driving ability: a review, *J Geriatr Psychiatry Neurol* 3(2):67-72, 1990.

Esiri MM: The basis for behavioural disturbances in dementia, *J Neurol Neurosurg Psychiatry* 61(2):127-130, 1996.

Grossman M, Mickanin J, Onishi K et al: An aspect of sentence processing in Alzheimer's disease: quantifier-noun agreement, *Neurology* 45(1):85-91, 1995.

Herskovits E: Struggling over subjectivity: debates about the "self" and Alzheimer's disease, *Med Anthropol Q* 9(2):146-164, 1995.

Hodges JR, Patterson K: Is semantic memory consistently impaired early in the course of Alzheimer's disease? *Neuropsychologia* 33(4):441-459, 1995.

Larson EB, Kukull WA, Katzman RL: Cognitive impairment: dementia and Alzheimer's disease, *Annu Rev Public Health* 13:431-449, 1992.

Lee VK: Language changes and Alzheimer's disease: a literature review, *J Gerontol Nurs* 17(1):16-20, 1991.

Lyketsos CG, Corazzini K, Steele C: Mania in Alzheimer's disease, *J Neuropsychiatry Clin Neurosci* 7(3):350-352, 1995.

Mielke R, Kessler J, Fink G et al: Dysfunction of visual cortex contributes to disturbed processing of visual information in Alzheimer's disease, *Int J Neurosci* 82(1-2):1-9, 1995.

Migliorelli R, Teson A, Sabe L et al: Anosognosia in Alzheimer's disease: a study of associated factors, *J Neuropsychiatry Clin Neurosci* 7(3):338-344, 1995.

Prince MJ: Predicting the onset of Alzheimer's disease using Bayes' theorem, *Am J Epidemiol* 143(3):301-308, 1996.

Randolph C, Tierney MC, Chase TN: Implicit memory in Alzheimer's disease, *J Clin Exp Neuropsychol* 17(3):343-351, 1995.

Raskind MA, Carta A, Bravi D: Is early-onset Alzheimer's disease a distinct subgroup within the Alzheimer disease population? *Alzheimer Dis Assoc Disord* 9(Suppl 1):S2-6, 1995.

Ripich DN, Petrill SA, Whitehouse PJ et al: Gender differences in language of AD patients: a longitudinal study, *Neurology* 45(2):229-302, 1995.

Sandson TA, Sperling RA, Price BH: Alzheimer's disease: an update, *Compr Ther* 21(9):480-485, 1995.

Stern Y, Jacobs DM: Preliminary findings from the predictors study: utility of clinical signs for predicting disease course, *Alzheimer Dis Assoc Disord* 9 Suppl 1:S14-18, 1995.

Terry RD: Biologic differences between early and late onset Alzheimer disease, *Alzheimer Dis Assoc Disord* 9 (Suppl 1):S26-27, 1995.

Trick GL, Trick LR, Morris P et al: Visual field loss in senile dementia of the Alzheimer's type, *Neurology* 45(1):68-74, 1995.

Clinical Diagnosis

James M Turnbull

Good judgement comes from experience,
but experience comes from bad judgement.

—John F Kennedy

In 1996, 1545 articles dealing with the subject of Alzheimer's disease appeared in scientific journals. Despite tremendous scientific interest and research, the diagnosis remains a clinical one before death. There are no specific antemortem markers for it.

In 1984 a work group on the diagnosis of Alzheimer's disease was established by the National Institute of Neurological and Communicative Disorders and Strokes (NINCDS) and the Alzheimer's Disease and Related Disorders Association (ADRDA). The clinical criteria for the diagnosis of probable, possible, and definite Alzheimer's disease were outlined. The diagnosis of probable Alzheimer's disease, it was stated, could be made with confidence if the dementia had a typical insidious onset with progression and no other systemic or brain diseases were present, which could account for the progressive memory loss and other cognitive deficits. Using the criteria for probable Alzheimer's disease, two recent large autopsy studies, one by Gearing and the other by Galasko, have reported confirmation rates of 87% and 90%, respectively.

Among the disorders that must be calculated are major depression, Parkinson's disease, multiinfarct dementia, drug intoxication, thyroid disease, vitamin B12 deficiency, subdural hematoma, occult hydrocephalus, Huntington's disease, brain tumors and chronic infections of the nervous system. The criteria for clinical diagnosis of Alzheimer's disease are shown in Box 8-1.

The diagnostic and statistical manual of the American Psychiatric Association was revised in 1994. It lists the diagnostic criteria for dementia of the Alzheimer's type (DAT) as multiple cognitive deficits manifested by impairment in short-term and long-term memory and at least one other area of higher cortical functioning. The latter include impairment in abstract thinking, judgment, or other executive functions, or disturbances such as aphasia (disorder of language), apraxia (inability to carry out motor activities despite intact comprehension and motor

Box 8-1
Criteria for Clinical Diagnosis of Alzheimer's Disease

1. The criteria for the clinical diagnosis of *probable* Alzheimer's disease include:
- Dementia established by clinical examination and documented by the Mini-Mental Test, Blessed Dementia Scale, or some similar examination, and confirmed by neuropsychological tests
- Deficits in two or more areas of recognition
- Progressive worsening of memory and other cognitive functions
- No disturbance of consciousness
- Onset between ages 40 and 90, most often after age 65
- Absence of systemic disorders or other brain disease that in and of themselves could account for the progressive deficits in memory and cognition

2. The diagnosis of *probable* Alzheimer's disease is supported by:
- Progressive deterioration of specific cognitive functions such as language (aphasia), motor skills (apraxia), and perception (agnosia)
- Impaired activities of daily living and altered patterns of behavior
- Family history of similar disorders, particularly if confirmed neuropathologically
- Laboratory results of normal lumbar puncture as evaluated by standard techniques
- Normal pattern of nonspecific changes in EEG such as increased slow-wave activity
- Evidence of cerebral atrophy on CT with progression documented by serial observation

function), or agnosia (failure to recognize or identify objects despite intact sensory function). To constitute a diagnosis of DAT, these impairments must interfere significantly with social or occupational functioning and represent a significant decline from a previous level of functioning. The course of DAT has a gradual onset and continuing cognitive decline, and the deficits are not due to any other central nervous system disorder, delirium, substance abuse, or major mental disorder such as schizophrenia or major depressive disorder.

The information needed to make the clinical diagnosis depends on the patient's medical history; neurological, psychiatric, and clinical examinations; neuropsychological tests; and laboratory studies.

MEDICAL HISTORY

It is paramount that information about the patient's medical history be obtained not only from the patient, but also from a collateral who knows the person well.

Box 8-1
Criteria for Clinical Diagnosis of Alzheimer's Disease—cont'd

3. **Other clinical features consistent with the diagnosis of** *probable* **Alzheimer's disease, after exclusion of causes of dementia and other than Alzheimer's disease, include:**
   - Plateaus in the course of progress of the illness
   - Associated symptoms of depression, insomnia, incontinence, delusions, illusions, hallucinations, catastrophic verbal, emotional, or physical outbursts, sexual disorders, and weight loss
   - Other neurologic abnormalities in some patients, especially with more advanced disease and including motor signs such as increased muscle tone, myoclonus, or gait disorder
   - Seizures in advanced disease
   - CT scan normal for age

4. **Features that make the diagnosis of** *probable* **Alzheimer's disease uncertain or unlikely include:**
   - Sudden, apoplectic onset
   - Focal neurologic findings such as hemiparesis, sensory loss, visual field deficits
   - Incoordination early in the course of the illness
   - Seizures of gait disturbances at the onset or very early in the course of the illness

Adapted from McKhann G et al: Clinical diagnosis of Alzheimer's disease: report of the NINCDS-ADRDA Work Group* under the auspices of Department of Health and Human Services Task Force on Alzheimer's Disease in *Neurology* 34:939-943, July 1984.

This approach is essential to establish the history that demonstrates the person has progressively deteriorated and to identify tasks that the patient can no longer perform adequately (e.g., those requiring sequential steps).

The history may disclose the difficulties the person has with memory, problems with activities of daily living, alterations in mood, delusions, and illusions. The collateral will often be able to identify the fact that the affected individual forgets appointments and errands, or is unable to find his way to an accustomed destination.

The collateral may report that the person is unable to use money and instruments of daily living such as the telephone. Other difficulties as described throughout this book will often be present.

Probably the most important part of the clinical examination is the mental status testing. This testing includes assessment of orientation, registration, attention, calculation, recent recall, comprehension, reading and writing, and the ability to draw or copy designs. Quantitative aids to the clinical examination include:

- The Mini-Mental State Examination (Box 8-2, Box 8-3)
- The Blessed Dementia Scale (Box 8-4)
- The Dementia Severity Rating Scale (Box 8-5)
- The Hachinski Ischemic Scale for estimating the likelihood of multiinfarct dementia (Box 8-6)

The psychiatric evaluation excludes various psychiatric disorders such as major depression, bipolar disorder, and schizophrenia.

The physical examination will particularly concentrate on examination of the sensory and motor systems, which will exclude other neurologic disorders such as Parkinson's disease and Huntington's disease.

DIFFERENTIAL DIAGNOSIS

The differential diagnosis of Alzheimer's disease can be remembered by using the mnemonic DEMENTIA.

D is for Drugs and Alcohol

In the evaluation of a person who is confused and suffering from memory loss, the first consideration should be any drugs that the individual is taking. One drug that frequently is overlooked in the elderly is alcohol. A significant number of elderly men and women have severe problems with alcohol. Women are particularly difficult to diagnose because they tend to be more circumspect in their drinking. Alcoholism is also more frequently associated with shame in women and is more difficult to treat. These individuals may have been drinkers who had stopped drinking because they were afraid they would not be able to keep their work schedule, or they may have drunk excessively on Friday or Saturday nights. Now that they do not need to go to work, they may start drinking earlier and earlier in the day. Some people adopt this behavior partly to drive away the symptoms of depression. However, over time, alcohol aggravates depression.

Another reason people drink excessively after retirement is boredom. Depression and boredom are two real problems for many individuals who have not planned for retirement.

➤ A history of the patient's use of alcohol is always important.

Since patients often deny drinking excessively, relatives should be asked about indirect evidence, such as empty bottles found in the garbage can or bottles around the house.

Most of the other drugs a patient might be taking are either prescribed or bought over the counter. Over-the-counter drugs frequently are not included in the drug history, because many elderly people do not consider such drugs medication. Yet the elderly are the largest single group of purchasers of such drugs, which include sleeping pills, laxatives, antihistamines, tonics, and antacids.

Text continued on p. 97

Instructions for Administration of Mini-Mental Status Examination

Orientation

1. Ask for the date. Then ask specifically for parts omitted, e.g., "Can you also tell me what season it is?" Score one point for each correct answer.
2. Ask in turn, "Can you tell me the name of this hospital?" (town, county, etc.) Score one point for each correct answer.

Registration

Ask the patient if you may test his/her memory. Then say the names of 3 unrelated objects, clearly and slowly, about one second for each name. After you have said all 3, ask the patient to repeat them. This first repetition determines his/her score (0-3), but keep saying them until he/she can repeat all 3, up to 6 trials. If all 3 are not eventually learned, recall cannot be meaningfully tested.

Attention and Calculation

Ask the patient to spell the word "world" backwards. The score is the number of letters in correct order (e.g., DLROW = 5, DLRW = 4, DLORW, DLW = 3, DRLWO = 1).

Recall

Ask the patient if he/she can recall the 3 words you previously asked him/her to remember. Score 0-3.

Language

Naming:	Show the patient a wristwatch and ask him/her what it is. Repeat for pencil. Score 0-2.
Repetition:	Ask the patient to repeat the sentence after you. Allow only one trial. Score 0 or 1.
3-Stage Command:	Give the patient a piece of blank paper and repeat the command. Score 1 point for each part correctly executed.
Reading:	On a blank piece of paper write the sentence, "Close your eyes," in letters large enough for the patient to see clearly. Ask him/her to read it and do what it says. Score 1 point only if he/she actually closes his/her eyes.
Writing:	Give the patient a blank piece of paper and ask him/her to write a sentence for you. Do not dictate a sentence; it is to be written spontaneously. It must contain a subject and verb to be sensible. Correct grammar and punctuation are not necessary.
Copying:	On a clean piece of paper, draw intersecting pentagons, each side about 1 inch, and ask him/her to copy it exactly as it is. All ten angles must be present and 2 must intersect to score 1 point. Tremor and ration are ignored.

● **Box 8-3**
Mini-Mental State Examination (MMSE)

Maximum Score	Score	
		Orientation
5	( )	What is the (year) (date) (day) (month)?
5	( )	Where are we? (state) (county) (town or city) (hospital) (floor)
		Registration
3	( )	Name 3 common objects (e.g., "apple," "table," "penny"). Take 1 second to say each. Then ask the patient to repeat all 3 after you have said them. Give 1 point for each correct answer. Then repeat them until he/she learns all 3. Count trials and record: Trials:
		Attention and Calculation
5	( )	Spell "world" backwards. The score is the number of letters in correct order (D_ L_ R_ O_ W_).
		Recall
3	( )	Ask for the 3 objects repeated above. Give 1 point for each correct answer. [Note: Recall cannot be tested if all 3 objects were not remembered during registration.]
		Language
2	( )	Name a "pencil," and "watch." (2 points)
1	( )	Repeat the following: "No ifs, ands, or buts." (1 point)
3	( )	Follow a 3-stage command: "Take a paper in your right hand, fold it in half, and put it on the floor." (3 points)
1	( )	Read and obey the following:
1	( )	Close your eyes. (1 point)
1	( )	Write a sentence. (1 point)
		Copy the following design. (1 point)

Total Score _____

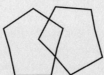

Adapted from Folstein MF, Folstein SE, McHugh PR: "Mini-Mental State": a practical method for grading the cognitive state of patients for the clinician, *J Psychiatr Res 1975* 12:196-198 and Cockrell JR and Folstein MF: Mini-Mental State Examination (MMSE), *Psychopharm Bull* 24 (4):689-692, 1988.

● Box 8-4

Blessed Dementia Scale

Each item scores 1 point except for the items noted.

1. Inability to perform household tasks
2. Inability to cope with small sums of money
3. Inability to remember short lists of items
4. Inability to find way outdoors
5. Inability to find way about familiar streets
6. Inability to interpret surroundings
7. Inability to recall recent events
8. Tendency to dwell in the past
9. Eating:
   - Messily, with spoon only
   - Simple solids, such as biscuits (2 points)
   - Has to be fed (3 points)
10. Dressing:
    - Occasionally misplaced buttons, etc.
    - Wrong sequence, forgets items (2 points)
    - Unable to dress (3 points)
11. Sphincter control:
    - Occasional wet bed
    - Frequent wet bed (2 points)
    - Doubly incontinent (3 points)
12. Increased rigidity
13. Increased egocentricity
14. Impairment of regard for feelings of others
15. Coarsening of affect
16. Impairment of emotional control
17. Hilarity in inappropriate situations
18. Diminished emotional responsiveness
19. Sexual misdemeanor (de novo in old age)
20. Hobbies relinquished
21. Diminished initiative or growing apathy
22. Purposeless hyperactivity

TOTAL SCORE_____

Scores range from 0 to 27. The higher the score, the greater the degree of dementia. A second part is the Information Score and contains items testing orientation and memory.

Modified from *Br J Psychiatry* 114:808, 1968. In Gallo JJ, Reichel W, Anderson L: *Handbook of geriatric assessment,* Rockville, MD, 1988, Aspen Publishers.

● **Box 8-5**
Dementia Severity Rating Scale

PATIENT NAME: _____ ID NUMBER _____

DATE: _____

PERSON COMPLETING FORM: _____

RELATIONSHIP TO PATIENT: _____

In each section, circle the number that most closely applies to the patient. Please circle only one number per section.

Memory
0 - Normal.
1 - Occasional "benign" forgetfulness of no consequence.
2 - Mild consistent forgetfulness with partial recollection of events.
3 - Moderate memory loss, more marked for recent events and severe enough to interfere with everyday activities.
4 - Severe memory loss; only well-learned material retained with newly learned material rapidly lost.
5 - Usually unable to remember basic facts such as the day of the week, month and/or year, when last meal was eaten, or the name of the next meal.
6 - Unable to test due to speech and language difficulty and/or ability to follow instructions.
7 - Makes no attempt to communicate and is no longer aware of surroundings.

Orientation
0 - Normal.
1 - Some difficulty with time relationships, but not severe enough to interfere with everyday activities.
2 - Frequently disoriented in time and sometimes disoriented to place.
3 - Almost always disoriented in time and usually disoriented to place.
4 - Unable to answer questions related to time of day or name of present location.
5 - Is unaware of questioner and makes no attempt to respond.

Judgment
0 - Normal
1 - Only doubtful impairment in problem-solving ability.
2 - Moderate difficulty in handling complex problems, but social judgment usually maintained.
3 - Severe impairment in handling problems, social judgment usually impaired.
4 - Unable to exercise judgment in either problem solving or social situation.

● **Box 8-5**
Dementia Severity Rating Scale—cont'd

Social Interactions/Community Affairs

0 - No alteration in ability to participate in community affairs.

1 - Only mild impairment, of no practical consequence, but clearly different from previous years. Still able to work (if applicable), but performance not up to previous standards.

2 - Unable to function independently in community activities, although still able to participate to some extent and, to casual inspection, may appear normal. Unable to hold a job or, if still working, requires constant supervision.

3 - No pretense of independent function outside of home. Unable to hold a job but still participates in home activities with friends. Casual acquaintances are aware of a problem.

4 - No longer participates in any meaningful way in home-based social activities involving people other than the primary caregiver.

Home Activities/Responsibilities

0 - Normal.

1 - Some impairment in activities such as money management and home maintenance, but no effect on the ability to shop, cook, or clean. Still watches TV and reads newspaper with interest and understanding.

2 - Unable to perform activities related to money management (bill paying, etc.) or complex household tasks (maintenance). Some difficulty with shopping, cooking, and/or cleaning. Losing interest in the newspaper and TV.

3 - No longer able to shop, cook, or clean without considerable help and supervision. No longer able to read the newspaper or watch TV with understanding.

4 - No longer engages in any home-based activities.

Personal Care

0 - Normal.

1 - Needs occasional prompting but washes and dresses independently.

2 - Requires assistance with dressing, hygiene, and personal upkeep.

3 - Totally dependent for help. Does not initiate personal care activities.

Speech/Language

0 - Normal.

1 - Occasional difficulty with word finding, but able to carry on conversations.

2 - Unable to think of some words, may occasionally make inappropriate word substitutions.

3 - No longer spontaneously initiates conversation but can usually answer questions using sentences.

Continued

Dementia Severity Rating Scale—cont'd

4 - Answers questions, but responses are often unintelligible or inappropriate. Able to follow simple instructions.
5 - Speech usually unintelligible or irrelevant. Unable to answer questions or follow verbal instructions.
6 - No response, vegetative.

Recognition
0 - Normal.
1 - Occasionally fails to recognize more distant acquaintances or casual friends.
2 - Always recognizes family and close friends but usually not more distant acquaintances.
3 - Alert, occasionally fails to recognize family and/or close friends.
4 - Only occasionally recognizes spouse or caregiver.
5 - No recognition or awareness of the presence of others.

Feeding
0 - Normal.
1 - May require help cutting food and/or has limitations as to the type of food, but otherwise, able to eat independently.
2 - Generally able to eat independently but may require some assistance.
3 - Needs to be fed. May have difficulty swallowing or requires feeding tube.

Incontinence
0 - Normal.
1 - Rare incontinence. Bladder incontinence (generally less than one accident per month).
2 - Occasional bladder incontinence (an average of two or more times a month).
3 - Frequent bladder incontinence despite assistance (more than once per week).
4 - Total incontinence.

Mobility/Walking
0 - Normal.
1 - May occasionally have some difficulty driving or taking public transportation, but fully independent for walking without supervision.
2 - Able to walk outside without supervision for short distances, but unable to drive or take public transportation.
3 - Able to walk within the home without supervision, but cannot go outside unaccompanied.
4 - Requires supervision within the home, but able to walk without assistance (may use cane or walker).
5 - Generally confined to a bed or chair. May be able to walk a few steps with help.
6 - Essentially bedridden. Unable to sit or stand.

From Clark CM and Eubank CM: *Alzheimer Dis Assoc Disord* 10 (1):36–39, 1996.

● Box 8-6
Hachinski Ischemic Scale

The score for each feature is noted in parentheses. A score of greater than 7 suggests a vascular component to the dementia.
1. Abrupt onset (2)
2. Stepwise deterioration (1)
3. Fluctuating course (2)
4. Nocturnal confusion (1)
5. Relative preservation of personality (1)
6. Depression (1)
7. Somatic complaints (1)
8. Emotional incontinence (1)
9. History of hypertension (1)
10. History of strokes (2)
11. Evidence of associated atherosclerosis (1)
12. Focal neurological symptoms (2)
13. Focal neurological signs (2)

Modified from *Arch Neurol* 32:634, 1975. In Gallo JJ, Reichel W, Anderson L: *Handbook of geriatric assessment*, Rockville MD, 1988, Aspen Publishers.

Many prescribed drugs cause confusion in the elderly. Particular offenders are psychoactive medications, (drugs that affect the mind), such as neuroleptic drugs, benzodiazepines, antidepressants, lithium, and hypnotic drugs. Such drugs have a prolonged action, especially in older patients because of the impaired functioning of their liver and kidneys. There also is evidence that the brain of older individuals is more sensitive to these drugs.

In a great number of nursing homes many residents take tranquilizers, although this practice often is more for the convenience of the staff rather than for the benefit of the resident. For example, many residents may have watched late-night television before entering the nursing home; however, institutional rules demand that residents retire at 9:00 p.m. The medication is prescribed to ensure that residents retire at this hour, as well as for other reasons. The ensuing sedation produces a state referred to as "mashed potato syndrome," so called because the resident is taking so many neuroleptic drugs that when lunch is served, the person falls face first into his mashed potatoes.

● Case Study—Drug-Induced Confusional State

In one case, a man was referred to a geriatric outreach program because two women had seen him standing naked on the balcony of an apartment building at 2:00 p m in midwinter. The women complained that he was a "flasher." The social worker and the physician who went to the apartment to investigate found an 80-year-old man sitting in almost total darkness with all the shades drawn. His medicine cabinet revealed that he was taking amitriptyline (Elavil), imipramine (Tofranil), haloperidol (Haldol), thioridazine

(Mellaril), promazine (Sparine, which has been removed from the market), chlorpromazine (Thorazine), and diazepam (Valium).The physician put all the drugs on the kitchen table and asked, "Now, Mr. Jones, which of these medications do you take?" Mr. Jones replied, "It depends on how I feel." The physician then asked, "Which ones did you take today?" The patient replied, "I took one of these, but I don't remember. I think I took two of the other ones because they work really good and help me, and I took one of the blue ones." The label on one of the containers revealed that the prescription had been written by a physician who had been dead for 5 years and was dead when the medication was refilled. The prescription read, "Valium 5 mg q.i.d., ad lib," meaning the prescription could be refilled an unlimited number of times, even after the physician's death.

Mr. Jones had seen several physicians since his doctor had died, but he had never been asked what medication he was taking or what drugs he had at home. He had never been instructed to throw away the old medication when a new one was added. This man's confusion was cured by discontinuing all his medication.

● Case Study—Patient Who Got His Medication from a Neighbor

It is also important to remember that some elderly patients borrow drugs from their neighbors. A 75-year-old man was seen in psychiatric consultation in a local hospital because of confusion that had begun in the previous five days. He was unable to answer questions, was confused and delusional, and looked very ill. He was totally disoriented. Despite an intensive workup, which included a computed tomographic (CT) scan of the head, lumbar puncture, and electroencephalogram (EEG), no cause could be found for his delirium. The patient was thought to have Alzheimer's disease, and a psychiatric consultation was requested. While this consultation was taking place, a neighbor who knew the patient well entered the room and was asked what she thought had happened to him. She said that the patient had been borrowing pills from her "for swelling of the ankles." Because one pill did not work, he had taken two and ended up taking three a day. It was discovered that the patient had borrowed a form of digitalis and was suffering from digitalis toxicity.

Many elderly people never throw away old medications because they are so expensive. Consequently, as in the case of Mr. Jones, these individuals may still be using medications that were prescribed months or years earlier without informing their current physician.

> Elderly patients should be encouraged to show their physicians all the medications they are taking, including over-the-counter drugs, and physicians should be diligent in questioning patients about their medication.

E Is for Eyes and Ears

Some people appear confused because they cannot hear or see well. Out of self-consciousness they often pretend that they can hear and may answer questions with totally irrelevant responses, thus giving the impression of having dementia. Also, some elderly people may be too vain to wear a hearing aid, and they may need to be confronted with the reality of their hearing problem to be convinced of their need for such an aid.

● Case Study—Deafness Presenting with Confusion

One such person was a psychiatrist in his eighties who was a close friend of mine. He did not want anyone to know he could not hear, yet whenever anyone had a conversation with him, particularly in a restaurant or other noisy place, he could not understand what was being said unless the speaker shouted. One day I said to him, "Everybody thinks you have

Alzheimer's disease. You appear demential simply because you won't wear your hearing aid." From that time on, he wore the hearing aid.

The other sensory area that is affected by aging is eyesight. When people start losing their vision, they may bump into things while walking across a room, making them appear to be confused. This problem is discussed further in Chapter 9.

M is for Metabolic, Endocrine Diseases, and Nutritional Deficiency

Patients with uncontrolled diabetes and hypothyroidism often display confusional states. Diabetes mellitus can become uncontrolled for a number of reasons, including infection, dietary indiscretion, failure to take necessary medication, and use of sugar-containing medicines such as cough syrups.

Any imbalance in serum electrolytes may be manifested as impaired mental functioning. Such an imbalance can be precipitated by a bout of diarrhea or by medications such as diuretic drugs and lithium, an agent used to correct mood disorders that is notorious for producing delirium through electrolyte disturbance.

Elderly people commonly do not eat wholesome meals and are likely to suffer from numerous nutritional deficiencies, as are patients who have had bowel surgery. Patients with such deficiencies display confusion and other signs of dementia. It is sometimes difficult to obtain a history of such surgery because the patient may have forgotten the relevant information, and records may not be readily available. Some patients may be starving and suffering from ketosis.

E Is For Emotional Disorders

Paranoid disorders and mood disorders are the two most common forms of psychiatric illness in the elderly that may be confused with Alzheimer's disease. Elderly individuals have a higher incidence of paranoid disorders than younger people.

Depression, which is common in the elderly, can be confused with Alzheimer's disease because it does not manifest itself in the classic manner.

Elderly patients who are depressed frequently have a list of somatic complaints and demonstrate emotional withdrawal or apparent confusion. The diagnosis of depression is made because of the abruptness of onset, lack of animation in the patient, loss of appetite, and insomnia.

N is for Neurological Disorders

Multiinfarct dementia is the second most common cause of dementia in older people. Unlike Alzheimer's disease, it is abrupt in onset and progresses in a stepwise fashion rather than a steady decline.

Hydrocephalus, usually found in newborn infants, can occur among the elderly, although only rarely (1-2% of dementias). This condition is associated with a clinical triad consisting of rigid gait, urinary incontinence, and impaired mental functions. The early diagnosis is important because the condition is reversible.

(Hydrocephalus is further discussed in Chapter 10.) Parkinson's disease, which generally manifests itself by affecting motor functions, can also be associated with impaired mental function.

T is for Tumors and Trauma

Two of the greatest advances in medical technology in the past 20 years have been CT scanning and magnetic resonance imaging (MRI). Although these methods are not very helpful in the diagnosis of early Alzheimer's disease, they do aid in diagnosing traumatic injury and tumors of the brain.

I is for Infection

Elderly people often appear to be confused when they have an infection, and the clinical picture may be further obscured if the individual does not have an elevated temperature. The two most common infections in the elderly that produce a dementia-like picture are pneumonia and urinary tract infections, which are discussed in Chapter 9. In the last decade it has been recognized that patients with AIDS often develop a dementia as part of the illness.

A is for Arteriosclerosis

Arteriosclerosis can lead to heart failure and insufficient blood supply to the heart or the brain. Patients with heart failure sometimes have bouts of confusion and frequently experience depression. These symptoms may masquerade as pseudodementia. Arteriosclerosis may also be responsible for strokes. If the stroke is massive and affects the motor area of the brain, the patient has paralysis. Lesser strokes, on the other hand, may not be noticed until so many have occurred and sufficient brain tissue has been destroyed that a dementia results. This condition is called multiinfarct dementia, and is discussed in Chapter 10.

MENTAL STATUS EXAMINATION

After the medical history, the next most important component of a patient evaluation is a mental status examination. The major purpose of this examination is to exclude other possible mental disorders. Like the differential diagnosis, the mental status examination has a handy mnemonic: AMSIT.

A Stands for Appearance, General Behavior, and Speech

The patient's appearance may point to impaired mental function. For example, a person who comes to the physician's office wearing three pairs of pants, has most of the buttons on his shirt undone, has not knotted his tie, and has soup stains down the front of his suit is not likely to have normal mental functions. Behavior is commonly easy to judge: Does the person sit still? Is he agitated? Does he keep moving around? During a combined interview, the patient's behavior toward the caregiver and the examiner is a useful indicator of brain function. Some patients are mute throughout the interview, yet they appear to understand what is happening. Others may lash out at the caregiver or appear to have no interest whatsoever in the proceedings.

M is for Mood, with Sadness or Elation, the Two Ends of the Spectrum, being of Particular Interest

Sometimes a person's relatives may believe that he has Alzheimer's disease if he is very excited, talks rapidly, cannot seem to get his words out fast enough, and is elated. However, such a condition is more likely to be a bipolar disorder than a dementia.

S Stands for Sensorium and Refers to the Person's Orientation to Time, Place, and People

A person loses sensorium in the reverse order in which it was learned. A child first learns to recognize his parents and other significant people, then where he lives, and lastly how to tell time. These skills are lost in reverse order, and therefore disorientation to time is the first to manifest itself.

I Represents Intellectual Functioning

The Mini-Mental Status Examination is a valuable tool for rapid evaluation of intellectual functioning. It consists of 30 questions, some that test sensorium and others that test arithmetic, abstract thinking, and memory. The test also indicates the severity of the disease. With a literate patient who has a high school education, a score of less than 24 is highly suggestive of impaired intellectual functions.

T Stands for Thinking Processes

Patients with Alzheimer's disease demonstrate changes in almost all the categories included under this section. Early in the disease most patients have difficulty focusing on a goal and often are circumstantial or tangential in their thinking; that is, when asked questions, they tend to give answers that may contain many extraneous details but that do not directly answer the question. Later in the course of the disease, much of a patient's thinking is illogical, incoherent, or both.

As a rule, delusions and hallucinations do not occur until Alzheimer's disease is fairly advanced.

The hallucinations frequently are visual and sometimes frightening, such as "seeing" smoke or flames when none exist. The delusions often focus on strangers being in the house or people from the past coming to visit, and they occur because the patient does not recognize familiar objects or people. Abstracting ability almost always is affected fairly early in the disease. The patient with Alzheimer's disease gives concrete responses when asked proverbs or when asked to state what is familiar about common objects. Social judgment frequently is impaired, and insight is almost always absent.

LABORATORY TESTS

A diagnostic accuracy of approximately 80% can be achieved through the purely clinical portions of the examinations; the addition of laboratory tests increases this rate to about 90%. The following tests are recommended (see also the glossary):
1. Blood count and vitamin B12 level
2. Comprehensive biochemical screening (autoanalysis of the blood)
3. Thyroid function tests, TSH (thyroid stimulating hormone) is at present the most sensitive indicator of thyroid dysfunction
4. CT scan or MRI of the brain
5. SPECT scan of the brain
Additional tests that may be useful in some instances include the following:
1. Human immunodeficiency syndrome (AIDS) virus test in susceptible patients
2. Electroencephalogram (EEG)
3. Electrocardiogram (ECG)
4. Lumbar puncture
5. Chest x-ray film
   Occasionally a patient must be referred for psychological testing. Neuropsychologists can be particularly helpful in differentiating Alzheimer's disease from other brain disorders that cannot be distinguished either by laboratory tests or the usual clinical measures. A group of tests known as the Halstead-Reitan Battery is especially helpful in making such distinctions. Tests of this type are discussed further in Chapter 3.

SUMMARY

The diagnosis of Alzheimer's disease currently is in a state of flux. Traditionally, this diagnosis has been made on clinical grounds with supporting laboratory data. However, some of the new techniques such as single photon emission computerized tomography, are proving valuable. It is also likely that in the near future biochemical markers will be identified to diagnose the condition without having to rely on examining the brain microscopically. For the time being, the diagnosis of Alzheimer's disease remains one of exclusion; all other conditions likely to present with impaired memory and cognitive deficits have to be excluded.

BIBLIOGRAPHY

American Psychiatric Association: *Diagnostic and statistical manual of mental disorders,* ed IV, Washington, DC, 1994.

Galasko D, Hansen LA, Katzman R et al: Clinical-neuropathological correlations in Alzheimer's disease and related dementia, *Arch Neurol* 51:888-895, 1994.

Gearing M, Mirra S, Hedreen JC et al: The consortium to establish a registry for Alzheimer's disease (CERAD). Neuropathological confirmation of the clinical diagnosis of Alzheimer's disease, *Neurology* 45:461-466, 1995.

Mayeux R: Commentary: Diagnostic problems in nursing home patients with dementia: Why we should and how we can improve accuracy, *Alzheimer Dis Assoc Disord* 1(Suppl 1):S184-S187, 1994.

McKhann G et al: Clinical diagnosis of Alzheimer's disease: report of the NINCDS-ADRDA Work Group, *Neurology* 34:939-944, July 1984.

Rasmusson DX, Brandt T, Steele C et al: Accuracy of clinical diagnosis of Alzheimer disease and clinical features of patients with non-Alzheimer disease neuropathology, *Alzheimer Dis Assoc Disord* 10(4):180-188, 1996.

Factors that Aggravate the Symptoms

Ronald C Hamdy
Larry B Hudgins

*To study the phenomena of disease without
books is to sail an uncharted sea, while
to study books without patients, is not to
go to sea at all.*

—William Osler

A generalized deterioration in functional activities of daily living is expected in patients with Alzheimer's disease. Progressive decline and gradual loss of higher cortical cognitive functions commonly spearhead the deterioration. However, in some patients the rate of declining function and disability may accelerate. When this occurs, reversible causes should be sought and actively treated because often the underlying Alzheimer's disease process is not the cause of this sudden physical and/or mental deterioration. In many instances some other specific disease is responsible. The presence of any factor that worsens the patient's mental and/or physical state should be detected since many such factors are reversible if treated early. If not detected in time, they may lead to further irreversible deterioration.

—•— Alzheimer's disease is associated with a gradual deterioration. A rapid deterioration is usually due to other causes.

A person's mental functions are controlled by the brain, which is made up of many nerve cells, or neurons. These are described in Chapters 2 and 3. Brain functioning depends on the number of brain cells, their integrity, and the efficiency of the blood circulation. Since neurons have no nutrition stores, they depend entirely on the circulation to provide them with adequate quantities of glucose, oxygen, and various other nutrients. Similarly, an efficient circulation removes from the brain any waste or toxic substances that have been formed by the brain cells through their metabolic activity.

The blood flow through the brain provides it with substances essential for its functioning and removes waste products. If the blood circulation is ineffective, not only will the nerve cells be deprived of various nutrients, but also various waste or toxic substances will accumulate in or around the nerve cells. The nerve cells cannot function properly under these conditions, and the patient's mental impairment may worsen. For instance, the patient may become confused, lethargic, apathetic, and drowsy, or may become irritable, violent, and aggressive. Since patients with Alzheimer's disease already have a reduced number of brain cells, they are particularly vulnerable to several factors that may interfere with the functions of the remaining nerve cells. In healthy older individuals these factors may not lead to any deterioration of the mental functions, but they may be of sufficient magnitude to affect patients with Alzheimer's disease. Factors responsible for a rapid deterioration include:

1. Sudden reduction in the number of neurons
2. Sudden decrease in the blood supply to the brain
3. Diminished quality of blood reaching the brain
4. Altered sensory perceptions
5. Drugs
6. Other influences

SUDDEN REDUCTION IN NUMBER OF NEURONS

To function properly, the brain must have a minimum number of healthy cells. In Alzheimer's disease brain cells progressively die. If the number of neurons is also suddenly reduced, the patient's mental state may deteriorate abruptly. Several conditions may be responsible for the loss of neurons, including:

• Strokes
• Subdural hematomas
• Space-occupying lesions inside the skull

Strokes

When a patient suffers a stroke, or cerebrovascular accident, the blood supply to a part of the brain is suddenly interrupted and the brain cells in that area die. Strokes have three main causes:

1. A THROMBUS, or blood clot, which forms inside the blood vessel and usually complicates preexisting abnormalities in the blood vessels themselves, such as arteriosclerosis or a stenotic (narrowed) lesion
2. An EMBOLUS, which is part of a blood clot that becomes detached and circulates in the bloodstream until it becomes impacted in one of the small arteries
3. A HEMORRHAGE, which occurs when a blood vessel ruptures. When this happens, not only is the blood flow to the involved area of the brain interrupted, but also blood accumulates in the brain, compressing and destroying neighboring brain cells

In approximately two thirds of patients older than 65 years who suffer strokes, the cause of the stroke is a thrombus. In the other one third, the stroke is the result of an embolus. Cerebral hemorrhages are rare in old age.

The signs of a stroke depend on its severity and which part of the brain is affected. Massive strokes, particularly those affecting the motor functions, have a dramatic presentation, with the patient developing speech difficulties or paralysis of an arm or leg.

Lesser strokes may not cause paralysis and therefore may go unnoticed. Such strokes may interfere only marginally with a patient's mental functions until so many have occurred and so much brain tissue has been destroyed that the patient's mental functions become severely impaired. This condition is the underlying process of multiinfarct dementia. Although a great deal of research is in progress to limit the extent of the deficits following a stroke, and even to reverse them, currently little can be done once a stroke has occurred. Several therapeutic measures, however, can be taken to prevent additional strokes, such as taking low-dose aspirin, controlling hypertension, reducing elevated cholesterol levels, and quitting smoking.

Subdural Hematomas

A subdural hematoma is a blood clot that forms following a hemorrhage that occurs inside the skull but outside the brain. Characteristically, subdural hematomas complicate head injuries. In most instances the trauma itself is relatively minor, such as a fall in the bathtub. Since the manifestations often are not obvious until a few days or even weeks later, by then the patient or caregivers may have forgotten all about it. Even if the trauma is severe enough to render the patient unconscious, he or she usually recovers consciousness and may appear normal for a few days or weeks before subtle changes develop. Patients with Alzheimer's disease, however, already have fewer brain cells and may have a much more dramatic presentation.

> Symptoms may not appear for a few days or even weeks. By that time the patient and relatives may have forgotten the incident.

Immediately after the injury, the patient may not appear any worse than usual, but a few days or weeks later the symptoms usually become more severe and may include a significant change in personality, apathy, lethargy, irritability, aggressiveness, and even violence.

The time gap between trauma and impairment of mental functions occurs because the initial hemorrhage is limited in size or because the bleeding stops. With time, however, the hemorrhage turns into a blood clot, which starts to draw fluid from the surrounding tissues (by osmosis) and grows larger. As the clot enlarges, pressure is exerted on the brain tissue, interfering with the activity of brain cells. The brain functions then deteriorate even further and overt symptoms develop. Subdural hematomas are also discussed in Chapter 10.

Space-Occupying Lesions in Skull

Unlike most other cavities in the body, the skull, or cranial cavity, has a constant volume that is largely occupied by the brain. If a patient develops an abscess or metastases (secondary cancer growths) in the brain, these space-occupying lesions can grow only at the expense of the brain cells, which first become compressed and later may be destroyed. Patients with Alzheimer's disease, who already have a reduced number of brain cells, are particularly vulnerable to space-occupying lesions in the skull.

SUDDEN DECREASE IN BLOOD SUPPLY TO BRAIN

As previously mentioned, the brain has no reserve capacity and therefore depends completely on the blood circulation for the oxygen, glucose, and other nutrients it needs. Even though enough neurons may be present for the brain to function at a certain level, mental functions can deteriorate as the blood flowing through the brain (cerebral blood flow) is reduced. Although the brain represents only approximately 2% of a person's body weight, it receives about 15% of the quantity of blood pumped by the heart and uses about 25% of the total inhaled oxygen. Any compromise in the blood flow to the brain is poorly tolerated in patients with Alzheimer's dementia, who already have a reduced number of brain cells.

Circulation of blood throughout the body is maintained by the heart. The quantity of blood pumped by the heart in each beat is known as the stroke volume. The quantity of blood pumped in one minute is known as the cardiac output and is derived by multiplying the stroke volume by the heart rate. A number of conditions can reduce the cardiac output, including myocardial infarctions and arrhythmias.

Myocardial Infarction

In myocardial infarction, part of the heart muscle is deprived of its blood supply and dies. If the area destroyed is large enough, the overall function of the heart may be disrupted and the amount of blood pumped during each contraction (stroke volume) will be reduced. The effect of this reduction may be magnified if the heart rate is changed (see the following discussion of arrhythmias). As a result, the heart will not be able to maintain an adequate cardiac output, leading to a decrease in the amount of blood that reaches various parts of the body, including the brain. If this condition occurs in a patient with Alzheimer's disease, whose brain functions are already jeopardized, mental functions are likely to deteriorate considerably.

In contrast to the classic symptoms of heart attack, older people may suffer a myocardial infarction without having any chest pain. This condition is known as a "silent myocardial infarction." The only sign of myocardial infarction in an older person may be a bout of confusion, dizziness, fainting, or a fall.

Arrhythmias (Irregularities of Heart Rhythm)

Elderly people are much more vulnerable to the effects of a change in heart rhythm, known as an arrhythmia, than are younger persons.

At rest, the heart of an older person beats approximately 65 times a minute, slightly faster than one beat per second. The heart functions in cycles, with each cycle consisting of a contraction (systole), during which the blood in the heart is forcefully ejected into the arteries, and a period of relaxation (diastole), during which blood returns to the heart through the veins. Systole is an active process, and diastole is generally a passive one that allows the heart muscles to relax and prepare for the next contraction. In normal healthy people, the amount of blood ejected during systole is the same as that received by the heart during diastole.

When the heart rate increases (tachycardia), both the systolic and the diastolic periods are shortened. At high rates, however, the diastolic period tends to be shortened even more than the systolic period. This change interferes with the amount of blood that fills the heart during diastole and in turn reduces the amount of blood pumped when the heart contracts (stroke volume). In an attempt to maintain a constant cardiac output, the heart beats even faster. At these very high rates, the cardiac output cannot be maintained and may actually fall because of the markedly shortened diastolic period.

Alternatively, an exceedingly slow heart rate (bradycardia), may compromise the cerebral blood flow to the point that the patient suffers episodes of syncope (fainting). If this situation occurs, a permanent cardiac pacing device may be necessary.

ALTERED QUALITY OF BLOOD REACHING BRAIN

Since the brain depends entirely on the blood for the oxygen and nutrients it needs to function properly, it is easy to see that even if the number of brain cells is adequate and the blood flow (circulation) is effective, mental functions may become impaired if the quality of the blood reaching the brain is not adequate. Because patients with Alzheimer's disease already have a reduced number of brain cells, they are particularly vulnerable to any such change. The quality of blood reaching the brain may be altered by:
• Reduced oxygenation of the blood
• Reduced blood glucose
• The presence of toxic compounds in the bloodstream

Hypoxemia (Reduced Amount of Oxygen in the Blood)

As the blood passes through the lungs, the hemoglobin molecules in the red blood corpuscles take up oxygen. The oxygenated blood returns to the heart, which pumps it to other parts of the body, including the brain. If the blood is not oxygenated adequately in the lungs, less oxygen will be carried to the rest of the body, including the brain. This state of reduced oxygenation of the blood is called hypoxemia.

Blood oxygenation in the lungs may be inadequate for a number of reasons, including:
• Respiratory tract infections (such as pneumonias and bronchitis)
• Pulmonary embolisms (small pieces of blood clots in the lungs)
• Chronic obstructive airway diseases (asthma and emphysema)
• Pulmonary neoplasia (cancer of the lungs)

- Pleural effusions (accumulation of fluid between the lungs and the chest wall)
- Pneumothorax (accumulation of air between the lungs and the chest wall)

Patients with Alzheimer's disease, particularly those in an advanced stage, may have neurological dysfunction that interferes with the swallowing reflex and leads to aspiration of the posterior pharyngeal or gastric contents into the lungs. In such patients the gag reflex is often lost, sensation is decreased, the swallowing muscles are often weak, and the cough reflex is inefficient or absent. As a result, aspiration and pneumonia will develop in the lowermost dependent parts of the lung and will result in rapid physical and mental deterioration of the patient.

Anemia also can decrease the amount of oxygen circulating in the blood. Because the number of red blood cells and the total quantity of circulating hemoglobin are reduced in persons with anemia, the amount of oxygen that can be carried by the blood also is reduced.

Hypoglycemia (Reduced Amount of Glucose in the Blood)

Since brain cells have no glucose stores, a sudden reduction in the blood glucose level leaves them unable to function properly, resulting in impaired mental functions. Hypoglycemia, or reduced blood glucose level, commonly occurs when a patient receives an overdose of insulin or when he receives a normal dose but skips a meal. Less frequently, orally administered hypoglycemic agents used to control diabetes mellitus may induce hypoglycemia. Sustained hypoglycemia may result in further brain cell death.

Severe and prolonged hypoglycemia may also result in a myocardial infarction (often silent), due to the release of adrenaline leading to tachycardia and coronary artery constriction.

Toxic Substances in Bloodstream

Even during normal functioning, the body produces many potentially toxic substances that are usually of no concern because they are changed into less toxic compounds or eliminated from the body. If the organs that transform or eliminate these substances (primarily the kidneys and liver) are impaired, the toxic compounds accumulate. Toxic substances may accumulate in the blood as a result of:
- Ineffective removal of toxic substances by the kidneys or liver
- Infections
- Ingested toxic substances, including medications

Impaired Renal Functions

One of the main functions of the kidneys is to rid the body of many toxic substances, especially the water-soluble ones, by excreting them in the urine. If the kidneys do not work properly, these toxic substances accumulate. Since renal functions are usually reduced in older persons, excess toxic metabolites, such as blood urea, cannot be fully excreted and can accumulate in the blood. Although all parts of the body are exposed to these toxic metabolites, the brain is particularly sensitive to them. They can cause changes in sensorium such as confusion, somnolence, and, occasionally, seizure. Causes of impaired renal functions include:

- Medications
- Dehydration
- Infections
- Obstruction to the flow of urine

Several factors can cause renal impairment, including drugs, particularly antihypertensive agents; nonsteroidal anti-inflammatory agents, analgesics, and some antibiotics. Dehydration is a common condition, especially in older patients whose sense of thirst often appears to be blunted. Infections and obstruction to the flow of urine as occurs in prostatic hypertrophy or as a result of renal or bladder stones (calculi) may also lead to impaired kidney functions. Compromised renal functions can lead to accumulation of drugs in the blood such as digitalis, oral hypoglycemic agents, seizure medication, and psychotropic agents.

Impaired Hepatic Functions

Whereas the kidneys eliminate toxic compounds that are soluble in water by excreting them in the urine, the liver eliminates water-insoluble or fat-soluble toxic compounds by excreting them with bile or by conjugating them with compounds that make them water soluble so that they can be excreted later by the kidneys. Alcohol abuse is one cause of impaired hepatic function. Hepatic impairment also may be caused by certain drugs, especially those metabolized (broken down) in the liver, such as most tranquilizers, sedatives, and other compounds that act on the central nervous system.

INFECTIONS

If a patient develops an infection, regardless of its location, toxic compounds are likely to accumulate in the body, circulate in the bloodstream, and reach the brain, possibly interfering with its functioning. This situation can produce an acute confusional state.

Chest Infections

If the infection is located in the lungs, not only do toxic products accumulate but also the amount of oxygen in the blood often is diminished since the lung congestion that complicates such infections interferes with the free passage of oxygen molecules. Chest infections are notorious for producing confusional states in elderly people. Although individuals who do not have Alzheimer's disease sometimes become confused as a result of chest infections, the confusion tends to be much more severe in patients with Alzheimer's disease or other dementing illnesses.

Chest infections frequently are difficult to diagnose in older people because most of the characteristic symptoms and signs seen in younger adults are absent. Such signs include fever, tachycardia (rapid heart rate), cough with expectoration of sputum, and the characteristic findings detected during the clinical examination and through x-ray films.

- Chest infections often present with confusion and are difficult to diagnose in older patients.

An older person who has a chest infection may not have a fever because the temperature-regulating center in the brain often does not function properly in old age and is less sensitive than in youth. This situation may be one reason why elderly people are more likely to develop hypothermia. Similarly, an increased heart rate may not be observed if some disorder in the heart's conduction tissue prevents it from increasing its rate. Cough and expectoration of sputum may be absent if the patient is dehydrated. Alternatively, cough and expectoration of sputum may have been present for a long time if the patient has a chronic obstructive airway disease. Similarly, the characteristic physical findings may be obscured by dehydration and by abnormal chest configuration due to kyphosis and kyphoscoliosis. The last two conditions can also mask the characteristic radiological features of chest infection.

A rapid respiratory rate may be the only sign of a chest infection in an older person.

One of the most important signs in the diagnosis of chest infections in old age is an increased respiratory rate. Unfortunately, this sign is often overlooked and, when considered, it is often approximated rather than carefully observed. A rapid respiratory rate may be the only sign of a chest infection in an older person. Ironically this single sign usually is the one that is given the least importance during the clinical examination and subsequent observation of the patient.

Subacute Bacterial Endocarditis

Subacute bacterial endocarditis is another cause of confusion and impaired mental functioning in old age, especially in patients with Alzheimer's disease. In this condition the heart valves are infected, and the heart may be unable to maintain an adequate cardiac output and circulation. Bacteria and their toxic products circulate in the blood, producing bacteremia or toxemia, which further interfere with the patient's mental functions. Subacute bacterial endocarditis is insidious in onset and progresses slowly. The diagnosis usually is not made until fairly late, when the disease has become well established.

ALTERED PERCEPTION OF ENVIRONMENT

The normal individual receives sensory input from the environment, processes the information, and develops a logical plan of action. To react appropriately to any situation, a person must be able to perceive, understand, and process several messages received from the environment. For example, a normal person who wakes up at 2 AM will not begin to prepare breakfast for the whole household. If the person does not know the time, he or she will check a clock, realize the time, and try to go back to sleep. Even if no clock is available, a guess might be made that it is too early to get out of bed, let alone fix breakfast. Poor vision, in contrast, may interfere with the ability to read the time on the clock accurately and may cause the person to think that it is time to get up.

Impaired Vision

Vision is the prime factor that determines a person's behavior in most instances. For example, if a person notices black particles in his food while eating, his immediate reaction depends on what he thinks the particles are. This reaction is mainly governed by visual acuity and ability to correlate what is actually seen with past visual experiences. Similarly, a person's reaction to someone who knocks on the door and identifies himself as a sales representative will be governed largely by the person's perception of the salesman and whether he "looks honest." On a more basic level, finding one's way to a rest room, for example, depends largely on visual acuity.

If the light rays that enter the eyes are abnormally distorted, as can happen with cataracts and glaucoma, the patient's perception of objects may be erroneous and may lead him to "see" things that are not really there, that is, to have illusions. This situation is particularly likely to happen if the patient is not fully conscious, as may occur if sedative or hypnotic preparations have been taken, or if the person awakens in the middle of the night or is confused for any other reason such as Alzheimer's disease.

Elderly people often have reduced visual and auditory acuity. About 1.4 million people in the United States are estimated to suffer from severe visual impairment. Of these, approximately 990,000 are older than 65 years. The three main diseases responsible for diminished vision are glaucoma, cataracts, and senile macular degeneration of the retina. In addition, the curvature of the cornea becomes less smooth and more irregular in old age, a condition known as astigmatism. Frequently, light that enters the eye may be refracted by deposits in the cornea, which are increasingly present in old age.

Although many elderly people wear eyeglasses, they are frequently inadequate. Older people have their eyeglasses checked at regular intervals of two to three years or whenever their eyesight seems to have deteriorated. Wearing dirty glasses obviously will further impair their already impaired vision. Caregivers, both professionals as well as lay, need to routinely ensure that eyeglasses are kept clean and cared for properly.

Impaired Hearing

Any deterioration in a patient's hearing may interfere with conversational ability. Since the patient may misinterpret questions, inappropriate answers are more likely to be given. Buzzing in the ears (because of wax or other diseases) may lead the patient to believe that someone is talking to him or her. If the eyesight is also poor, a shadow may be interpreted as a person talking.

As an individual ages, visual and auditory acuity gradually deteriorate. If the patient also has a sudden decline in eyesight or hearing, he or she may become or appear to have become confused or disoriented and to have impaired mental functions. The individual thus may not be able to perceive his environment accurately and may make errors of judgment. Before the patient's mental functions are assessed, it is important to make sure that there is no significant hearing loss. Otherwise, the results of the test may be false. Some improvement may occur with hearing aids, as indicated by audiometric testing. Another common problem is excessive cerumen, or wax, in the external canal. This cerumen buildup may become impacted and may be difficult to remove with irrigation alone. However, once the wax has been removed, a remarkable improvement in hearing may be noted. Batteries in hearing aids need to be regularly checked and the device itself routinely examined to ensure it is in good working condition.

Sudden Change in Surroundings

A sudden change in surroundings can be confusing to older people, especially those suffering from Alzheimer's disease. Such confusion frequently occurs when a patient is first admitted to a nursing home or other similar institution where she may not recognize the surroundings. This situation is particularly likely when a patient wakes up at night and encounters a strange environment. During the day he or she may recognize the environment, but in the dark after just awakening, the patient may not remember at once the new situation. This type of confusion may also be noted when a patient with Alzheimer's disease is taken away from a familiar environment to spend a few days with a relative.

Pain and Discomfort

In a patient who is confused, pain and discomfort may significantly increase the degree of confusion and mental functions. For example, the patient may be unable to understand or describe his pain or discomfort.

Common causes of discomfort include a full bladder, urinary incontinence, a full rectum, constipation, fecal incontinence, and decubitus ulcers. Hunger and thirst also are uncomfortable sensations, as are being too hot or too cold and lying on crumpled sheets with foreign objects such as food debris. Pain can be caused by a number of diseases (e.g., osteoarthritis), leg cramps, and infections.

DRUGS

Primum non nocere! Nowhere in health care is the first tenet of the field—*Primum non nocere* (first do no harm)—more apt than in geriatric medicine. In regard to medications, the smallest dose possible should be tried first, and then increased if necessary. Since elderly patients are very sensitive to medications, adverse drug reactions occur often.

Prescribed medications can aggravate mental impairment. Drugs that act on the central nervous system, such as hypnotics, sedatives, tranquilizers, antihistamines, and cold remedies, are particular offenders. Many of these medications can be purchased over the counter without a physician's prescription. Considerable evidence exists that older people are much more susceptible to the effects of these drugs than younger patients. An older person's body cannot eliminate the drug through either excretion by the kidneys or breakdown by the liver as quickly as a younger person can. Thus these drugs should be given in the smallest effective dose. If necessary, the dosage can be adjusted according to the patient's response. Also, short-duration drugs are preferable since older patients tend to metabolize and excrete drugs more slowly than normal.

Many over-the-counter drugs contain compounds that can sedate a patient. Besides sleeping preparations, such drugs include many cold remedies, antiallergic medications, and even some antacids and antidiarrheal mixtures. If these drugs are given to the patient in large doses or in conjunction with other medications, drug overdose may result and the patient's confusional state may worsen. Some histamine (H2) blockers such as cimetidine interfere with the breakdown of other medications in the liver and may result in an increased blood level of these medications.

It must also be remembered that alcohol is a powerful sedative that often potentiates the action of many other drugs. Drinking an excessive amount of alcohol may cause discomfort by increasing the volume of urine produced, thereby distending the bladder, and by precipitating dehydration.

Many routinely prescribed drugs may interfere with a patient's mental activities, for example, by altering the blood electrolytes (diuretics), precipitating anemia (drugs that irritate the gastrointestinal mucosa and cause bleeding from the gastrointestinal tract), inducing heart failure, precipitating cardiac irregularities, and reducing the blood pressure or the blood glucose level.

Because drug-induced confusion and impaired mental function are so common in old age, the physician, nurse, and family caregivers must be aware of all medications that the patient is taking, whether prescribed, bought over the counter, or borrowed from others.

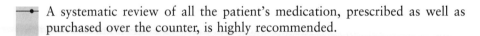

A systematic review of all the patient's medication, prescribed as well as purchased over the counter, is highly recommended.

OTHER INFLUENCES

Physical Restraints

Physical restraints are often used to control patients who demonstrate abnormal behavior and to prevent injury. Restraints are necessary for only a very small number of patients and generally are overused. Injudicious use of restraints aggravates a patient's irritability, frustration, and confusion. Physical restraints are discussed further in Chapter 17.

Sleep Deprivation

Sleep deprivation is a known and common cause of confusion, not only in older patients with Alzheimer's disease, but in any age group.

Coexisting Medical Conditions

Many diseases can cause confusional states, particularly in elderly people. Some of these diseases were described earlier in this chapter. It is important to ensure that no medical condition is responsible for a patient's deteriorating mental state before the assumption is made that the deterioration is secondary to Alzheimer's disease.

Because patients with Alzheimer's disease may suffer from other diseases that can considerably worsen their mental and physical impairment, caregivers must be aware of this fact and need to report any sudden deterioration to the physician, who will try to identify the cause. Often the cause is reversible, and the patient's condition may improve once the disorder has been identified and treated. Alzheimer's disease progresses slowly and insidiously and seldom is the cause of sudden deterioration in a patient's condition.

BIBLIOGRAPHY

Burney-Puckett M: Sundown syndrome: etiology and management, *J Psychosoc Nurs Ment Health Serv* 34(5):40-43, 1996.

Carter GL, Dawson AH, Lopert R: Drug-induced delirium, *Drug Saf* 15(4):291-301, 1996.

Casey DA, DeFazio JV Jr, Vansickle K et al: Delirium. Quick recognition, careful evaluation, and appropriate treatment, *Postgrad Med* 100(1):121-124, 128, 133-134, 1996.

Cole MG, Primeau F, McCusker J: Effectiveness of interventions to prevent delirium in hospitalized patients: a systematic review, *Can Med Assoc J* 155(9): 1263-1268, 1996.

Hall GR, Wakefield B: Acute confusion in the elderly, *Nursing* 26(7):32-38, 1996.

Johnson JC: Delirium in the elderly, *Emerg Med Clin North Am* 8(2):255-265, 1990.

Klein-Schwartz W, Oderda GM: Poisoning in the elderly: epidemiological, clinical, and management considerations, *Drugs Aging* 1(1):67-89, 1991.

Liptzin B: Delirium, *Arch Fam Med* 4(5):453-458, 1995.

McDougall GJ: A review of screening instruments for assessing cognition and mental status in older adults, *Nurse Pract* 15(11):18-28, 1990.

Neelon VJ, Champagne MT, Carlson JR et al: The NEECHAM confusion scale: construction, validation and clinical testing, *Nurs Res* 45(6):324-330, 1996.

Orticio LP: Confusion and the patient on an intensive topical ocular antibiotic regimen: a case analysis, *J Ophthalmic Nurs Technol* 9(4):145-151, 1990.

Oxman TE: Antidepressants and cognitive impairment in the elderly, *J Clin Psychiatry* 57 Suppl 5:38-44, 1996.

Rasin JH: Confusion, *Nurs Clin North Am* 25(4):909-918, 1990.

Rummans TA, Evans JM, Krahn LE et al: Delirium in elderly patients: evaluation and management, *Mayo Clin Proc* 70(10):989-998, 1995.

Stewart RB, Hale WE: Acute confusional states in older adults and the role of polypharmacy, *Annu Rev Public Health* 13:415-430, 1992.

Tess MM: Acute confusional states in critically ill patients: a review, *J Neurosci Nurs* 23(6):398-402, 1991.

Thompson L, Wood C, Wallhagen M: Geriatric acute myocardial infarction: a challenge to recognition, prompt diagnosis, and appropriate care, *Crit Care Nurs Clin North Am* 4(2):291-299, 1992.

Trzepacz PT: Delirium, Advances in diagnosis, pathophysiology and treatment, *Psychiatr Clin North Am* 19(3):429-448, 1996.

Whatley LJ, Bradnock J: Treatment of the classical manifestations of dementia and confusion, *Br Med Bull* 46(1):169-180, 1990.

Other Dementias

Jorge G Ruiz

*That is the essence of science: ask an imperti-
nent question, and you are on the way to a
pertinent answer.*

—Jacob Bronowski

Dementia is the result of an irreversible decline in mental functions. Although
Alzheimer's disease is a common and important cause, there are many other
conditions that may lead to dementia. It is important to identify these conditions
because in some cases the decline in mental functions can be stopped and even
reversed. Even if no improvement is expected, it is relevant to make an accurate
diagnosis of the cause of dementia because of the different prognostic and
psychosocial implications. The purpose of this chapter is to briefly review other
causes of dementia apart from Alzheimer's disease.

VASCULAR DEMENTIAS

Vascular dementias are the result of an interference with the blood flow to the
brain. When this occurs, the brain cells are deprived of nourishment and die.
There is usually a relative preservation of personality and the frequent
occurrence of depression.

Vascular dementia is the second most common type of dementia in the elderly
in western societies, and is probably responsible for about 10% to 30% of all
cases of dementia. The incidence of dementia increases linearly with increasing
age. Both sexes are about equally affected, despite the increased incidence of
stroke in men. Unlike Alzheimer's disease, the onset of vascular dementia is
usually abrupt, the rate of deterioration is stepwise, and neurological signs are
usually detected during the clinical examination.

These signs vary according to the part of the brain deprived of blood supply,
and can be broadly grouped into cortical and subcortical signs. Among the

117

former, localized muscle weakness, aphasia, and agnosia are the most recognizable. In the latter group, apathy, slow mental processes, emotional incontinence, abulia, and psychomotor retardation are more common. The neurological examination also usually reveals gait abnormalities, bilateral asymmetric deficits, rigidity, hyperreflexia, spasticity, and extensor plantar reflexes. Risk factors predisposing to vascular dementia include:

- Hypertension
- Cardiovascular disease
- Smoking
- Hyperlipidemia
- Excessive alcohol consumption
- Diabetes mellitus
- Lower educational background
- Older age
- History of previous strokes

Neuropsychological studies show that when compared with patients with Alzheimer's disease, those with vascular dementia have more deficits in areas of planning, sequencing, and verbal fluency. Patients also often exhibit severe anosognosia and emotional lability. In addition, whereas patients with Alzheimer's disease have difficulties understanding grammatical structures, those with vascular dementia have difficulties recognizing words, naming, and repeating.

Brain imaging studies are useful in diagnosing vascular dementias; electroencephalograms (EEG), for instance, may show focal abnormalities in parts of the brain.

CLINICAL SYNDROMES

Three clinical syndromes are recognized:

Lacunar Dementia

Lacunae are defined as small cerebral infarcts that lie in the deeper subcortical parts of the brain and result from the occlusion of penetrating branches of the larger cerebral arteries. Dementia in these patients is caused by multiple lacunar infarcts disseminated through the brain tissue and especially white matter or by a single lacunar infarction in a critical area of the brain associated with cognition.

The presence of mood lability with occasional outbursts of rage, forced laughing or crying, or depression; lack of initiative or spontaneity; psychomotor retardation; primitive reflexes; incontinence; small stepped gait; and dysarthria are common findings.

Binswanger's Disease

This type of dementia is usually seen in patients with hypertension over the age of fifty years. It is characterized by a slowly progressive dementia with memory problems, confusion, loss of initiative and interest, and slowing of the thought process. In some cases focal deficits are apparent such as neglect, apraxia or aphasia, bilateral pyramidal signs and pseudobulbar palsy. Other findings include disorientation, poor recall of recent events, and nonfluent, spontaneous speech. Other features sometimes observed include subcortical signs such as parkinsonism, gait disorder, and urinary incontinence.

The cause of Binswanger's disease is not well understood but hypertension seems to be an important culprit. Episodes of hypotension related to antihypertensive use or hypoperfusion states such as heart failure or dehydration can reduce the blood flow through the brain and lead to infarcts in the white matter, without there being an actual interference with the blood flow as occurs in cases of strokes.

Post-Stroke Dementia, Multiinfarct Dementia

Many patients become demented after their first stroke, while others do so only after multiple infarcts. Aphasia is a common finding. Although the Hachinski Ischemia Scale is commonly used to differentiate multiinfarct dementia from other types of dementias, autopsy studies have raised some questions about its validity.

TREATMENT AND PREVENTION OF VASCULAR DEMENTIAS

Currently, the only therapeutic alternative for the management of patients with vascular dementia is an aggressive treatment of the risk factors predisposing to this condition, especially hypertension. Investigators have shown a delayed progression of vascular dementia in those patients in which adequate blood pressure control was achieved. Treatment of diastolic hypertension reduces the incidence of stroke by about 40%. Treatment of isolated systolic hypertension in persons aged 60 years and older reduces the incidence of stroke by more than one third.

On the other hand, energetic blood pressure control in older patients to levels achieved in younger individuals can be hazardous. The use of potent antihypertensive medication can cause reduced cerebral blood flow and cause impaired cognitive function in older patients.

The management of vascular dementias can be targeted towards three different groups of patients:
- Those at risk of developing vascular dementia, but who are cognitively and physically intact
- Those who have mild cognitive impairment
- Those who have dementia

Patients with Risk Factors for Vascular Dementia

Therapeutic modalities for individuals at risk for vascular dementia include:
- Smoking cessation
- Exercise
- Diet control for patients with hyperlipidemia, diabetes, or obesity

- Judicious use of antihypertensives
- Lipid-lowering agents
- Antiplatelet agents or anticoagulants for patients with atrial fibrillation
- Estrogen Replacement Therapy (ERT) in women

Four factors independently increase the risk of strokes: previous stroke or transient ischemic attack, diabetes mellitus, history of hypertension, and advancing age. It is therefore important to control hypertension and diabetes mellitus. Other drugs are also effective in reducing the risk of strokes in certain patients.

The use of the anticoagulant warfarin prevents ischemic strokes in patients with atrial fibrillation. Physicians, however, are often reluctant to prescribe this therapy for patients 60 years of age and older because of the associated risk of bleeding. To avoid hemorrhages, the dose of warfarin should be carefully titrated by regular blood tests. Warfarin also interacts with a number of other medications that can increase its anticoagulant effect. Patients on warfarin therefore should not be given any medication without first consulting their physicians.

Aspirin prevents platelet aggregation, and is the treatment of choice to prevent the recurrence of strokes (also called the secondary prevention of embolic strokes). Although warfarin is superior to aspirin in nonrheumatic atrial fibrillation, aspirin is an efficient alternative when anticoagulant is contraindicated.

The drug ticlopidine also reduces the risk of strokes in patients who have previously sustained a stroke. It is useful in patients who cannot tolerate aspirin.

The present evidence suggests that lack of Estrogen Replacement Therapy (ERT) is associated with an increased risk for dementia in elderly women. ERT therefore may eventually prove to be a useful prophylactic agent for reducing the risk of vascular dementia among postmenopausal women.

Predementia Stage

This group includes patients with only mild cognitive impairment, and those who have experienced transient ischemic attacks, stroke, or silent cerebral ischemia. The suggested approach includes a maximization of therapeutic regimens for these conditions, such as anticoagulation for atrial fibrillation or other sources of embolization, antiplatelet agents such as aspirin, and carotid endarterectomy.

Dementia Stage

The use of antidepressants, antihypertensives, cholinergic agents, nerve growth factors, and antiplatelet agents may help the prognosis of patients in this group. In vascular dementia, risk factor control plus antiplatelet therapy such as aspirin have been shown to reduce the development of cerebral infarctions, to increase brain perfusion, and to stabilize or even improve cognitive test performance, despite age-related cerebral atrophy.

Several drugs have been investigated for the treatment of cognitive deficits in vascular dementia.

Propentoxifilline: Propentoxifilline has been useful in the treatment of vascular dementia. Clinical trials showed clinically relevant, statistically significant efficacy in the domains of cognitive function, global function, and activities of daily living in patients with vascular dementia. Therapeutic effects were observed as early as after the first 3 months of treatment, and the symptomatic effect lasted at least 12 months and was very well tolerated.

Nimodipine: Studies have confirmed the therapeutic efficacy and safety of nimodipine, a calcium antagonist selective for the central nervous system in the treatment of vascular dementias. Several studies have shown a highly significant improvement of the global functional state. In hypertensive patients, nimodipine had a synergistic effect with other antihypertensive drugs.

Buflomedil: The efficacy of buflomedil was monitored in patients suffering from mild vascular dementia using rating scales and neuropsychological tests. The findings of the study indicate that buflomedil improved the symptoms of vascular dementia; the most significant improvement was recorded in patients who had received it for the longest period. The efficacy of buflomedil may be due to its effects on platelet aggregation and improvement in blood flow distribution to the ischemic brain and oxygenation of brain tissue.

Alpha-glycerylphosphorylcholine and cytosine diphosphocholine: Both treatments produced a definite symptomatic improvement and showed a very good tolerability. The results suggest that in most tests Alpha-glycerylphosphorylcholine possessed a statistically higher efficacy and an overall more satisfactory activity assessed by both patients and investigators compared with cytosine diphosphocholine.

DEMENTIA DUE TO PARKINSON'S DISEASE

Approximately one quarter of the patients with Parkinson's disease have dementia. The life expectancy of such patients is reduced when compared with nondemential patients with Parkinson's disease. Some evidence suggests an increase in the last 30 years in the prevalence of dementia in patients with Parkinson's disease.

> Common features of the dementia associated with Parkinson's disease include a high incidence of depressive symptoms, cognitive slowing or bradyphrenia, and language disturbances such as dysarthria and hypophonia with absence of aphasia.

Patients with Parkinson's disease and dementia also often demonstrate impairment of visuospatial skills even without involvement of motor speed and manual dexterity, and problems with executive functions (abstract thinking, planning, ability to benefit from feedback, judgment, and initiative). There are also defects in attention and vigilance, with up to one third of patients having either hallucinations or delusions, or both. Insomnia, confusion, agitation, personality changes, and self-care problems are not uncommon, and often present management difficulties. Many patients with Parkinson's disease and dementia experience psychosis, with major behavioral, cognitive, and functional problems.

Atypical neurologic features for idiopathic Parkinson's disease such as early occurrence of autonomic failure, symmetrical disease presentation, and only moderate response to a dopamine agonist also are associated with more severe

---

—● Risk Factors Associated with the Development of Dementia in Patients with Parkinson's Disease Include:

- Being older than 70 years of age
- Female gender
- Developing confusion or psychosis on levodopa-containing medication such as Sinemet
- Having a "mask face" as a presenting sign
- Family history
- Depression
- Hypertension
- Psychological stress
- Severity of the extrapyramidal syndrome
- Low educational and socioeconomic status

---

dementia of a higher frequency rate and with lower scores on cognitive rating scales.

—● Longitudinal studies suggest a faster cognitive decline in Parkinson's disease patients who are depressed than in non-depressed patients.

Management of Dementia Due to Parkinson's Disease

There are no current therapeutic strategies specifically targeting the cognitive deficits in demented patients with Parkinson's disease. Experimental approaches include MAO-B inhibitors, calcium channel blockers, cholinesterase inhibitors, and cholinergic agonists.

The management of such patients includes the treatment of symptoms associated with dementia, such as behavioral disturbances, depression, and intercurrent medical conditions. The propensity of these patients with dementia to develop drug-induced psychotic symptoms is well recognized. Drug-induced psychosis may exacerbate cognitive disturbances, contributing to worsening dementia.

The psychotic patients had significantly more insomnia, confusion, agitation, personality changes, and self-care problems and were noted by their caregivers to be significantly more unmanageable at home than their nonpsychotic counterparts.

On cognitive scales, psychotic patients were significantly more impaired. Psychotic symptoms in patients with Parkinson's disease dementia are associated with major behavioral, cognitive, and functional problems. The reduction of dose or discontinuation of antiparkinsonian agents may be necessary to achieve symptom control. Furthermore, the initiation of antiparkinsonian agents in demented patients with Parkinson's disease must be evaluated thoroughly, given the high incidence of behavioral disturbances and mental changes in such patients.

If psychotic symptoms arise, management is usually complicated by the use of neuroleptic agents such as phenothiazine, risperidone, and haloperidol, which can worsen the patient's motor symptoms, limiting its utility in demential patients with Parkinson's disease. New psychoactive medications such as Clozapine or Remox-ipride offer reasonable alternatives. Electroconvulsive therapy (ECT) has been used for the treatment of psychiatric complications in Parkinson's disease, but patients with dementia have a higher frequency of post-ECT delirium. The judicious use of anticholinergic agents cannot be overemphasized. In elderly patients with mild Parkinson's disease and no evidence of cognitive deficits, the use of anticholinergic agents resulted in a dementia syndrome characterized by memory disturbance, personality changes, abnormal behavior, and lethargy, with the dementia disappearing after the discontinuation of these medications.

DEMENTIA DUE TO DIFFUSE LEWY BODY DISEASE

Diffuse Lewy body disease (DLBD) is a clinical entity characterized by:
• Mild extrapyramidal features
• Progressive dementia
• Visual hallucinations
• Relatively acute onset
• Fluctuating course

The initial presentation can be diverse. The dementia is rarely found in younger people, with the majority of cases developing in elderly people.

A characteristic feature of this disease is its often fluctuating course. The clinical presentation is characterized by dementia with an insidious and gradual, but fluctuating, course accompanied by cortical features such as aphasia, apraxia, and agnosia. There is memory impairment, and there are problems with visuo-spatial abilities. Some elements of subcortical involvement can also be observed, namely decreased attention and verbal fluency deficits. Extrapyramidal characteristics include rigidity, bradykinesia, shuffling gait, and a flexed posture. Other neuropsychiatric abnormalities include transient clouding of consciousness or loss of consciousness, psychosis, delusional and paranoid ideation, and hallucinations, predominantly visual but also auditory. Frequent and repeated falls commonly occur.

Hallucinations occur frequently in Diffuse Lewy body disease. They appear to be related to an extensive cholinergic deficit in the temporal neocortex and a resulting imbalance between decreased cholinergic and relatively preserved serotonergic activities. Neurochemical analyses of the temporal cortex have revealed a distinction between hallucinating and nonhallucinating patients in both cholinergic and monoaminergic transmitter activities. In contrast with the cholinergic enzyme choline acetyltransferase, which was more extensively reduced in hallucinating individuals, serotonergic S2 receptor binding and both dopamine and serotonin metabolites were significantly decreased in nonhallucinating cases. These results suggest that an imbalance between monoaminergic and cholinergic transmitters is involved in hallucinogenesis in the human brain.

Less common features are myoclonus, chorea, dystonia, orthostatic hypotension, aphasia, corticospinal tract signs, dysphagia and cachexia.

An important characteristic is the sensitivity of these patients to neuroleptic agents. When patients with DLBD receive neuroleptic drugs for behavioral disturbances, they can develop severe and irreversible extrapyramidal side effects and, in some cases, neuroleptic malignant syndrome. There is evidence of a reduced survival rate in patients with DLBD who receive neuroleptics. The disease is characterized by relentless progression, with a duration of approximately 6 years, followed by death.

Neuropsychological studies reveal severe impairment of attention, deficits in verbal fluency, impaired visuo-spatial performance, and difficulty writing from dictation.

Electroencephalograms are frequently abnormal in these patients, with slowing of posterior background rhythms and often frontally dominant burst patterns. CT scans and MRI of the brain may only show moderate to severe cerebral atrophy.

Lewy bodies are rounded, eosinophilic, intracytoplasmic neuronal inclusions composed of altered neurofilaments. In Diffuse Lewy body disease, Lewy bodies can be found in a widespread distribution in the cerebral cortex and in the brainstem, diencephalic nuclei, and basal ganglia. The presence of a protein called Ubiquitin in areas of the hippocampus is very specific for Lewy body disease and serves to differentiate pathologically this condition from Alzheimer's disease. A variable degree of senile degenerative change is also present in the forms of numerous senile plaques and minimal neurofibrillary tangles in most cases. Neither the clinical nor the neuropathological features of this group are typical of Parkinson's or Alzheimer's disease but suggest a distinct neurodegenerative disorder, part of the Lewy body disease spectrum, in which mental symptoms predominate over motor disabilities.

The syndrome is more frequently identified in men than in women over the age of 60 years. Several autopsy studies have revealed a prevalence of Diffuse Lewy body disease of between 12% to 27%, making it the second most common type of dementia after Alzheimer's disease. These figures, however, have been met with some skepticism, and new operational criteria to be used in longitudinal studies will clarify the real incidence and frequency of this disorder.

Management of Diffuse Lewy Body Disease

Because of the similarity of DLBD to Parkinson's disease, levodopa has been used to treat the motor abnormalities frequently seen in this disorder. Although motor function improved under treatment with levodopa, cognitive deficits were not affected by the use of this drug.

The possible common etiology between Lewy body disease and Alzheimer's disease may be a target for nicotinic cholinergic agonists as a new developing area for therapeutic intervention. Loss of cholinergic receptors has been reported not only in Alzheimer's disease but also in Diffuse Lewy body disease. Clinical studies suggest that compounds that act to stimulate nicotinic receptors may improve learning and memory in a variety of models of cognitive impairment in animals.

Early clinical studies have suggested positive effects on cognition of nicotine in human beings with and without Alzheimer's disease. Nicotinic compounds may slow the progression of Alzheimer's disease, as suggested by preclinical models of cell death as well as by epidemiological evidence of a protective effect of smoking in Alzheimer's disease and Parkinson's disease patients. Diffuse Lewy body disease patients with extremely low cholinergic activity were responders in therapeutic trials of the cholinesterase inhibitor tacrine, and the combined data suggest that cholinergic therapy may be particularly relevant to patients with Lewy body type dementia.

DEMENTIA DUE TO HIV DISEASE

Dementia caused by infection of the brain with the HIV virus may affect up to one third of patients with AIDS. In a prospective study to determine the incidence of clinical dementia, patients with AIDS and AIDS-related complex were examined neurologically and neuropsychologically every 6 months for 2 years of follow-up. Although no patient was clinically dement ial at baseline, 28% of them developed dementia during the 2 years of observation. Progression to dementia was associated with neuropsychological deterioration and with worsening MRI appearances.

The overall prevalence of dementia in adult AIDS patients is estimated to range from 7.3% to 11.3%. Risk factors for more rapid development of dementia include:

• Lower hemoglobin and body mass index 1 to 6 months before the onset of AIDS
• More constitutional symptoms
• Older age at AIDS onset

The number of AIDS patients over age 60 has risen steadily in the past decade, and 10% of acquired immunodeficiency syndrome cases now are reported in people 50 years of age or older. The number of transfusion-acquired AIDS cases probably will soon peak. Homosexual and bisexual behavior remains the predominant risk factor for AIDS until the seventh decade.

HIV-1 infection is characterized by multiple neurological syndromes occurring at all stages of infection. Dementia due to HIV disease, however, is the most devastating central nervous system consequence of AIDS because of its insidious nature, poor prognosis, and associated functional impairment. The median survival of patients with dementia due to HIV disease is approximately 6 months.

A clinical triad of progressive cognitive decline, motor dysfunction, and behavioral abnormalities typifies dementia due to HIV disease.

Cognitive impairment usually precedes motor difficulties and the rate of progression is usually variable, characterized by impaired attention and concentration, forgetfulness or excessive preoccupation with other topics, and difficulties understanding written material. Speech is usually well preserved until the later stages, when it becomes monotonous and slow with word finding difficulties and eventual progression to mutism. Slowing of thought processes and deterioration of executive function ability become evident with advancing illness.

Motor dysfunction includes fine and coarse tremors, poor balance, gait disturbances with loss of coordination, and frequent falling. Walking eventually requires assistance due to clumsiness and the eventual development of paresis of lower extremities. Fine motor movements become clumsy and slowed, and patients have difficulties with handwriting. Bowel and bladder incontinence may later develop, as well as myoclonus and seizures.

— The most remarkable behavioral changes comprise apathy resulting in social withdrawal and reduced work production.

Clinical depression and anxiety are also commonly found in subjects with this type of dementia, and psychosis and agitation can also be seen. Patients with mild dementia due to HIV disease perform markedly worse in the cognitive areas of executive function, memory, and complex attention but not in affect or the cognitive areas of simple motor function, orientation, language, or visuospatial construction.

AIDS in the elderly can present in several different ways, many times atypically, often manifesting as an undetected dementia. The risk of dementia is greater in older patients and intravenous drug users than in homosexual and bisexual men and in patients with lower CD4+ cell counts. The risk of developing dementia was almost double for women than for men.

Disease progression appears to be more rapid in the elderly, although the observed shorter survival time may result from a delay in diagnosis. Consistent with many other disease presentations in the elderly, symptoms of HIV infection such as fatigue, anorexia, weight loss, and decreased physical and cognitive function are often nonspecific. The diagnosis can be confirmed by appropriate laboratory studies. However, the diagnosis of HIV encephalitis or AIDS dementia complex (ADC) is often complicated by the frequent coexistence of opportunistic infections.

Theories regarding the cause of HIV-associated dementia have centered around the elaboration of substances that may be toxic to neurons, oligodendrocytes, or myelin. These potential toxins include HIV proteins, cellular metabolites, and cytokines. Current evidence suggests that there are large numbers of macrophages/microglia cells present in the nervous system of patients infected with HIV, which produce substances toxic to the brain cells.

There is a significant correlation between the number of macrophages in brain tissue and the severity of dementia. The presence of macrophages and microglia is indeed a better correlate with HIV-associated dementia than is the presence and amount of HIV-infected cells in the brain, supporting the concept that the pathogenesis of HIV-associated dementia is likely due to indirect effects of HIV infection on the brain.

Based on new studies, HIV-1-infected macrophages can initiate neurotoxicity, which is then amplified through cell-to-cell interactions with astrocytes. Substantial numbers of astrocytes are actively or latently infected with HIV-1. Astrocyte infection may then lead to neuronal dysfunction directly or through loss of supporting growth factors, dysregulation of neurotransmitter reuptake, or loosening of the blood-brain barrier, permitting further seeding of HIV-1 in the nervous system.

Treatment and Management of HIV-induced Dementia

Experience with available antiviral agents suggests that dementia due to HIV disease can be effectively prevented and treated, at least for some period, and that assessment of this condition is indeed a valuable approach for measuring antiviral therapy.

Zidovudine: Zidovudine is an inhibitor of HIV replication that may have a beneficial effect on patients with ADC. Zidovudine was found to be effective in preventing the onset of dementia due to HIV disease in some studies, but other studies did not find such a protective effect. Following the introduction of zidovudine, some investigators reported a major decline in the incidence of AIDS dementia complex, and recent results from the Multicenter AIDS Cohort Study revealed that the incidence has probably stabilized or declined slightly. It has been demonstrated in clinical studies that patients with ADC may improve with zidovudine treatment, and that the development of ADC is rare in patients receiving the nucleoside analogue on a long-term basis. Supporting evidence has also come from neuropathological studies, which have demonstrated that zidovudine decreases HIV-specific neuropathological abnormalities.

Methylphenidate: Methylphenidate has been used in several clinical studies in men with late-stage HIV disease in an attempt to improve decreased memory and attention span, diminished concentration, apathy, and slowing. Several noncontrolled studies in clinical settings have reported good results in improving both affective and cognitive symptoms associated with HIV disease. Side effects have been relatively mild, and patient satisfaction with treatment has been high. However, no studies have been conducted in early-stage HIV disease. Methylphenidate treatment of cognitive changes in men with HIV/AIDS holds significant promise to improve the quality of life for persons living with HIV/AIDS.

Haloperidol or Chlorpromazine: Treatment with either haloperidol or chlorpromazine in relatively low doses resulted in significant improvement in the symptoms of delirium as measured by the Delirium Rating Scale. In contrast, no improvement in the symptoms of delirium was found in the lorazepam group. Cognitive function, as measured by the Mini-Mental State, improved significantly for patients receiving chlorpromazine. Treatment with haloperidol or chlorpromazine was associated with an extremely low prevalence of extrapyramidal side effects. All patients receiving lorazepam, however, developed treatment-limiting adverse effects.

High-potency neuroleptics can cause neuroleptic malignant syndrome. Patients with dementia due to HIV disease appear to have an increased likelihood of developing acute onset parkinsonism and dystonia when treated with dopamine antagonists. It has been hypothesized, based on clinical evidence, that hypersensitivity to these drugs in dementia due to HIV disease is probably related to direct invasion of the basal ganglia by the HIV virus and a secondary alteration in dopaminergic mechanisms.

━━● AIDS patients are more susceptible to extrapyramidal symptoms than are psychotic patients without AIDS.

In a retrospective chart review of 804 men younger than 50 years, the likelihood and severity of extrapyramidal symptoms in patients with AIDS and psychotic patients without AIDS who had taken dopamine-blocking drugs was 2.4 times as high among the AIDS patients as among the comparison group.

DEMENTIA DUE TO PICK'S DISEASE

Pick's disease is a rare type of dementia that is frequently confounded with Alzheimer's dementia. Disinhibition is frequently the earliest clinical presentation of Pick's disease, often preceding cognitive deficits by many years.

Disinhibited behavior includes sexually inappropriate behavior, wandering unclothed, touching or kissing strangers, impulsive behavior, childlike behavior, and urinating in inappropriate places. Hyperorality is an evidence of temporal lobe involvement and is manifested by eating or drinking uneatable objects, putting food or inedible objects in the mouth without swallowing, eating other people's food, or chronically chewing one's own body parts such as fingers or hands.

The age of onset is about 58 years with a mean duration of illness of about 10 years. Up to three quarters of patients with Pick's disease present with personality changes such as apathy, social impropriety, decreased personal hygiene, obsessive behavior, indecisiveness, and laxity. Emotional characteristics commonly seen include emotional lability and depression. Alterations in language include anomia with or without dysarthria and decreased verbal output. Other characteristic behaviors comprise roaming behavior, traveling with the apparent purpose of exploration such as walking or driving away searching and examining a new area, and returning to the point of departure.

Patients with Pick's disease often develop speech abnormalities more often than patients with Alzheimer's disease. Their speech is characterized by reduced verbal output sometimes progressing to mutism, echolalia, reiterative speech, and dysarthria.

> When patients present with a progressive aphasia characterized by anomia, Pick's disease should be considered as a possible diagnosis.

In Pick's disease, there is usually preservation of receptive speech. Aggressive behavior is also seen. In most cases, memory for recent events is quite normal, but sometimes an amnestic syndrome is closely related with an unusually severe atrophy of the hippocampus.

The disease is characterized by a circumscribed fronto-temporal atrophy. The diagnosis can be established by brain imaging studies. The CT scan shows the fronto-temporal cortical atrophy and atrophy of the caudate nucleus. Furthermore, CT scans and MRI reveal lobar atrophy in the frontal lobes, temporal lobes, or both in almost half the cases of Pick's disease. SPECT and PET studies reveal decreased perfusion in the bilateral frontal regions in Pick's disease, while MRI and/or CT show mild to moderate cerebral atrophy.

There is a scarcity of data concerning the epidemiology of this disorder. Most series are small, and it is difficult to estimate incidence and prevalence since it is a rare disorder. Some researchers have calculated that Pick's disease accounts for 1%

to 2% of all cases of dementia. Most cases are sporadic, but there is evidence of familial transmission in a few cases.

The pathogenesis of Pick's disease is not known, and there are no therapeutic alternatives for patients with Pick's disease, but symptomatic treatment for behavioral disturbances and other manifestations of dementia is probably similar to other dementias.

NORMAL PRESSURE HYDROCEPHALUS

Normal pressure hydrocephalus (NPH) is a clinical syndrome characterized by the triad of:
• Dementia
• Urinary incontinence
• Gait disturbances

The cognitive disturbances include slow mental processing, impaired recall, difficulties with planning of complex actions, and no evidence of cortical dysfunction. Although most patients present with the classic triad, various combinations of symptoms are also seen. Gait is characterized by a slow shuffling with wide-based ataxia often associated with hyperreflexia, incoordination of the lower extremities in the standing position, and decreased speed of taking strides. The onset of gait disturbance prior to cognitive impairment has been associated with a more favorable response to shunt surgery, while a long duration of dementia has been shown to be a poor prognostic sign.

Urinary incontinence may be accompanied by fecal incontinence. Incontinence and long disease duration are associated with poor prognosis and response to surgical procedures. Age by itself is not an indicator of bad response to shunt.

In the elderly patient, these symptoms may be overlooked or discounted if the clinician is not well versed in this condition. Normal pressure hydrocephalus has classically been described as an idiopathic disorder. Recent studies, however, indicate that this syndrome may be associated with deep white matter infarction. Other symptoms that can be seen in the patient with normal pressure hydrocephalus are aphasia, dyspraxia, cerebellar dyspraxia, tremor, Babinski's sign, rigidity, and hypokinesia.

> Brain imaging is the cornerstone in the diagnosis of normal pressure hydrocephalus.

CT scans reveal moderate to marked enlargement of the lateral ventricles out of proportion to the degree of enlargement of cerebral sulci and the basal cisterns, accompanied by enlargement of the third and fourth ventricles. The temporal horns are usually more expanded than in atrophy and the overall ventricular system has a distended, bullous configuration. Still there is no clear-cut way of distinguishing this presentation from that of plain cerebral atrophy, although the presence of a dilated third ventricle should be highly suggestive of hydrocephalus. MRI does not give any additional information to that obtained with CT. SPECT is a useful supplement in the diagnosis of NPH versus normal aging, and may also help to identify patients not likely to benefit clinically from surgery.

Management of Normal Pressure Hydrocephalus

Patients with normal pressure hydrocephalus may respond to surgery, provided it is initiated in a timely manner. The cerebrospinal fluid tap test is often used to identify patients who will respond favorably to surgery. During this test, about 40 ml of cerebrospinal fluid are withdrawn, and the patient's condition is compared before and afterwards. An improvement is suggestive of a good response to surgery.

Idiopathic normal-pressure hydrocephalus remains difficult to treat. There is controversy in the literature as to whether any of the cardinal manifestations of the disease predicts a good outcome after shunt surgery. The clinical response to shunting is extremely variable, with rates ranging from 25% to 91%. Shunt complication rates occur in up to half the cases, and serious morbidity or mortality rates are up to 7%.

In our recent study, improvement was highest in the group of patients whose NPH was caused by a subarachnoid hemorrhage. Old age was not correlated to poorer response to shunt surgery, and up to 11% of the elderly patients were able to leave long-term care institutions with a 36% reduction of assistance needed for activities of daily living. The variability in proportion of response to shunting, complications of shunt surgery, and mortality seems to depend on many factors, including the experience of the surgeon and center performing the operation, differing clinical selection criteria for surgery, criteria for the types of complications, timing of surgery, nonstandardized outcome criteria, duration of follow up, and selection and publication biases. The most frequent surgical complications are infection, mechanical shunt dysfunction, subdural hematoma, intracerebral hemorrhage, ischemic strokes, and seizures.

In a study on patients with normal-pressure hydrocephalus, 96% of those shunted on the basis of intracranial pressure monitoring demonstrated a clear postshunting improvement at one year with a statistically significant correlation between high-wave relative frequency and the grade of improvement. At the same time, 66.6% of shunted patients showed a significant improvement in cognitive functions. Complications of shunting were successfully managed without residual deficits in this series.

CREUTZFELDT-JAKOB DISEASE

During the last ten years infectious diseases such as scrapie in sheep and bovine spongiform encephalopathy (BSE), or mad cow disease in cattle, have received increased attention. The appearance of mad cow disease in Great Britain has increased the fear that humans can develop Creutzfeldt-Jakob disease (CJD) through their intake of contaminated meat. The infectious agent is a prion that probably has a pure protein structure and lacks DNA.

Creutzfeldt-Jakob Disease is an invariably fatal dementing illness characterized by loss of higher levels of brain functions, resulting in dementia and ataxia. Epidemiological surveillance of CJD done in the United Kingdom to identify changes in the occurrence of this disease after the epidemic of bovine spongiform encephalopathy in cattle raise the possibility that it is causally linked to BSE.

The clinical diagnosis of sporadic Creutzfeldt-Jakob disease relies on the evaluation of rapidly progressive dementia, ataxia, myoclonus, changes in the electroencephalogram, and other neurological signs.

The definite diagnosis requires neuropathological techniques. There is no practical and reliable premortem test for Creutzfeldt-Jakob disease and the related transmissible spongiform encephalopathies.

The electroencephalogram is highly suggestive of CJD if periodic sharp wave complexes are seen. The MRI appearance of Creutzfeldt-Jakob disease reveals specific findings of moderate to marked bilateral, symmetrically increased signal intensity in the putamen and caudate nucleus. Single photon emission computed tomography (SPECT) may be helpful for premortem diagnosis of CJD, but its sensitivity and specificity need further investigation.

It is estimated that Creutzfeldt-Jakob disease occurs at about a rate of approximately 1 new case per 2 million persons per year worldwide, but in large metropolitan areas it can approximate 1 new case per 1 million people. The increased number of cases may be due to better case ascertainment. The mean age at onset of this disease is about 60 years, with men being as equally affected as women. Familial cases constitute 5% to 10% of the total number of cases and seem to be genetically determined. The disease progresses rapidly and usually ends in death in about 4 to 6 months.

Creutzfeldt-Jakob's discase is a transmissible encephalopathy that occurs mainly sporadically, but also in an inherited and infectious form. The inherited form may be caused by various mutations in the prion protein gene on chromosome 20. These mutations are found in the familial form and reveal an autosomal dominant inheritance pattern.

The infectious form seems to be rare in humans and is largely due to iatrogenic transmission during various medical procedures, including the administration of human gonadotrophin and growth hormone, some neurosurgical procedures, corneal transplants, and EEG electrodes implantation. An epidemiologic follow-up of 6284 recipients of pituitary-derived Human Growth Hormone (HGH) found seven neuropathologically confirmed cases of CJD in this population. The median duration of HGH therapy of 100 months in the CJD cases was significantly longer than 41 months for all patients starting treatment before 1970; thus, the duration of pituitary HGH therapy appears to be a major risk factor for CJD. No therapy is yet known for this condition.

DEMENTIA DUE TO PROGRESSIVE SUPRANUCLEAR PALSY

Progressive supranuclear palsy (PSP) is characterized by:
• Supranuclear gaze palsy
• Neck dystonia
• Parkinsonism
• Pseudobulbar palsy
• Gait imbalance with frequent falls
• Frontal lobe-type dementia

In the advanced typical case when supranuclear gaze palsy and other main features are present, the diagnosis is relatively easy. Diagnostic problems, though, are frequent in the early stages due to the variable clinical presentation and in those atypical cases in which gaze palsy does not develop or that present as a severe dementia disorder or as an isolated akinetic-rigid syndrome. PSP is a significant cause of parkinsonism and its etiology remains obscure.

DEMENTIA DUE TO HUNTINGTON'S DISEASE

Huntington's disease (HD) is an inherited neuropsychiatric degenerative process characterized by:
• Movement disorder
• Dementia
• Depression

Visuospatial processing capacity, as well as the ability to perform spatial manipulation, are markedly affected in patients with HD. In contrast, consistency of spatial judgment appears to remain relatively intact in these patients. HD is also associated with mood disorders, personality changes, irritable and explosive behavior, a schizophrenia-like illness, suicidal behavior, sexuality changes, and specific cognitive deficits. Cognitive symptoms of concentration difficulties and lassitude are prominent. The duration of symptoms is significantly associated with the declining ability to mentally perform spatial manipulations.

Dementia in HD is probably of purely subcortical origin. The diagnosis of HD is aided by genetic testing, neuroimaging, and neuropsychological testing. Neuropsychological findings include impaired mental flexibility and concentration, deterioration of verbal and procedural memory, diminished nonverbal memory, and slowing of both fine and gross motor functions. MRI reveals fronto-temporal atrophy and atrophy of the corpus striatum in particular.

There is striking atrophy and neuronal loss in the neostriatum, particularly in the caudate nucleus, which has rich connections to the limbic system. HD results in organic mental disorders from dysfunction of prefrontal-subcortical circuits coursing through the caudate nuclei.

Treatment approaches to Huntington's disease have been confined to palliative care with secondary symptom management and psychotherapeutic support. Family education and genetic counseling should also be considered.

DEMENTIA DUE TO OTHER GENERAL MEDICAL CONDITIONS

Subdural Hematoma

Subdural hematomas are among the most common forms of intracranial hemorrhage in the elderly and are a surgically reversible cause of dementia. Subdural hematoma may be acute, subacute, or chronic. Acute subdural hematomas have a clear temporal relationship between the history of trauma and onset of symptoms, but the presentation of subacute and chronic hematomas can develop over a period of weeks and months.

The clinical presentation of chronic subdural hematoma is usually ill-defined and can be frequently overlooked. It is usually characterized by confusion and disorientation, memory deficits and full-blown dementia syndrome, headaches, hemiparesis, personality changes, hallucinations, and sometimes seizures. Although there is usually a history of head trauma, many times there is no evidence of traumatic injury. Physical examination may reveal signs of intracranial hypertension such as papilledema. Aphasia may be present in up to a fifth of cases, and cranial nerve palsies, especially of the third and sixth cranial nerves, are sometimes seen. Hemiparesis and gait disturbances are also seen.

The incidence of chronic subdural hematomas is highest in the sixth and seventh decades. Elderly individuals are especially predisposed to developing subdural hematomas due to underlying brain atrophy and vein fragility. The use of anticoagulant agents can also be a contributing factor. Brain imaging studies are needed to confirm the presence of a subdural hematoma. Early recognition of a subdural hematoma is important, given its treatability and potential reversibility.

Hypothyroidism

Hypothyroidism is traditionally known as a potentially reversible cause of dementia. Nevertheless, a review of 2781 cases from studies of etiology in dementia revealed only one case of reversible dementia due to hypothyroidism. Although it is generally accepted that dementia symptoms in hypothyroidism can be significantly reduced, many questions about the therapeutic efficacy remain unexplained. It has not been systematically investigated which psychopathological symptoms respond well to thyroid hormone replacement, how long the treatment should last, and whether duration of symptoms or severity of dementia have an influence on the degree of remission of psychopathological impairment.

According to present knowledge, symptoms of mental impairment begin insidiously and progress slowly. They may precede the typical somatic manifestations of thyroid dysfunction. Among the most frequent manifestations are recent memory loss and difficulty concentrating. Psychological tests reveal problems with abstraction, attention, and memory. The frequency of this type of dementia is not known.

Alcohol-Induced Dementia

Chronic alcoholism results in brain damage and dysfunction, leading to a constellation of neuropsychiatric symptoms, including cognitive dysfunction, the Wernicke-Korsakoff Syndrome, alcoholic cerebellar degeneration, and alcoholic dementia.

Alcohol and its metabolite acetaldehyde are directly neurotoxic. Alcoholics are thiamine deficient as a result of poor diet, gastrointestinal disorders, and liver disease. In addition, both alcohol and acetaldehyde have direct toxic effects on thiamine-related enzymes in the liver and brain. Alcoholics frequently develop severe liver disease, which per se results in altered thiamine homeostasis, in cognitive dysfunction, and in neuropathologic damage to astrocytes. The latter may result in the loss of neuron-astrocytic trafficking of neuroactive amino acids and thiamine esters, which are essential to CNS function. These findings suggest that alcohol-related dementias may be more common than previously suspected in the distribution of dementias in long-term care facilities.

BIBLIOGRAPHY

Vascular Dementias

Bennett DA, Wilson RS, Gilley DW et al: Clinical diagnosis of Binswanger's disease, *J Neurol Neurosurg Psychiatry* 53:961-965, 1990.

Caplan LR: Binswanger's disease. Revisited, *Neurology* 45:626-633, 1995.

Censori N, Manara O, Agostinis C et al: Dementia after first stroke, *Stroke* 27:1205-1210, 1996.

Cucinotta D, Aveni-Casucci MA, Pedrazzi F et al: Multicentre clinical placebo-controlled study with buflomedil in the treatment of mild dementia of vascular origin, *J Int Med Res* 20:136-149, 1992.

Di Perri R, Coppola G, Ambrosio LA et al: A multicentre trial to evaluate the efficacy and tolerability of alpha-glycerylphosphorylcholine versus cytosine diphosphocholine in patients with vascular dementia, *J Int Med Res* 19:330-341, 1991.

Gorelick PB, Mangone CA: Vascular dementias in the elderly, *Clin Geriat Med* 7:599-615, 1991.

Hachinski V: Preventable senility: a call for action against the vascular dementias, *Lancet* 340:645-648, 1992.

Hachinski VC, Lassen NA, Marshall J: Multi-infarct dementia a cause of mental deterioration in the elderly, *Lancet* ii:207-209, 1974.

Hommel M, Besson G: Clinical features of multiple lacunar and small deep infarcts, *Adv Neurol* 62:181-186, 1993.

Kertesz A, Clydesdale S: Neuropsychological deficits in vascular dementia vs. Alzheimer's disease. Frontal lobe deficits prominent in vascular dementia, *Arch Neurol* 51:1226-1231, 1994.

Kontiola P, Laaksonen R, Sulkava R et al: Pattern of language impairment is different in Alzheimer's disease and multi-infarct dementia, *Brain Lang* 38:364-383, 1990.

Lopez OL, Larumbe MR, Becker JT et al: Reliability of NINDS-AIREN clinical criteria for the diagnosis of vascular dementia, *Neurology* 44:1240-1245, 1994.

Meyer JS, Obara K, Muramatsu K et al: Cognitive performance after small strokes correlates with ischemia, not atrophy of the brain, *Dementia* 6:312-322, 1995.

Mortel KF, Meyer JS: Lack of postmenopausal estrogen replacement therapy and the risk of dementia, *J Neuropsychiatry Clin Neurosci* 7:334-337, 1995.

Parnetti L, Senin U, Carosi M et al: Mental deterioration in old age: results of two multicenter, clinical trials with nimodipine. The Nimodipine Study Group, *Clin Ther* 15:394-406, 1993.

Phillips SJ, Whisnant JP: Hypertension and the brain. The National High Blood Pressure Education Program, *Arch Intern Med* 152:938-945, 1992.

Rother M, Kittner B, Rudolphi K et al: HWA 285 (propentofylline)—a new compound for the treatment of both vascular dementia and dementia of the Alzheimer type, *Ann N Y Acad Sci* 17:404-409, 1996.

Skoog I: Risk factors for vascular dementia: a review, *Dementia* 5:137-144, 1994.

Skoog I, Lernfelt B, Landahl S et al: 15 year longitudinal study of blood pressure and dementia, *Lancet* 1141-1145, 1996.

Starkstein SE, Sabe L, Vazquez S et al: Neuropsychological, psychiatric, and cerebral blood flow findings in vascular dementia and Alzheimer's disease, *Stroke* 27:408-414, 1996.

Starr JM, Whalley LJ: Senile hypertension and cognitive impairment: an overview, *J Hypertens* 10 (Suppl 2):S31-S42, 1992.

Van Swieten JC, Caplan LR: Binswanger's disease, *Adv Neurol* 62:193-211, 1993.

Wetterling T, Kanitz RD, Borgis KJ: Comparison of different diagnostic criteria for vascular dementia (ADDTC, DSM IV, ICD 10, NINDS-AIREN), *Stroke* 27:30-36, 1996.

Zimetbaum P, Frishman W, Aronson M: Lipids, vascular disease, and dementia with advanced age, *Arch Intern Med* 151:240-244, 1991.

Parkinson's Disease Dementia

Aarsland D, Tandberg E, Larsen JP et al: Frequency of dementia in Parkinson disease, *Arch Neurol* 53:538-542, 1996.

Cedarbaum JM, Gandy SE, McDowell FH: "Early" initiation of levodopa treatment does not promote the development of motor response fluctuations, dyskinesias, or dementia in Parkinson's disease, *Neurology* 41:622-629, 1991.

Greene P, Cote L, Fahn S: Treatment of drug-induced psychosis in Parkinson's disease with clozapine, *Adv Neurol* 60:703-706, 1993.

Jacobs DM, Marder K, Cote LJ et al: Neuropsychological characteristics of preclinical dementia in Parkinson's disease, *Neurology* 45:1691-1696, 1995.

Jagust WJ, Johnson KA, Holman BL: SPECT perfusion imaging in the diagnosis of dementia, *J Neuroimaging* 5 (Suppl 1):S45-52, 1995.

Levin BE, Tomer R, Rey GJ: Cognitive impairments in Parkinson's disease, *Neurol Clin* 10:471-485, 1992.

Marder K, Tang MX, Cote L et al: The frequency and associated risk factors for dementia in patients with Parkinson's disease, *Arch Neurol* 52, 1995.

McFadden L, Mohr E, Sampson M et al: A profile analysis of demented and nondemented Parkinson's disease patients, *Adv Neurol* 69:339-341, 1996.

Mendis T, Mohr E, Gray P et al: Symptomatic relief from treatment induced psychosis in Parkinson's disease: an open-label pilot study with Remoxipride, *Mov Disord* 1994:197-200, 1994.

Mindham RHS, Biggins CA, Boyd JL et al: A controlled study of dementia in Parkinson's disease over 54 months, *Adv Neurol* 60:470-474, 1993.

Mohr E, Mendis T, Grimes JD: Late cognitive changes in Parkinson's disease with an emphasis on dementia, *Adv Neurol* 65:97-113, 1995.

Naimar D, Jackson E, Rockwell E et al: Psychotic symptoms in Parkinson's disease patients with dementia, *J Am Geriatr Soc* 44:296-299, 1996.

Nishiyama K, Mizuno T, Sakuta M et al: Chronic dementia in Parkinson's disease treated by anticholinergic agents. Neuropsychological and neuroradiological examination, *Adv Neurol* 60:479-483, 1993.

Ross HF, Hughes TA, Boyd JL et al: The evolution and profile of dementia in Parkinson's disease, *Adv Neurol* 69:343-347, 1996.

Sano M, Stern Y, Williams J et al: Coexisting dementia and depression in Parkinson's disease, *Arch Neurol* 46:1284-1286, 1989.

Sawada H, Udaka F, Kameyama M et al: SPECT findings in Parkinson's disease associated with dementia, *J Neurol Neurosurg Psychiatry* 55:960-963, 1992.

Starkstein SE, Mayberg HS, Leiguarda R et al: A prospective longitudinal study of depression, cognitive decline, and physical impairments in patients with Parkinson's disease, *J Neurol Neurosurg Psychiatry* 55:377-382, 1992.

Stern Y, Marder K, Tang MX et al: Antecedent clinical features associated with dementia in Parkinson's disease, *Neurology* 43:1690-1692, 1993.

Tison F, Dartigues JF, Auriacombe S et al: Dementia in Parkinson's disease: a population-based study in ambulatory and institutionalized individuals, *Neurology* 45:705-708, 1995.

AIDS Dementia

Bacellar H, Munoz A, Miller EN et al: Temporal trends in the incidence of HIV-1 related neurologic diseases: Multicenter AIDS Cohort Study. 1985-1992, *Neurology* 44:1892-1900, 1994.

Breitbart W, Marotta R, Platt MM et al: A double-blind trial of haloperidol, chlorpromazine, and lorazepam in the treatment of delirium in hospitalized AIDS patients, *Am J Psychiatry* 153:231-237, 1996.

Brown GR: The use of methylphenidate for cognitive decline associated with HIV disease, *Int J Psychiatry Med* 25:21-37, 1995.

Glass JD, Wesselingh SL, Selnes OA et al: Clinical-neuropathologic correlation in HIV-associated dementia, *Neurology* 43:2230-2237, 1993.

Goebel FD: Combination therapy from a clinician's perspective, *J Acquir Immune Defic Syndr Hum Retrovirol* 10 (Suppl 1):S62-68, 1995.

Karlsen NR, Reinvang I, Froland SS: A follow-up study of neuropsychological functioning in AIDS-patients. Prognostic significance and effect of zidovudine therapy, *Acta Neurol Scan* 91:215-221, 1995.

Lipton SA, Gendelman HE: Dementia associated with the acquired immunodeficiency syndrome, *N Engl J Med* 332:934-940, 1995.

Maruff P, Currie J, Malone V et al: Neuropsychological characterization of the AIDS dementia complex and rationalization of a test battery, *Arch Neurol* 51:689-695, 1994.

McArthur JC, Hoover DR, Bacellar H et al: Dementia in AIDS patients: incidence and risk factors. Multicenter AIDS Cohort Study, *Neurology* 43:2245-2252, 1993.

Portegies P: Review of antiretroviral therapy in the prevention of HIV-related AIDS Dementia Complex (ADC), *Drugs* 49 (Suppl 1):25-31, 1995.

Portegies P, de Gans J, Lange JM et al: Declining incidence of AIDS dementia complex after introduction of Zidovudine treatment, *Brit Med J* 299:819-821, 1989.

Portegies P, Enting RH, de Gans J et al: Presentation and course of AIDS dementia complex: 10 years of follow-up in Amsterdam, The Netherlands, *AIDS* 7: 669-675, 1993.

Power C, Selnes OA, Grim JA et al: HIV Dementia Scale: a rapid screening test, *J Acquir Immune Defic Syndr Hum Retrovirol* 8:273-278, 1995.

Price RW, Sidtis JJ: Evaluation of the AIDS dementia complex in clinical trials, *J Acquir Immune Defic Syndr* 3 (Suppl 2):S51-60, 1990.

Robertson KR, Hall CD: Human immunodeficiency virus-related cognitive impairment and the acquired immunodeficiency syndrome dementia complex, *Semin Neurol* 12:18-27, 1992.

Rosci MA, Pigorini F, Bernabei A et al: Methods for detecting early signs of AIDS dementia complex in asymptomatic HIV-1-infected subjects, *AIDS* 6:1309-1316, 1992.

Wallace JI, Paauw DS, Spatch DH: HIV infection in older patients: when to suspect the unexpected, *Geriatrics* 48:61-64, 69-70, 1993.

Pick's Disease

Mendez MF, Selwood A, Mastri AR et al: Pick's disease versus Alzheimer's disease: a comparison of clinical characteristics, *Neurology* 43:289-292, 1993.

Diffuse Lewy Body Dementia

Byrne EJ, Lennox G, Lowe J et al: Diffuse Lewy body disease: clinical features in 15 cases, *J Neurol Neurosurg Psychiatry* 52:709-717, 1989.

Hansen L, Salmon D, Galasko D et al: The Lewy body variant of Alzheimer's disease: a clinical and pathologic entity, *Neurology* 40:1-8, 1990.

Ince PG, McArthur FK, Bjertness E et al: Neuropathological diagnoses in elderly patients in Oslo: Alzheimer's disease, Lewy body disease, vascular lesions, *Dementia* 6:162-168, 1995.

Kalra S, Bergeron C, Lang AE: Lewy body disease and dementia. *Arch Intern Med* 156:487-493, 1996.

Kosaka K: Dementia and neuropathology in Lewy body disease, *Adv Neurol* 60:456-463, 1993.

Kuzuhara S, Yoshimura M: Clinical and neuropathological aspects of diffuse Lewy body disease in the elderly, *Adv Neurol* 60:464-469, 1993.

McKeith I, Fairbairn A, Perry R et al: Neuroleptic sensitivity in patients with senile dementia of Lewy body type, *Brit Med J* 305:673-678, 1992.

McKeith IG, Fairbairn AF, Perry RH et al: The clinical diagnosis and misdiagnosis of senile dementia of Lewy body type (SDLT), *Br J Psychiatry* 165:324-332, 1994.

Perry EK, Haroutunian V, Davis KL et al: Neocortical cholinergic activities differentiate Lewy body dementia from classical Alzheimer's disease, *Neuroreport* 5:747-749, 1994.

Perry RH, Irving D, Blessed G et al: Senile dementia of Lewy body type. A clinically and neuropathologically distinct form of Lewy body dementia in the elderly, *J Neurol Sci* 95:119-139, 1990.

Normal Pressure Hydrocephalus

Benzel EC, Pelletier AL, Levy PG: Communicating hydrocephalus in adults: prediction of outcome after ventricular shunting procedures, *Neurosurgery* 26:655-660, 1990.

Editorial, Normal-pressure hydrocephalus, *Lancet* 335:22, 1990.

Greenberg JO, Shenkin HA, Adam R: Idiopathic normal pressure hydrocephalus: a report of 73 patients, *J Neurol Neurosurg Psychiatry* 40:336-341, 1977.

Larsson A, Wikkelso C, Bilting M et al: Clinical parameters in 74 consecutive patients shunt operated for normal pressure hydrocephalus, *Acta Neurol Scand* 84:475-482, 1991.

Lund-Johansen M, Svendsen F, Wester K: Shunt failures and complications in adults as related to shunt type, diagnosis, and the experience of the surgeon, *Neurosurgery* 35:839-844, 1994.

Malm J, Kristensen B, Karlsson T et al: The predictive value of cerebrospinal fluid dynamic tests in patients with the idiopathic adult hydrocephalus syndrome, *Arch-Neurol* 52:783-789, 1995.

Pappada G, Poletti C, Guazzoni A et al: Normal pressure hydrocephalus: relationship among clinical picture, CT scan and intracranial pressure monitoring, *J Neurosurg* 30:115-128, 1986.

Petersen RC, Mokri B, Laws ER: Surgical treatment of idiopathic hydrocephalus in elderly patients, *Neurology* 35:307-311, 1985.

Raftopoulos C, Deleval J, Chaskis C et al: Cognitive recovery in idiopathic normal pressure hydrocephalus: a prospective study, *Neurosurgery* 35:397-404, 1994.

Raftopoulos C, Massager N, Baleriaux D et al: Prospective analysis by computed tomography and long-term outcome of 23 adult patients with chronic idiopathic hydrocephalus, *Neurosurgery* 38:51-59, 1996.

Sand T, Bovim G, Grimse R et al: Idiopathic normal pressure hydrocephalus: the CSF tap test may predict the clinical response to shunting, *Acta Neurol Scand* 89:311-316, 1994.

Stein SC, Langfitt TW: Normal-pressure hydrocephalus: predicting the results of cerebrospinal fluid shunting, *J Neurosurg* 41:463-470, 1974.

Vanneste J, Augustijn P, Dirven C et al: Shunting normal-pressure hydrocephalus: do the benefits outweigh the risks? A multicenter study and literature review, *Neurology* 42:54-59, 1992.

Creutzfeld-Jakob Disease

Fradkin JE, Schonberger LB, Mills JL et al: Creutzfeldt-Jakob disease in pituitary growth hormone recipients in the United States, *JAMA* 265:880-884, 1991.

Hsiao K, Meiner Z, Kahana E et al: Mutation of the prion protein in Libyan Jews with Creutzfeldt-Jakob disease, *N Engl J Med* 324:1091-1097, 1991.

Hsich G, Kenney K, Gibbs CJ et al: The 14-3-3 brain protein in cerebrospinal fluid as a marker for transmissible spongiform encephalopathies, *N Engl J Med* 335:924-930, 1996.

Kretzschmar HA: Human prion diseases (spongiform encephalopathies), *Arch Virol* 7(Suppl.):261-293, 1993.

Kretzschmar HA, Ironside JW, DeArmond SJ et al: Diagnostic criteria for sporadic Creutzfeldt-Jakob disease, *Arch Neurol* 53:913-920, 1996.

Steinhoff BJ, Racker S, Herrendorf G et al: Electroencephalogram (EEG) remains the most helpful laboratory diagnostic tool; serial recordings are necessary if the initial EEG finding is nonspecific. Accuracy and reliability of periodic sharp wave complexes in Creutzfeldt-Jakob disease, *Arch Neurol* 53:162-166, 1996.

Wientjens DP, Davanipour Z, Hofman A et al: Risk factors for Creutzfeldt-Jakob disease: a reanalysis of case-control studies, *Neurology* 46:1287-1291, 1996.

Will RG, Ironside JW, Zeidler M et al: A new variant of Creutzfeldt-Jakob disease in the UK, *Lancet* 347:921-925, 1996.

Progressive Supranuclear Palsy

Tolosa E, Valldeoriola F, Marti MJ: Clinical diagnosis and diagnostic criteria of progressive supranuclear palsy (Steele-Richardson-Olszewski syndrome), *J Neural Transm Suppl* 42:15-31, 1994.

Huntington's Disease

Mendez MF: Huntington's disease: update and review of neuropsychiatric aspects, *Int J Psychiatry Med* 24:189-208, 1994.

Mohr E, Brouwers P, Claus JJ et al: Visuospatial cognition in Huntington's disease, *Mov Disord* 6:127-132, 1991.

Other Dementias

Butterworth RF: Pathophysiology of alcoholic brain damage: synergistic effects of ethanol, thiamine deficiency and alcoholic liver disease, *Metab Brain Dis* 10:1-8, 1995.

Carlen PL, McAndrews MP, Weiss RT et al: Alcohol-related dementia in the institutionalized elderly, *Alcohol Clin Exp Res* 18:1330-1334, 1994.

Clarnette RM, Patterson CJ: Hypothyroidism: does treatment cure dementia? *J Geriatr Psychiatry Neurol* 7:23-27, 1994.

Cunha UG, Rocha FL, Peixoto JM et al: Vitamin B12 deficiency and dementia, *Int Psychogeriatr* 7:85-88, 1995.

Shetty KR, Duthie EH: Thyroid disease and associated illness in the elderly, *Clin Geriatr Med* 11:311-325, 1995.

Traynelis VC: Chronic subdural hematoma in the elderly, *Clin Geriatr Med* 7:583-598, 1991.

Victor M: Alcoholic dementia, *Can J Neurol Sci* 21:88-99, 1994.

Unit Three

3

We need new resources as new difficulties spring up to challenge modern man. Important choices become imperative.

—Pope John Paul II

Management

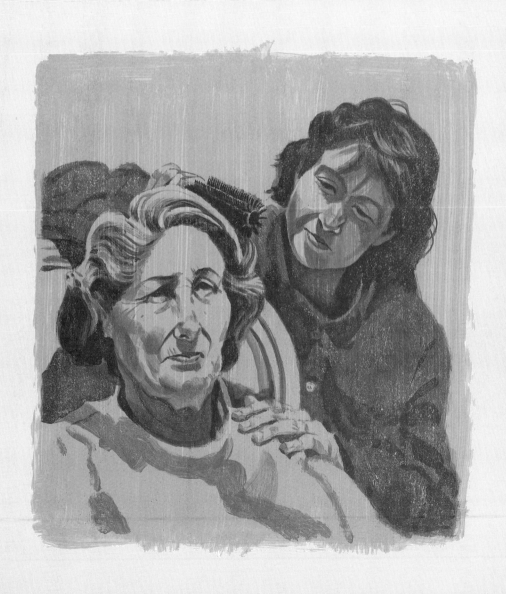

General Principles of Management

Lynda C Abusamra

The battle against polypharmacy, or the use of a large number of drugs (of the action of which we know little, yet we put them into bodies of the action of which we know less), has not been brought to a finish.

—William Osler

Effective management of patients with Alzheimer's disease is dependent on many things. Good interpersonal relationships between caregivers and patients, and whether the person is a family caregiver or a professional caregiver are fundamental to effective care. These relationships must occur in a supportive environment, whether that environment is home, a respite care center, a day care, a long-term care facility, or an acute care agency. The "fit" between the patient and his or her environment must be arranged to maximize the patient's functioning. Attention to these factors, along with an appropriate balance of activity and quiet, can positively maximize the patient's functional repertoire. Potential dysfunctional and/or disruptive behaviors can be kept to a minimum.

INTERPERSONAL RELATIONSHIPS BETWEEN CAREGIVERS AND PATIENTS: TREATING THE PERSON

Although persons with Alzheimer's disease have cognitive deficits and may have concurrent depression, personality changes, and gradual impairment in other functional abilities and domains, most patients retain a sense of humor and emotional sensitivity until relatively late in the disease process. Thus, it is of paramount importance to remember to treat the *person* who has this chronic, progressive, debilitating disease, rather than merely treating the chronic *disease*. In the course of caregiving, it is easy to focus on the negative behaviors and weaknesses of the patient while ignoring or discounting the positive strengths and events that occur in the course of a day. Recent research suggests that

143

—● Basic Principles for Treating the Person

1. Respect for the person
2. Validating personhood
3. Maintaining eye contact
4. Employing distraction
5. Alternating activity and quiet time
6. Responding to the emotional content of the message
7. Employing nonverbal communication when possible
8. Attending to the level of environmental stimulation
9. Using behavioral means to connect with the patient's past

---

persons with Alzheimer's disease, at least early in the course of the illness and probably even when moderately impaired, are able to reliably and consistently indicate preferences for daily living routines and activity. This research suggests that there are basic principles that are effective in the management of patients with Alzheimer's disease. Plans and interventions should and can be successfully modified to accommodate the desires and wishes of patients. The box above suggests ways to focus on the person receiving care. An individualized approach to caregiving can add to the quality of life for the patient as well as the caregiver and result in maximizing the functional capabilities of the patient.

THE NEED FOR INDIVIDUALITY

The importance of respect for the patient as an individual who is afflicted with a serious debilitating disease cannot be overstated. Each patient with Alzheimer's disease brings with him or her a lifetime of personal experience that influences the manifestations of the disease process in individual ways. While there may be physical and behavioral similarities between patients, no two are ever really alike. Even in the presence of Alzheimer's disease when personality changes occur, many of the patient's previous personality characteristics remain. Recent research suggests that while personality changes do take place in the course of the disease, the direction or constellation of these changes occurs in a fairly predictable way, so it becomes worthwhile to consider and prescribe individualized modes of care.

Alzheimer's disease is of such consequence that without adequate support, the disease can devastate an entire family. For family caregivers, there is the bittersweet knowledge of "the person that was." The incidence of depression is high among both family and professional caregivers. Using an approach that responds to the person with Alzheimer's disease as an individual can "lighten the load" and alleviate some depression.

—■ This one key strategy involves knowing the patient's personal history and trying to link present behaviors and expressions to his or her past.

This technique is often calming and soothing to the patient. If caregivers are sensitive to the idea that the patients may be trying to rework a past failure, disappointment, or other significant event in their lives, the behavioral manifestation may even make sense to the caregivers when viewed through the patients' eyes.

ESTABLISHING GOOD COMMUNICATION

Tips for good communication with patients:
- Talk away from distractions and noise.
- Maintain eye contact.
- Talk softly.
- Use simple familiar words and short, simple sentences.
- Ask yes/no questions.
- Allow plenty of time for patient to process information and give a response.
- Try repeating information in the same way. If this fails, try using different words to say the same thing.
- Visually demonstrate what you are saying.
- Stay calm and patient.
- Ask those who know the patient best about nicknames, possible meaning of a repeated word, family terms, etc.
- Don't argue or attempt to reason.
- Don't talk in a condescending tone.
- Use gentle touch.
- Connect with the past.
- Use music with which the patient is familiar.

Dysfunction in activities of daily living and behavioral difficulties in patients with Alzheimer's disease often stem from the utter frustration of not being able to communicate, as well as not being able to interact socially in a way that is rewarding and meaningful. Since these individuals generally can and do still respond to the emotional or affective content of communication interactions, inappropriate or ineffective communications between caregivers and patients can trigger dysfunction and inappropriate behavioral responses.

People commonly communicate messages that focus on cognitive content. In light of the decreased cognitive abilities of the patient, it may be necessary for caregivers to learn new strategies for communicating with people with Alzheimer's disease. For professional caregivers, the personal history of the patient is usually lacking. However, when nurses' aides were given short personal histories of their patients, the change in their attitudes toward their patients was reflected in seeing their patients as more adaptable, more able to set goals, and as having more interpersonal skills. It also had a positive impact on their patients' care.

Professional caregivers need to be taught to communicate and respond empathetically and with sensitivity and genuineness in light of the person's past skills and accomplishments. When caregivers are taught how to respond, are supported in their efforts, and are challenged to make a difference in the daily lives of their patients, the rewards are abundant for both caregivers and patients. The self-esteem of both parties is increased, which in turn comforts the patient and empowers the caregivers, increasing morale and leading to better levels of care.

When interacting verbally with patients with Alzheimer's disease, it is vital to remember that they do have cognitive deficits. Arguing with the patient or attempting to reason with him or her is ineffective. These two activities only serve to frustrate and aggravate the patient and may frustrate the caregiver as well. The best strategy to use in a verbal altercation is distraction. Quietly, gently, and in a soothing voice an attempt should be made to direct the patient's attention elsewhere. Maintaining eye contact and approaching the person directly, in full view without being confrontational, are helpful.

Other specific strategies include using nonverbal communication and other sensory modalities to enhance communication.

➤ The sense of touch is primary, emerging long before language.

A gentle touch on the arm or the side of the face can help establish contact with the patient (Figure 11-1). Gentle massage of the shoulders can also be comforting and relieve tension. At home, caregivers and patients alike can be taught to benefit from this activity. Providing taste sensations familiar to the patient from long ago can trigger pleasant associations and allow the patient to relive past experiences and provide a meaningful jolt to the memory. Music is a very effective way to establish communication with the patient, especially when the music is chosen from an earlier period of the patient's life. Most individuals with Alzheimer's disease can sing along with others long after they have lost their ability to communicate with words. Music can be used as an individual activity between patient and caregiver, or in a group with concurrent simple motor activity.

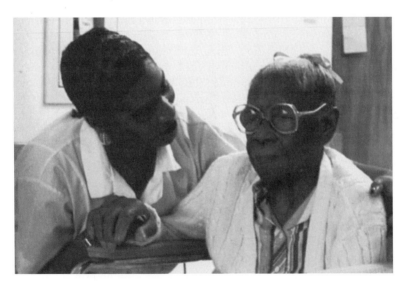

Figure 11-1.   The nursing assistant uses touch to calm a person with Alzheimer's disease. (Sorrentino SA et al: *Mosby's textbook for long-term care assistants*, St Louis, 1994, Mosby.)

MAINTAINING A SUPPORTIVE ENVIRONMENT

Keys to maintaining a supportive environment:
• Keep the environment simple.
• Avoid clutter.
• Provide environmental cues and labels.
• Incorporate all senses to keep in touch with the environment.

In whatever setting the patient resides, the environment should be arranged so that it is neither too stimulating nor too boring. At home, it may be helpful to conduct an environmental checkup for safety hazards and other recommendations to create the most ideal environment that is practical. In other settings, creativity must be employed to overcome barriers that cannot be changed but may be possible to modify. For instance, in long-term or acute care facilities, it may not be possible to eliminate the noise of call lights and intercoms, but the noise may be masked by soft music of the patient's choice and by making sure doors are closed.

Large, open, and cluttered spaces are often difficult and confusing places for patients. Having so much space and so many objects around becomes overstimulating for patients. The environment should be made as simple and as "user friendly" as possible. Controlling the number and type of stimuli in the environment of the person with Alzheimer's disease will help to maximize functioning and attention, and decrease agitation. The environment should provide information and orienting cues, such as signs on bathroom doors, labels on patient drawers and closets, clocks, and calendars. Placing objects in the environment that stimulate other senses (rather than just visual) can be therapeutic for the patient. Wall hangings that can be handled by the patients provide a way to stimulate the sense of touch. Due to age changes that compromise vision, make sure that lighting is adequate and glare is reduced.

MAINTAINING CONSISTENCY AND ROUTINE

Routine is soothing to the patient. A stable, consistent environment must be maintained.

Generally, a reasonably consistent routine for carrying out daily activities such as mealtime, bathing, and toileting, as well as consistency in the patient's environment, should be maintained. People with dementing conditions require a certain amount of routine and structure on which they can depend. When faced with changing situations, activities, caregivers, and/or environments, the patient with Alzheimer's disease has great difficulty adapting to the change and often responds with a stresslike reaction. Providing this consistency helps to reduce the stress the patient experiences.

Early in the course of the disease, the patient can participate in usual daily activities with little or no difficulty. But as the disease progresses, patients will have different requirements and preferences, so the day should be appropriately structured to meet his or her needs. Basic health needs for hygiene, nutrition, and sleep must be met. These types of activities are best achieved when a routine and schedule have been established. The patient begins to "learn" from the repetition of the same activity carried out in the same manner. However, there does need to be enough flexibility in the caregiver to permit adapting schedules and activities to accommodate the changing moods and needs of the patient. The same is true for the patient's environment. Furniture and belongings should remain stable. When changes are made, such as rearranging furniture, hanging new pictures, or changing a patient's room location, stress is created since the environment is less familiar.

ACTIVITY AND EXERCISE

Simple physical activity and exercise is healthy. Quiet time activities should be simple and individualized.

Physical activity for the person with Alzheimer's disease is important for several reasons. First, it can help the patient maintain mobility, muscle strength, balance, and bone mass. General conditioning is especially important because these individuals have a fall rate three times as high as cognitively intact elders. Although exercise may not prevent falls, conditioning may reduce potential injuries. Second, sleeping problems that become more serious as the disease progresses can be somewhat alleviated by exercise-induced physical fatigue. Third, it can help promote bowel regularity and aid in the prevention of constipation. Planned exercise can also reduce aimless wandering behavior, and if engaged in by both the patient and the caregiver as a shared activity, it can reduce stress and alleviate depression. Any physical activity should be interspersed with quiet activities in order not to overfatigue the patient or the caregiver.

Quiet time activities are somewhat dependent on the capabilities of the patient. Knowing the person allows the caregiver to judge which activities are safe for participation and which ones are not. With supervision, the patient should be encouraged to try a variety of activities. However, too much assistance can unnecessarily deprive the individual of autonomy. Caregivers should help, but not take over, as the person maintains as wide a behavioral repertoire as possible. Here are a few activities that might be tried:
• Use a readily available "play dough" (made out of flour, salt and water—can be colored with food coloring if desired) to mold figures or just squish in one's hand.
• String brightly colored beads or even old buttons.
• Provide old scraps of fabric to make beautiful collages.
• Provide laundry for folding.
• Indoor gardening can be pleasurable.

There are many other simple activities that can be used for quiet times (See Chapter 19). The above ideas are but a few of the kinds of things that can be done. The important part of engaging in simple activities is the *process*. The impaired elder has the opportunity "to do" something and to feel as if he is still a contributing person. The product is of less consequence than the activity itself.

SUMMARY

The personalized care and management of patients with Alzheimer's disease is challenging. It is a task that requires creativity, patience, endurance, and support.

Caregivers need to continually assess the patient's abilities as the disease progresses and adjust the level of assistance provided to match the patient's changing needs and capabilities. The general principles discussed above, when used on a regular basis, will help keep the patient functioning on his own for as long as possible.

BIBLIOGRAPHY

Cotrell V, Schultz R: The perspective of the patient with Alzheimer's disease: a neglected dimension of research, *Gerontologist* 33(2):205-211, 1993.

Davies HD: Dementia and delirium. In Chenitz WC, Stone JT, Salisbury SA, editors: *Clinical gerontological nursing: a guide to advanced practice*, Philadelphia, 1991, WB Saunders.

Kolanowski AM, Whall AL: Life-span perspective of personality in dementia, *Image: J Nurs Schol* 28:315-320, 1996.

Kovach CR, Henschel H: Planning activities for patients with dementia, *J Gerontol Nurs* 22(9):33-38, 1996.

Lawton MP: Competence, environmental press and the adaptation of old people. In Lawton M, Windley P, Byerts TO, editors: *Aging and the environment: theoretical approaches*, New York, 1982, Springer-Verlag.

Lewis K: How to foster self determination: practical ways nursing home staff can empower residents, *Health Prog* 76(8):42-44, 1995.

Maxfield MC, Lewis RE, Cannon S: Training staff to prevent aggressive behavior of cognitively impaired elderly patients during bathing and grooming, *J Gerontol Nurs* 22(1):37-43, 1996.

Pietrukowicz M, Johnson M: Using life histories to individualize nursing home staff attitudes toward residents, *Gerontologist* 31(1):102-106, 1991.

Robinson A, Spencer B, White L: *Understanding difficult behaviors*, Ann Arbor, 1989, Geriatric Education Center of Michigan.

Management of Difficult Behaviors

Mary M Lancaster
Lynda C Abusamra
Warren G Clark

It is not enough for the physician to do what is necessary, but the patient and the attendants must do their part as well, and circumstances must be favorable.

—Hippocrates

Difficult behaviors associated with Alzheimer's disease often produce significant stress in caregivers. Behaviors discussed in this chapter are not applicable to all Alzheimer's patients; indeed, some patients may never experience any of them. When these behaviors present they are usually time-limited: as the disease progresses, they often disappear. Whenever difficult and problem behaviors arise, they demand special attention.

Helping patients and caregivers with any of these behaviors requires careful identification and definition of the problem, thoughtful planning for intervening, and consistency in carrying out a plan of action. Good communication between caregivers and patients is a must and requires reflection and support. Communication with the patient is often not easy because of the degree of cognitive impairment. A quiet environment, repeating information, use of touch, visual reinforcement, and use of speech patterns familiar to the patient enhance the communication process.

MEANING OF BEHAVIOR

Difficult or problem behaviors typically are grounded in one of three areas:
1. The tasks or activities the patient faces appear insurmountable.
2. There is a communication breakdown.
3. Something in the environment is provoking the patient.

For the patient with Alzheimer's disease, an insurmountable task is anything that is too complicated to perform, is no longer familiar, or one that requires learning. When faced with a task that seems insurmountable, the patient frequently reacts by "acting out" his frustrations.

Communicating with the Alzheimer's patient is often difficult. Patients forget the meaning of words and often experience difficulty in expressing themselves. Eventually, all speech and language abilities become severely impaired. Caregivers set the tone when communicating. If the caregiver is upset, angry, or frustrated, the patient will often experience the same emotional tone. A calm, gentle, reassuring approach in communicating is one of the most valuable tools a caregiver can possess. When the communication between the caregiver and the patient breaks down, the outcome is often displayed through difficult behaviors. Some useful tips for better communication are listed in Chapter 11.

For a patient with Alzheimer's disease the environment can be confusing and distracting. There may be too much noise or activity surrounding the patient, poor lighting, unfamiliar surroundings, or even temperature extremes. Overstimulation and/or understimulation can increase the patient's sense of disorientation and confusion. This often leads to frustration and anxiety, which is then manifested through a display of disruptive or difficult behavior.

Whatever the cause of the patient's reaction or behavior, there is always some meaning to it; however, the caregivers might not always be able to figure out the meaning. Most often in Alzheimer's disease, the patient is expressing some underlying physical or emotional need that is not being met. The behavior is often the only way of expressing the need or emotion. Caregivers need to be able to separate the behavior from the patient and attempt to figure out the underlying emotional tone and what the patient may really be "saying" or "getting" from her actions. It may be a form of stress release, a way to express fear or anxiety, or a means of getting a reward or attention.

PROBLEM-SOLVING BEHAVIOR MANAGEMENT

Defining the Problem

The problem-solving method of behavior management requires a clear definition of the problem and identification of precipitating and aggravating factors. This approach, which requires time for observing the behavior and data gathering, may lead to specific interventions for dealing with the behavior. Carefully defining the behavior is half the work of managing the problem. The more specific information one has about a behavior, the more likely a management plan will emerge. There are specific questions caregivers should address (see box on p. 152) when trying to define a behavior. All persons rendering care to the patient should be involved in the problem-solving process so everyone will carry out the same behavior plan. When identifying and defining the behavior, always be as specific and concrete as possible.

When considering antecedents or triggers, caregivers should always think first about the possibility of physical causes (hunger, pain, cold, etc.) since these are the most easily managed by addressing the physical issue. Defining the consequences of the behavior helps to identify caregiver reactions, reactions of others, and the patient's reactions. This leads to the next step of the behavior management process—defining the desired change or outcome.

● Steps in Defining the Problem

1. Who actually has the problem or behavior (patient or caregivers)?
2. Exactly (specifically) what is the problem/behavior?
3. What does the behavior mean to? or accomplish for the patient?
4. Where does the behavior occur?
5. When does it occur (time and frequency)?
6. Who is around/involved?
7. What happens just before the problem/behavior (i.e., triggers, antecedents)?
8. Is there a pattern or sequence?
9. What are the consequences of the behavior?

Defining the Desired Change or Outcome

This process allows caregivers to think about what they would rather see or experience. It also allows reflection on whether there really is a need to take action. Is the patient endangering himself or others? Is the behavior infringing on the rights of others? One possible outcome is to change the meaning of the behavior. This usually requires the caregiver to change his or her view about the behavior. For example, instead of seeing the patient who constantly "shadows" the caregiver as annoying, the caregiver could see the behavior as providing a constant companion and comfort for the patient.

A second possible outcome is to change the response to the behavior. This again is caregiver driven as illustrated in the following example:

Mrs. M is always repeating the same questions to her daughter. In fact, the daughter is becoming exasperated with telling her mother that she just answered the exact questions. The daughter has recently started ignoring her mother, which has only exacerbated the situation. A friend of the family suggested that the daughter write down the answers to the questions on a piece of paper and give it to her mother. This way she could refer her mother to the answer sheet whenever the questions surfaced. Although this did not eliminate the problem, it changed the daughter's response to her mother's behavior.

Finally, caregivers can work to change the behavior itself. This may be to increase or decrease the frequency of the behavior, to substitute another less difficult behavior, or to totally eliminate the behavior. Selecting one of these options requires change on the part of the patient and is often the most difficult to achieve.

Developing a Plan of Action

When the above steps have been completed, caregivers can begin to determine a plan of action for dealing with the behavior. All persons working with the patient need to be involved in the planning. Consistency in the implementation of the plan is absolutely necessary if a positive outcome is to be realized and for evaluating the effectiveness of the actions taken. Each person must react in the same manner to the patient's behavior. When one or two persons deviate from the plan, the patient may become more confused by the mixed responses. Caregivers must also realize that when dealing with difficult behaviors, the ability to be flexible is an asset. Early on in the disease process it becomes more and more evident that the only thing known for certain about patients with Alzheimer's disease is that their responses in situations and activities are variable. Caregivers cannot count on one thing working for the patient all the time. During the development of the action plan, caregivers are encouraged to be creative in coming up with possible interventions. Most of what has been learned about dealing with difficult behaviors has been through the creativity, persistence, and hard work of caregivers.

Evaluating the Effectiveness of the Action Plan

Once a plan of action has been implemented, it needs to be given enough time to work. Change comes slowly in most people; this is even more true for the patient with Alzheimer's disease. Caregivers should not expect a major change in the patient to occur over a few days; it may take several weeks. Caregivers need to meet together to brainstorm and discuss the intervention plan. What has the outcome been? Does the plan seem to have worked? Does it need more time? Do we need to go back and change some things? Assessing the action plan provides an objective view of what has transpired. Finally, caregivers must also realize that failure is a possibility. Instead of viewing everything as wasted time and energy when the plan fails, caregivers should examine the situation and try to determine the cause of failure. Or, they may need to go back to the drawing board and start again.

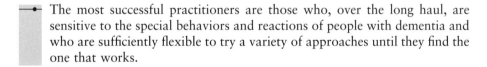

The most successful practitioners are those who, over the long haul, are sensitive to the special behaviors and reactions of people with dementia and who are sufficiently flexible to try a variety of approaches until they find the one that works.

KEYS TO BETTER CARE

Basic Intervention Techniques

Before discussing specific behaviors and their causes and interventions, some basic techniques commonly used to handle difficult and disruptive behaviors will be outlined. These techniques are not anything special and do not require training, but rather ones we all use in our daily lives. Numerous researchers have found that reacting in a simple, calm, matter-of-fact manner, yet demonstrating control of the situation is usually the best way to respond when patients act out. Plenty of patience and understanding go into effective handling of disruptive and difficult behaviors, as well as trial and error. An important fact to remember is that the patient suffers short-term memory impairment and is easily distracted. Caregivers should use these deficits to their advantage when intervening.

Management Strategies

Diversion or Distraction: moving or shifting the patient's attention from one stimuli to another.

Example:
While reminiscing about days gone by, the patient becomes anxious and agitated. By diverting attention to the beautiful flowers in the room, the patient seems to forget what was upsetting him or her and calms down.

Removal: separating the patient from the situation or stimulus.

Example:
The caregiver found that by having the patient eat alone, rather than in the kitchen with the family, his appetite and intake increased.

Redirection: moving or shifting energy from one activity to another.

Example:
A female patient who had been a seamstress all her life is using scissors to cut up everything in sight. Her daughter redirected her mother's cutting energy into something useful and less destructive—making paper dolls for her kindergarten class.

Task breakdown: separating an activity into smaller and simpler segments or steps. This is most commonly used in daily personal care activities, but can also be used for recreational activities such as craftwork.

Stimulus control: limiting choices for the patient.

Example:
Instead of taking her father through the cafeteria line where food choices could be overwhelming (and possibly cause a catastrophic reaction), the daughter seats her father at the table and has his meal brought to him.

Environmental manipulation: controlling certain aspects of the environment such as noise, lighting, and temperature.

Example:
Increasing the level of light indoors as the sun is setting helps many patients who typically experience increased agitation at this time of day remain calmer and less disoriented.

Reassurance: providing a sense of safety and security. This is most effective when fear and anxiety are the root cause of the behavior.

Example:
By routinely taking a couple of minutes every two hours to visit with the patient, the night nurse finds the patient did not yell out as loudly or as often.

Setting limits: taking control of the situation and not allowing certain actions/activities to happen, i.e., walking onto a busy highway. Setting limits/saying "no" are used as a last resort or when the patient is at immediate risk of injuring herself or others.

Validation as a Means of Communication and Problem Solving

One of the most frustrating processes for caregivers and patients is establishing effective communication. When verbal abilities decline, other methods of communicating may be instituted, but often with limited success. Such communication methods include reality orientation, reminiscence, life review, remotivation, diversion, and behavior modification. Most of these techniques rely on functional memory, which is impaired in Alzheimer's disease. A more useful strategy involves using validation to affirm the patient afflicted with Alzheimer's disease.

Validation is a method of communicating with empathy to help elderly persons, such as those with Alzheimer's disease, to regain dignity, reduce anxiety, and prevent withdrawal. The physical and developmental aspects of aging cannot be separated, and many disruptive behaviors can be related to failed resolution of past conflicts.

Feil's techniques of validation that can be used to facilitate communication include:
• Centering
• Using non-threatening words to build trust
• Rephrasing
• Using polarity
• Imagining the opposite
• Reminiscing
• Maintaining genuine close eye contact
• Using a clear, low, loving tone of voice
• Touching
• Using music

Centering. Centering is a technique that involves the caregiver's willingness to lay aside negative emotions in order to listen empathetically and to be receptive to the feelings of the patient. The caregiver stops all inner dialogue and focuses on breathing deeply and exhaling completely after each breath. The centering process takes about three minutes. This exercise frees the mind and allows the caregiver to focus on the patient. This technique is especially useful with the maloriented, time-confused, or repetitive mover stages.

Using non-threatening words to build trust. Using non-threatening words to build trust is an effective strategy because the focus is on the events rather than on the patient. Patients have little desire or capacity to understand why they behave the way they do and will usually retreat when confronted with emotion-laden content. Some personal knowledge of the patient's history helps the caregiver understand what is triggering the behavior.

Example:
If a female patient complains about someone assaulting her, try asking such questions as, "What does this person look like? When does this person bother you? Is it all the time?"

This approach eventually allows the caregiver to discover a way to exchange meaningful information with the patient.

Rephrasing. Rephrasing allows the caregiver to restate the meaning of whatever question or statement the patient has made in such a way as to validate the patient rather than argue with or demean him.

Example:
The patient says, "I am so angry today." The caregiver responds in a reassuring tone, "You're so angry today?" This approach allows the patient to express anger or dismay, while on a deeper level, recognizes his failing abilities.

Using polarity. In using polarity, the caregiver asks the patient to express the worst instance that he can imagine about his complaint.

Example:
In validating a patient who complains about the food being inedible, the caregiver asks, "Is it the worst food you have ever tasted?" This statement allows the patient to freely express emotion, thereby relieving some anxiety.

Imagining the opposite. To imagine the opposite, the caregiver asks the patient to express instances of when an event or problem does not occur.

Example:
When a patient states, "That witch came by last night," the caregiver can respond by asking if there are nights when he has not seen the witch. A response from the patient like, "Only when you are here," should prompt the caregiver to explore further. The caregiver might ask, "You mean if I were here all the time, the witch would not come?" The patient might respond, "I don't know. The only other time I was alone was after my wife died," to which the caregiver could respond, "What did you do after your wife died?" From that point the caregiver has helped the patient move beyond the fear to another time that can be further explored.

Reminiscing. Reminiscing can be used with the words "always" and "never" to bring to mind similar events from the past.

Example:
If a patient is having trouble eating or sleeping, the caregiver might ask, "Have you always had trouble sleeping?" This may trigger past episodes in the patient's memory when similar problems occurred. Such triggers can help the patient recall what might have worked in the past.

Maintaining close eye contact. Maintaining close eye contact helps the patient feel safe, recognized, and loved. A clear, low, soft, nurturing tone of voice can often trigger memories of loved ones and earlier happy experiences, thereby reducing stress.

Touching. Touching is another technique used to establish communication and to problem solve. Touching is most effective when used with the time-confused person. It is an effective way to establish emotional contact. However, touch should be used with caution and only with those patients who are comfortable with gentle touch.

Music. Music can be an effective communication link. Often when speech is impoverished, the ability to sing familiar songs remains intact. Using this as a means to communicate can help to reduce anxiety, divert attention, and preserve some quality of life for the patient.

The above techniques provide a variety of ways caregivers can help improve communication with Alzheimer's patients. These strategies are most effective when used by one person to establish a relationship with a patient with dementia.

IDENTIFICATION OF SPECIFIC BEHAVIORS

Agitation and Restlessness

Agitation is a state of extreme restlessness or irritability often characterized by pacing, hitting, yelling, or resistance. This state can be produced by medications, physical discomfort, anxiety, fatigue, sleep loss, insecurity, sensory overload, sensory deprivation, or sensory distortion such as that produced by cataracts. Agitation in the patient also may result from impatience or irritability on the part of the caregiver.

The first approach to the agitated patient is assessment of any physical cause of discomfort or pain, such as fecal impaction, systemic or localized infection, dehydration, urinary retention, osteoarthritis, or fractures (even in the absence of obvious trauma). Attention to the possibility of hunger or thirst and ensuring adequate sleep also are important.

Second, the environment should be surveyed to ensure an appropriate level of sensory stimulation and to determine the presence of any apparent irritants. Third, if attempts at task completion are thought to be the cause of the agitation, the patient should be observed while performing routine activities of daily living to identify contributing factors.

Finally, regardless of whether the caregivers' stress is considered a contributing factor, education should concentrate on teaching caregivers how their own emotional state affects their patients. This can be accomplished during staff meetings, support group meetings, or home visits to family caregivers. Supportive supervision and the opportunity for discussion of frustrations may assist caregivers dealing with agitation and restlessness.

Aggression and Combativeness

True aggression and combativeness are relatively rare in patients with Alzheimer's disease. However, when such behaviors occur, they are frightening to caregivers. The patient's aggression may be verbal, consisting of cursing or threats, or physical, including grabbing, pinching, hitting, or biting. It may be directed at caregivers or other persons. Aggression may be an isolated event, or it may occur with regularity. Close contact activities such as bathing or delivery of medications may precipitate aggression.

Aggression may reflect long-standing personality traits of the patient, or it may be completely out of character. It can be provoked by caregivers through adherence to an overly rigid daily routine for patient care or through a lack of adequate structure in the daily routine. Aggression may be an extension of the agitated behavior already described, especially when the underlying causes have not been adequately addressed and have been allowed to escalate. Patients may misinterpret routine activities as being invasive or threatening and respond aggressively out of self-defense. Physical aggression may result when patients no longer have the capacity for verbal expression of their frustrations.

Example:

Mr. J., a 67-year-old man, was admitted to the nursing home 2 months ago because his family was finding it increasingly difficult to care for him. The diagnosis of Alzheimer's disease had been made 5 years previously.

A widower, Mr. J. was confused in regard to the whereabouts of his wife. He wandered all day and frequently asked for his wife. The only time he was calm was during visits from his family, which occurred primarily on Sundays. Although the staff appreciated the calm that these visits brought, they noticed that Mr. J. became more agitated when the family left, following them to the door and attempting to leave with them. When the staff tried to lead him away, he would become belligerent and combative. This behavior sometimes resulted in his receiving medication, which served primarily to make him drowsy. On one occasion a staff member was injured when she fell while trying to avoid Mr. J.'s attempt to strike her.

The clinical nurse specialist was asked to advise the staff about methods of reducing Mr. J.'s aggressive episodes. She observed the behaviors described here and interviewed his family to hear their suggestions and gain their support for an intervention. With the staff and the family, she then devised a care plan in which the family would notify the staff 15 minutes before their intended time of departure from visits. The family would plan to leave a small memento with Mr. J. at each visit. A staff member would then begin discussing the memento with him, encouraging some brief reminiscing. The family would say good-bye quietly in the visiting room, and Mr. J. would not be allowed to walk them to the door. The staff member would remain with him for approximately 10 minutes after their departure. This intervention appeared to distract the patient from his feelings of abandonment without altering the nature of the family's visits. No further incidents of combative behavior occurred, and the staff noted that Mr. J.'s efforts to find his wife gradually decreased.

The strategies suggested for agitation and restlessness also should be applied to the care of the aggressive or combative patient. The aggressive patient always should be approached in a calm, low-key manner, and explanations of all activities should be given. Caregivers should be flexible in scheduling daily care and should allow the patient a sense of control over his body and personal space. Distraction can be an effective tool in breaking a cycle of escalating aggression. Situations known to provoke combative episodes should be avoided, and this approach should be followed by all those who care for the patient. The aggressive patient's environment, whether home or institution, should be free of objects that could be used to physically harm herself or others. Medications can be effective in calming agitated patients and interrupting the escalation of aggression (see Chapter 14). Since the use of physical restraints tends to increase the patient's confusion and aggressive behavior, they should be avoided in patients with Alzheimer's disease. The example above depicts a successful strategy for dealing with aggression.

Catastrophic Reactions

A catastrophic reaction is a disproportionate response to the stimuli eliciting the reaction. An example is the patient who begins to scream and throw things because he or she cannot tie shoes. Catastrophic reactions may be manifested by uncontrollable crying, extreme agitation, screaming, combativeness, or temper tantrums.

Catastrophic reactions occur in response to the patient's inability to handle a multitude of incoming stimuli. Decreased capacity to inhibit emotional responses contributes to an outpouring of affect in response to even minimal stimuli. These reactions can be frightening to both the patient and the caregiver. If the patient must make a choice between several options or must attend to several requests at the same time, such catastrophic responses may result. Attempting tasks that are too complex or trying to respond to "why" questions also may overwhelm the patient. Even trivial incidents such as spilling a drink can trigger a catastrophic reaction.

Prevention of catastrophic reactions should be a part of the care plan for any patient prone to them. Avoiding the circumstances known to trigger these reactions usually can be achieved through careful planning. The patient's environment and tasks demanded of him or her should be simplified. Distraction is most useful if the reaction is already in progress. Involvement in music- or food-related activities is frequently used for distraction. Caregivers must be cautioned not to overreact to the patient, thus increasing the potential for escalation of catastrophic reactions.

Vocalization/Screaming

Screaming behaviors can occur in patients with Alzheimer's disease who are very confused and have little ability to communicate. These behaviors are most disruptive to the environment, and they may include frequent repeated use of the same word or phrase. The patient's vocalization may or may not be understandable to the caregiver. Such behavior is most frequently related to visual or auditory deficits. Physical discomfort, sensory overload, fear, anxiety, boredom, or fatigue also may trigger this reaction in patients with Alzheimer's disease. Sometimes patients will react adversely to certain caregivers but not others. They may associate these individuals with bad memories from their past. Screaming may be reinforced by caregivers' responses that unintentionally reward the patient.

Caregivers must assess and correct any physical problems noted. Sensory input should be maximized through the use of hearing aids, eyeglasses, and careful use of touch. Massage and other attempts at relaxation may be helpful. Medications can be used with patients who are thought to be experiencing distortions of reality (see Chapter 13). Providing environmental stimuli such as soft music or television also may help. Contact with these patients must be maintained on a regular basis to help reduce the possibility of fear, feelings of abandonment, or loneliness. Relatives and volunteers who sit with such patients on a regular basis can assist greatly in reducing this type of behavior. Below is an example of an intervention for screaming.

Example: Dealing with Screaming
Mr. A., a 75-year-old man, has been living in a skilled nursing facility for the past 4 years. Complicating his early Alzheimer's disease is a previous cardiovascular accident that resulted in expressive aphasia. Mrs. A. visits her husband daily at mealtimes and feeds him. She also reads to him while holding his hand until he falls asleep.

On her way to visit one day, Mrs. A. was involved in a serious accident and broke her right tibia and left hip. Mrs. A. has been in the hospital for 3 weeks and is now being transferred to a rehabilitation hospital for therapy. When Mr. A. was notified about his wife's accident, his condition began to deteriorate. He became bedridden and would not assist with any activities of daily living. Mr. A. also has begun yelling and screaming. These vocalizations occurred for extended periods and were loud and incessant. This behavior has become very disturbing to everyone—staff, patients, and visitors.

When his condition worsened, Mr. A. was moved to the front of the building in a semiprivate room. His yelling, however, was audible to anyone entering the building. At the request and concern of the nursing staff, the treatment team has been called together to devise a plan to address Mr. A.'s screaming behavior.

The team conducted a thorough assessment of the situation and reached the following conclusions:

1. Screaming is Mr. A.'s current method of communication, and must be viewed by the staff as communication rather than meanness or harassment.
2. Mr. A. is reacting to the loss of his wife's visits plus numerous other physical and social losses.
3. Mr. A. has discovered that screaming brings attention, even if it is negative attention.
4. Through screaming, Mr. A. is trying to exert some control over his life.
5. The screaming occurs primarily in the late afternoon, when Mr. A. needs to use the toilet or is overly fatigued.
6. The previous tactics used by the staff to control Mr. A.'s screaming (e.g., telling him to stop, being firm, and stating that he would not get what he wanted by screaming) have become ineffective.

After discovering this information about the situation, the team developed and implemented the following plan:

1. No more changes are to be made in Mr. A.'s environment (e.g., his room will not be changed again).
2. Routines are to be established with Mr. A.'s input and the same staff are to provide his care on a daily basis to establish consistency in his life.
3. The activities director is to work with Mr. A. to add new activities to his daily life.
4. A friendly visitor program is to begin for Mr. A. and will involve the same two volunteers coming on a daily basis. The volunteers will be advised to try to establish a routine similar to the one Mrs. A. established.
5. Mr. A. is given a bell to ring if he needs something. Otherwise, he will be checked on at least every 2 hours.
6. Staff received in-servicing on the plan and were instructed to respond quickly to his bell calls but not to his yelling.

Two months later, Mr. A. is using the bell to call for assistance. He yells out occasionally, but this behavior tends to occur when unavoidable changes are made in his routines. The staff feel very good about working together to make this change without the need to give Mr. A. sedatives.

Eating Difficulties

Sometimes patients with Alzheimer's disease exhibit disruptions in normal eating patterns. The difficulties can stem from disruptive stimuli at mealtimes.

Example: Dealing with Abnormal Eating and Drinking Behaviors

The husband of one of our patients observed that when eating in a restaurant sometimes his wife would eat everything on her plate. On other occasions, however, she would not eat anything. While searching for an explanation, he discovered that when his wife faced the wall she cleaned the plate and that when she faced the staff, other customers, or the cash register she failed to eat at all. The distractions offered by the busy restaurant produced a failure to eat.

━● Principles for Dealing with Inappropriate Sexual Behavior

1. Protect the privacy of the patient, family, and visitors.
2. Do not make a big issue about the undesired behavior.
3. Handle any incident in a matter-of-fact manner.
4. Educate caregivers about the meaning of the behavior.
5. Determine the most likely reason or cause of the behavior.
6. Provide appropriate attention and affection to the patient.
7. Set limits when needed. May need to give patient more time alone.
8. If necessary, use distraction.
9. Use clothing that is not easily removed.
10. Reinforce appropriate attention-seeking behavior.

Inappropriate Sexual Behaviors

Sexual behaviors first must be defined on the basis of appropriateness. Such behaviors are determined to be inappropriate if the behavior is dysfunctional; serves no useful, healthy purpose; and does not fit within the setting or environment. Such behaviors may include masturbating, undressing, and touching in public. However, very often behaviors of a sexual nature are determined as inappropriate because they bother or embarrass the caregivers or others.

Sexuality and the Elderly

To be able to understand and intervene effectively in instances of inappropriate sexual behavior in patients with Alzheimer's disease, it is necessary to first develop a realistic attitude and knowledge base with regard to the sexual attitudes, feelings, and behaviors of older adults. Older men and women describe both similar and different degrees of sexual interest, participation, and satisfaction for a range of sexual behaviors. The combination of sexual variables of self-esteem, intimacy and sexual knowledge, attitudes, interest, participation, and satisfaction accounts for differences between men and women more than gender differences on any single variable. Viewing sexual health from a holistic perspective, the greatest predictors for continued sexual interest and activity are reasonably good health and the desire for continued intimacy. For older women the primary reason for lack of sexual activity is the absence of a suitable partner.

Considerations in Patients with Alzheimer's Disease

With this brief background in mind, it becomes relatively easy to begin to understand what might underlie the inappropriate sexual behaviors of Alzheimer's patients. Their sexual feelings and desires may remain quite intact, while their ability to express those feelings and their judgment relative to them have become impaired. Because of their dementia, many patients with Alzheimer's disease lose the ability to determine the appropriate time, place, or way to express sexual needs and desires. The patient may no longer recognize his surroundings, may have lost the ability to inhibit certain actions, or may have no other available mechanism for sexual gratification. This understanding at a very basic level may allow caregivers to be comfortable enough with their own feelings about the behavior to explore the inappropriate sexual behavior further. The goal, in whatever setting the inappropriate behavior occurs, should be to protect the patient and others (families, visitors, staff) from discomfort and embarrassment.

Meaning of the Behavior

An understanding of the basis and meaning of the behavior to the patient is needed to develop the most effective strategy for addressing the inappropriate sexual behavior. A careful physical assessment may reveal that masturbation in men is related to an underlying urinary tract infection or pruritus, while such behavior in women may be related to urinary tract infections, vaginitis, or a prolapsed uterus. Inappropriate sexual behavior may be a stress response to institutionalization or some other situation the patient finds overwhelming. It might be helping to relieve a sense of fear or threat, perceived loss of control, loss of a familiar environment or caregiver, frustration with tasks, misperceptions of caregivers, or simply fatigue. Some unwanted "sexual acting out" is found among many older persons and not limited just to those who are cognitively impaired.

The cause of inappropriate sexual behavior may be the need for intimacy. Older persons have often suffered multiple losses and may feel lonely and isolated. All humans have a need for intimacy. Inappropriate sexual behaviors may occur as a result of trying to establish intimacy through touch. This need for touch and intimacy seems central to the problem. Every attempt should be made on the part of caregivers to make the patient feel wanted, needed, and desired.

Context of the Behavior

With some self-examination concerning one's own degree of comfort about sexuality and inappropriate sexual behaviors, the next step is to examine the behavior and the context in which it occurs. If physical causes have been ruled out, the most common reason for such behaviors in the home is probably related to conflict between the caregiver and the patient. The caregiver may be inattentive to the patient's sexual needs due to stress, depression, or fatigue. An appropriate intervention might be to provide some respite for the caregiver, who can then recover some lost energy and cope more positively with the patient. The caregiver should be given the opportunity to express feelings about the sexual behaviors of the patient and to discuss feelings surrounding sexuality in older adults. This can provide the opportunity to dispel myths and to realize that others encounter similar problems and that such behaviors are not shameful. The caregiver can be taught to provide the gentle touches, kisses, and hugs that will provide an increased sense of intimacy to the patient.

Management of Sexual Behaviors

In long-term care and acute care settings, it is vital to establish a comprehensive plan for dealing with unwanted/inappropriate sexual behaviors. The staff must be educated about what the behaviors may represent, and encouraged to explore their own attitudes and feelings about sexuality in older adults. Education will help to increase the caregivers' comfort level with the behaviors. This is important to accomplish, because when caregivers are uncomfortable or upset with behaviors, generally the patients' undesired behaviors escalate. General measures for intervention also include providing privacy, bringing the patient a robe if the caregiver is unable to lead him to a private area, toileting at-risk patients on a regular basis, labeling rooms and areas to help patients locate appropriate privacy, and allowing patients to keep personal items in their rooms. Providing a relaxing massage or going for a walk and holding the patient's hand can provide the therapeutic touch that so many Alzheimer's patients need. When possible, at-risk patients should have a private room.

When inappropriate behavior is thought to be due to disturbance in memory and judgment, the patient should be oriented to person and place if possible. Short, simple commands should be used to direct the patient to his room or to redirect the behavior. If unwanted behavior persists, alternative clothing (pullover shirts, pants without zippers, clothes on backwards) can be used.

Cognitive impairment in conjunction with the decreased impulse control may require that limits be set for behavior that is acceptable and that is unacceptable. Caregivers should provide reassurance of acceptance to the patient, problem-solve to avoid triggers for unacceptable behaviors (environmental manipulation), and reward the patient for appropriate behavior. In most cases, the general interventions suggested in the case studies below, in combination with specific interventions based on the cause of the problem, will successfully address the problem of inappropriate sexual behavior. Caregivers should monitor the patient's response to the interventions, and if unsuccessful, reassess for other causes and institute alternative interventions. Any behavioral management of inappropriate sexual display must recognize the embarrassment and disgust potentially produced in the caregivers, who must be provided an opportunity to talk about their feelings. This can be accomplished during staff meetings and support groups.

Example: Dealing with Inappropriate Sexual Behaviors

Mr. L., a 65-year-old-man, was committed to a state psychiatric hospital after exposing himself to his 11-year-old niece in her bedroom. This behavior had happened at least twice and occurred while the niece's mother was at home. Mr. L. had been diagnosed as having Alzheimer's disease several years previously and had been cared for at home by his family. His wife worked during the day, and various family members watched Mr. L. during these times. Mr. L.'s wife had become increasingly tired and discouraged, and had lost interest in sexual relations over the past year. Mr. L. had no previous history of sexually deviant behavior and seemed confused and unable to remember the incidents. His family was embarrassed, angry, and in conflict about how to respond to his aberrant behavior.

In the hospital Mr. L. had been very restless, had made sexually explicit remarks to female staff members, and was reported by his family to be increasingly confused. The treatment staff developed a plan for setting firm limits on Mr. L.'s behavior, while simultaneously allowing him privacy for masturbation, which he did about three times a week. A staff psychologist met with Mrs. L. to encourage her to discuss her feelings about the loss of her independence and support from her husband. The family was able to provide her additional support, allowing her to rest and recognizing the degree of stress she had experienced. Mrs. L. was gradually able to again express affection toward her husband.

After 6 weeks of hospitalization with no episodes of exposing himself, Mr. L. began to receive day passes to go back to his home. A plan was developed to prevent him from being allowed to be alone with young children and to give him periods of privacy on a daily basis. There were no further incidents of exposure, and Mr. L. was discharged after 8 weeks of treatment.

Paranoid Thinking

Paranoid thinking is exhibited by mistrust and suspicion regarding certain persons or aspects of an individual's environment. In extreme cases this type of thinking can be delusional; the patient may have fixed false beliefs concerning plots to kill him or her, injure family members, or harm loved ones in other ways. The patient may respond to these delusions as if they were real and thus may be a danger to self or others.

Distortions of reality can occur with any type of dementia, or they may be a secondary effect of sensory deprivation or medications. Some of the symptoms of physical decline, such as malnutrition, dehydration, anemia, or infection, may contribute to the problem. In all such cases the decreased ability to receive and interpret stimuli leads to misinterpretations of ordinary situations.

Patients with Alzheimer's disease who experience paranoid thinking need a secure environment and consistent responses from caregivers. They should not be directly challenged about their thinking but should be offered frequent assurance of their own security. Maintaining a well-lit and non-threatening environment can help reduce the patient's anxiety. Simple explanations of all activities should be offered, and the patient should be allowed to inquire about and examine any aspect of his care for more information. If the patient has family or friends who are able to calm his fears or distract him, their help should be enlisted in providing care. Sometimes the availability of telephone contact with a family member can be reassuring to a patient. If feasible, patients should have their hearing and vision checked periodically. Paranoid thinking is linked to impaired sensory input. Antipsychotic medications can be effective, but they should be administered with close supervision (see Chapter 13).

Depression and Apathy

Differentiating depression from dementia can be difficult (see Chapter 8). Patients with early-stage Alzheimer's disease may recognize their poor prognosis and feel extremely sad and hopeless. Although suicide is rare in patients with Alzheimer's disease, certain highly publicized recent cases may reflect a growing acceptance of this act as an alternative. More common is the occurrence of a sense of hopelessness that may be shared by the caregivers. In patients with Alzheimer's disease, depression may be associated with biochemical changes occurring in the brain. A common symptom among patients who cannot communicate their feelings effectively is a tendency to withdraw and become apathetic. This response may contribute to some of the problem behaviors described previously.

When patients with Alzheimer's disease are experiencing severe depressive symptoms, such as thoughts of death or inflicting self-harm, they should be assessed for the potential for suicide. If a psychiatric evaluation indicates that such potential is high, treatment in a psychiatric facility is indicated. However, all persons caring for patients with Alzheimer's disease should try to minimize the patient's opportunity for self-harm by providing close observation and an environment with few objects that can be used as weapons. Depressed patients often respond to an environment that promotes physical comfort and the opportunity for performing simple, familiar, and meaningful tasks. Cheerful reminiscence and favorite music also can raise the patient's spirits. Antidepressant medications also may improve the patient's mood and sleep pattern (see Chapter 13).

Example: Dealing with Depression and Apathy

Mrs. C., an 80-year-old woman, resided at a continuing care center for 9 years following the death of her husband. She experienced signs of dementia for several years and was diagnosed with Alzheimer's disease shortly after the initial onset of symptoms. She functioned fairly well, living in her own apartment until approximately 3 months ago, when her son and some friends noticed that she was becoming increasingly withdrawn and was eating less.

Recently Mrs. C. had lost seven pounds and had a recurrence of sleep disturbance similar to the type she had experienced after her husband's death. The physical examination was unremarkable. After psychiatric consultation, administration of a tricyclic antidepressant was recommended. After 3 months of treatment, including several changes in the dosage of the medication, Mrs. C. had improved only marginally.

An occupational therapist was consulted to recommend activities that might interest and stimulate Mrs. C. A plan was developed so that she would attend a partial day treatment program that focused on socialization and provided a lunch. Initially Mrs. C. expressed reluctance, but eventually she began to attend regularly. In addition, she was referred to a music reminiscence group conducted at the center. At these group sessions she discussed feelings stimulated by the music and was able to acknowledge some fears related to loneliness. She was then asked to join a telephone support network within the center and began to anticipate calls from her new friends. Mrs. C.'s level of participation in activities of daily living stabilized at a level that was higher than before the onset of symptoms, and her weight returned to normal. She remained on a small dose of antidepressant medication, which she felt helped her sleep better.

Sleep Disturbances

Sleep patterns change with aging so that older persons not only generally sleep fewer hours, but spend less time in deep, restful sleep and also less time in REM (dream) sleep. They may experience times of wakefulness during the night that lead to daytime sleepiness. Superimposed on these age-associated changes in sleep are the abnormal, disruptive changes in sleep associated with Alzheimer's disease. As a result, patients with Alzheimer's disease spend a high percentage of sleep in stage 1 (light sleep) and less time in stages 3 and 4 (deep sleep), and experience more arousals and awakenings, all of which parallel the severity of the dementia. Some patients with Alzheimer's disease are awake during the nighttime hours and sleep during the daytime. Others sleep fitfully for very brief periods, giving the appearance of constant wakefulness. Some may even suffer from sleep-related respiratory disorders.

Sundowning is a phenomenon often associated with sleep disorders. It is probably related to a circadian rhythm disturbance. It is commonly described as a period of increased agitation, restlessness, and some disorientation, usually occurring in the early evening from about 3 or 4 PM to around 8 PM. Helping the patient who is experiencing sundowning usually requires manipulating the patient's environment. Interventions for managing sundowning include a short nap around 1 PM for no more than one hour to combat fatigue, increasing the light level in the home or facility in mid to late afternoon, providing orienting cues throughout the day, and closing curtains and blinds to eliminate the possibility of the patient seeing the outside darkness. Some facilities have instituted a "light room," where patients are taken for 1 to 2 hours for the purpose of reestablishing a more appropriate wake-sleep cycle. This has met with some success and may become more widely used in the near future.

Physical restraints are known to increase the patient's confusion and restlessness, and should be avoided. Providing close supervision of the patient is necessary during episodes of sundowning. Finally, psychotropic medications may be needed to help calm the patient if all other measures fail. These medications should be used in small doses and under the direction of the physician.

Both sleep/wake disturbances and sundowning affect the quality and quantity of sleep for both patient and caregivers. These behaviors can become very frustrating and tiresome for caregivers. Although the patient usually can fall asleep when the need arises, this option is not always available to the caregiver.

The fact that the patient is awake at night is not the problem, as he will sleep when the need arises. The problem is what the patient does during these waking times. He may get up and begin to resume daytime activities, turning on the lights and wandering around disturbing others. Some patients may have periods of wakefulness during which they demonstrate panic because they cannot recognize their nighttime surroundings. Institutionalization (long-term care and acute care settings) also can have an effect on sleep patterns because of increased noise, medications, pain, and unfamiliar surroundings and routines.

Management of Sleep Disruptions

Generally pharmacologic treatment is of little use, and may be contraindicated because of potential adverse side-effects. Behavioral strategies are much more likely to provide at least partial relief for any sleep difficulties. In order to help a patient reestablish normal sleep patterns, the caregiver should begin by investigating any factors that might keep the patient awake. Such factors include pain, medications, fear and insecurity, noise, and increased lighting. Eliminating any of these factors may be all that is necessary to help the person sleep. A nightlight is often useful in helping the patient with dementia feel more secure during the night.

Secondly, the patient's daily schedule of activity should be observed. Patients who have difficulty sleeping should be kept active during the day and not permitted to spend a good portion of the day sitting and napping. Exercise such as walking will help the patient to expend energy and be more fatigued at bedtime. Exercise also often has the added benefit of reducing agitation and stimulating verbal abilities. If patients are unable to walk, chair or even bed exercises can be used as well as alternative activities such as emptying and rearranging drawer contents, stacking newspapers, or folding clothes. It is very important to establish a bedtime routine or ritual so that the patient will realize that it is time to go to bed. Such a routine may involve bathing, putting on pajamas, having a light snack including warm milk, brushing teeth, and toileting. Going through this same routine every night will help the patient recognize what behavior is expected.

Coffee, cigarettes, tea, and soda drinks containing caffeine should be avoided late in the day because of their stimulant effect. Diuretics should be administered early enough in the day to avoid the need for the patient to get up several times at night to void. Reassurance and soft, pleasant music may be comforting to the patient and aid in sleep onset. Finally, if the patient continues to get up and wander at night, making sure he has a safe place to wander is imperative. Alarms can be placed on the patient's bed to alert caregivers to the fact that the patient is getting out of bed.

In the home setting, caregivers must have the opportunity to obtain adequate amounts of sleep. Encouraging the caregiver to elicit the help of another person to watch the patient while he or she rests is one approach. Helping the caregiver to understand the patient's behavior and to rest whenever the patient rests is vitally important. Sleep medications and tranquilizers used by caregivers should be done judiciously and only under the direct supervision of a physician. Caregivers need to be educated regarding the side effects of these medications.

Example: Dealing with Sleep Disturbances

Mrs. W., a 72-year-old widow, moved in with her daughter, Joyce, approximately 6 months ago after a hospitalization for pneumonia. Diagnosed as having Alzheimer's disease 8 years earlier, Mrs. W. appears to have been in the second stage for approximately 4 1/2 years. Her level of confusion and disorientation increased significantly when she entered the hospital, and her condition has remained about the same. Joyce has come to the local Alzheimer's support group for help because, as she puts it, "Mom becomes like another person after supper. She doesn't recognize me, she disrupts everything, and nothing seems to calm her down until she falls asleep. She always seems so much better in the morning." The group members, many of whom have been through the same type of experience, begin to discuss the problem with Joyce.

The group facilitator initiates the conversation by asking Joyce to describe a typical day. During the discussion, it is discovered that Mrs. W. is not provided the opportunity for a nap in the early afternoon, but she does sleep well at night. Joyce also comments on how hungry her mother seems to be at suppertime. In addition, it seems that Mrs. W.'s behavior became worse in October, when the time changed.

The facilitator explained to Joyce that her mother appears to be manifesting "sundowning." An explanation of this behavior with some general information and guidelines is given, and a plan is devised to assist Mrs. W. with functioning in the late afternoon and early evening. This plan is as follows:

1. To avoid extreme fatigue, Mrs. W. will take a 1-hour nap at 1 PM. Joyce is cautioned not to allow her mother to sleep too long since a long nap may interfere with nighttime sleep.
2. To help relieve the apparent hunger and possible low glucose level, Joyce is to provide her mother with a high-carbohydrate snack at 4 PM.

3. To maintain the same level of illumination in the house, Joyce will turn on the lights 2 hours before sundown. She also will close the curtains 1 hour before sundown so that her mother does not notice the changing light level outside.
4. Joyce will try to engage her mother in a low-stimulation (quiet) activity immediately after supper.

After 2 months Joyce reported that although her mother still exhibited increased confusion at nighttime, the frequency and the degree of confusion and disruption had decreased significantly. She also commented that she was very thankful that this improvement was accomplished without medication.

Repetitious Behaviors

Repetitious behaviors occur on a continuous basis and generally serve no functional purpose. Most of the time these behaviors are benign, posing no danger to the patient or the caregiver. However, they can be very annoying and may cause a great deal of frustration for caregivers. Some examples of repetitious behaviors frequently encountered are questioning, following the caregiver, or performing one task over and over again.

Patients in the later stages of Alzheimer's disease have significant memory loss. Many of the activities the patient engages in may be caused by the fact that he cannot remember having completed the task. The patient also may not remember that he has just been given the answer to a question. Constant questioning about the whereabouts of a certain person or continually following a caregiver may be a demonstration of the patient's concern or insecurity. Repeatedly performing a task may result from boredom, the inability to carry a task to completion, or an attempt on the part of the patient to feel as if he is helping the caregiver. Some medications can cause the patient to have "nervous" energy that is expended through repetitive actions.

Managing Repetitious Behaviors

In dealing with repetitious behaviors, the primary emphasis is on helping caregivers understand that the patient is not behaving in a certain way just to annoy them. Caregivers need to know that the behaviors commonly occur and are part of the dementia process. If the patient is showing signs of fear or insecurity, the cause of these feelings should be determined. Providing reassurance through a calm manner and the use of touch can be helpful. Distracting the patient with a favorite activity may help to break the pattern of the behavior. Sometimes ignoring the behavior will stop it because no reinforcement is provided. If the behavior is benign, such as folding and unfolding clothes, there is no reason to attempt to stop it. However, if the behavior is causing a problem (e.g., constantly moving or hiding objects or watering plants), caregivers should attempt to substitute a less problem-prone task.

Memory aids such as clocks, calendars, and notes can help to orient the patient to surroundings and events, and provide him with the information he is seeking. Engaging the patient in simple conversation may satisfy the need for interaction. Using television, music, or videotapes appropriate for the patient's cognitive ability may provide a distraction for the patient. Finally, giving the patient a chore that she can still perform will add a sense of control to her life and bolster self-esteem.

SUMMARY

Dealing successfully with problematic behaviors requires collaboration among caregivers (both family members and health professionals), creative thinking, and problem-solving techniques. Although not every patient with Alzheimer's disease will experience the behaviors discussed here, most will experience at least one or two. Since these behaviors often cannot be attributed to a specific cause, a complete investigation of the circumstances surrounding the behaviors is necessary. Health professionals play a major role in assisting caregivers to understand the patient's behaviors and the effects they are having on their lives. Providing caregivers with this understanding and possible interventions to use can help give them a sense of control over problems and relieve some of the stress associated with caring for someone with Alzheimer's disease.

BIBLIOGRAPHY

Abrams WB, Beers MH, Berkow R, editors: Sleep disorders associated with dementia. In *Merck Manual of Geriatrics,* Whitehouse Station NJ, 1995, Merck Research Laboratories.

Banazak DA: Difficult dementia: six steps to control problem behaviors, *Geriatrics* 51(2):36-42, 1996.

Birren JE, Sloane RB, Cohen GD, editors: *Handbook of mental health and aging,* San Diego, 1992, Academic Press.

Bliwise DL, Hughes M, McMahon PM et al: Observed sleep/wakefulness and severity of dementia in an Alzheimer's disease special care unit, *J Gerontol,* Series A: Biological and Medical Sciences 50A(6):M303-M306, 1995.

Burney-Puckett M: Sundown syndrome: etiology and management, *J Psychosoc Nurs Ment Health Serv* 34(5):40-43, 1996.

Chou KR, Kaas MJ, Richie MF: Assaultive behavior in geriatric patients, *J Gerontol Nurs* 22(11):30, 1996.

Feil N: *The validation breakthrough: simple techniques for communicating with people with Alzheimer's-type dementia,* Baltimore, 1993, Health Professions Press, Inc.

Freeman S: Community management of the agitated patient: interventions for the caregiver, *Caring* 14(7):44-45, 1995.

Johnson BK: Older adults and sexuality, *J Gerontol Nurs* 22(2):6-15, 1996.

Kovach CR, Henschel H: Planning activities for patients with dementia: a descriptive study of therapeutic activities on special care units, *J Gerontol Nurs* 22(9):33-38, 1996.

Lewis K: How to foster self-determination: practical ways nursing home staff can empower residents, *Health Prog* 76(8):42-44, 1995.

Little JT, Satlin A, Sunderland T et al: Sundown syndrome in severely demented patients with probable Alzheimer's disease, *J Geriatr Psychiatry and Neurol* 8(2):103-106, 1995.

Matteson MA, Linton A: Wandering behaviors in institutionalized persons with dementia, *J Gerontol Nurs* 22(9):39-46, 1996.

Maxfield M, Lewis RE, Cannon S: Training staff to prevent aggressive behavior of cognitively impaired elderly patients during bathing and grooming, *J Gerontol Nurs* 22(1):37-43, 1996.

Namazi KH, Zadorozny CA, Gwinnup PB: The influences of physical activity on patterns of sleep behavior of patients with Alzheimer's disease, *Int J Aging Hum Dev* 40(2):145-153, 1995.

Philo SW, Richie MF, Kaas MJ: Inappropriate sexual behavior, *J Gerontol Nurs* 22(11):17-22, 1996.

Potts HW, Richie MF, Kaas MJ: Resistance to care, *J Gerontol Nurs* 22(11):11, 1996.

Ruppert RA: Caring for the caregiver, *Am J Nurs Practitioner* 96(3):40-45, 1996.

Satlin A, Volicer L, Stopa EG et al: Circadian locomotor activity and core-body temperature rhythms in Alzheimer's disease, *Neurobiol Aging* 16(5):765-771, 1995.

Snyder M, Egan EC, Burns KR: Interventions for decreasing agitation behaviors in persons with dementia, *J Gerontol Nurs* 21(7):34-40, 1995.

vanSomeren EJW, Mirmiran M, Swaab DF: Non-pharmacological treatment of sleep and wake disturbances in aging and Alzheimer's disease: chronobiological perspectives, *Behav Brain Res* 57(2):235-253, 1993.

Vollen KH: Coping with difficult resident behaviors takes TIME, *J Gerontol Nurs* 22(8):22-26, 1996.

Werner P, Hay DP, Cohen-Mansfield J: Management of disruptive vocalizations in the nursing home, *Nurs Home Med* 3(9):217-225, 1995.

White MK, Kaas MJ, Richie MF: Vocally disruptive behavior, *J Gerontol Nurs* 22(11):23, 1996.

Psychopharmacology in Dementia

James M Turnbull

I do not want two diseases,
one nature made,
one doctor made.

—Napoleon Bonaparte

The diagnosis of Alzheimer's disease is more dependent on intellectual impairment and memory loss than on behavioral change. However, it is the behavioral disturbances that greatly affect the quality of life not only for the patient but also for the family and the caregivers. These behavioral changes, described in detail in other chapters of this book, include agitation, wandering, screaming, aggression, violence, and inappropriate sexual acting out.

—• Drugs used to treat these behaviors do not affect the overall course of Alzheimer's disease. They are merely symptomatic treatments.

A close relationship exists between depression and dementia, one that is classically illustrated by the most tragic of Shakespeare's characters, King Lear. The early stages of Alzheimer's disease are frequently associated with the characteristic signs and symptoms of a mood disorder, including anhedonia (loss of pleasure in things that were formerly enjoyed), insomnia, low mood, crying spells, hopelessness, change in appetite, lethargy, and even thoughts of suicide. The frequency of depressive disorders in patients with dementia may be as high as 20%.

Phamacotherapy of behavioral disturbances and depression is both appropriate and in some cases life saving, but it is also fraught with danger. The physiological changes that take place with aging affect the pharmacokinetics and pharmacodynamics of drugs. Most patients older than 75 are taking more than one medication, which leads to problems with compliance, drug-drug interactions, and iatrogenic illness. Frequently, a close look at the combination of drugs a patient is taking is the key to explaining the appearance of new symptoms.

Since drug metabolism takes place in the liver, which may have reduced perfusion, it is important to choose drugs that have low hepatotoxicity and simple metabolic profiles (i.e., are inactive by a one-step process rather than two or more steps). The cytochrome P450 system is an important factor to be considered, particularly when prescribing antidepressants.

Renal function and perfusion also decline with age, and drugs such as lithium, nortriptyline, and fluoxetine, in which renal excretion is an important elimination route, are likely to have a prolonged effect. The pharmacodynamics of medications also changes with age because of a decrease in the number of receptors and in neurotransmitter levels. Target organs, particularly the brain, also undergo structural changes.

Two important steps should precede the prescription of any psychoactive drug to a patient with dementia. The first step is a thorough assessment of the problem, including the differential diagnosis mentioned in Chapter 8. The second is to evaluate what nonpharmacologic management has already been attempted.

ANTIPSYCHOTICS

Neuroleptic drugs are almost exclusively used for the treatment of psychotic disorders in younger patients, for example, conditions such as schizophrenia, bipolar disorder, delusional disorder, and psychotic depression. In the older population the set of indications for neuroleptics tends to be broader and less well defined. Therefore strict Omnibus Budget Reconciliation Act (OBRA) guidelines have been developed for the use of these drugs in nursing homes. The major drugs included in this category are listed in Table 13-1. In almost all cases the starting dose is half that of the dose for younger adults.

There are several indications for use of neuroleptics in the patient with dementia. Aggression, restlessness, delusions, hallucinations, and some forms of inappropriate sexual behavior are more responsive to this class of drugs than symptoms such as persistent wandering or screaming.

The introduction of what are described as "atypical" or "novel" antipsychotics has changed prescribing practices for the treatment of delusions, hallucinations, and other symptoms and signs of a thought disorder. These new agents, clozapine, risperidone, and olanzepine, have a far more favorable side effect profile than older agents.

High potency, low-dose neuroleptics, such as pimozide and fluphenazine, are likely to produce extrapyramidal side effects. Low potency, high-dose drugs, such as chlorpromazine and thioridazine, are strongly sedating and anticholinergic, and they produce orthostatic hypotension. Drugs in the middle range of potency, such as thiothixene and perphenazine, are often selected. Despite numerous studies on treatment, there are no clear guidelines regarding the length of treatment. It is advisable to provide drug "holidays" at regular intervals. Such drug-free periods provide information about the need to continue administration of neuroleptics. Symptoms often remit spontaneously as a result of environmental changes or progression of the dementia. Regular review should also include administration of the Abnormal Involuntary Movement Scale (AIMS) test (Table 13-2).

Text continued on p. 177

Table 13-1

Selected Antipsychotic Drugs

Class/Generic Name	Trade Name	Dose Equivalent (mg)	Usual Daily Oral Adult Dose (mg)	Single Parenteral Adult Dose (mg)	Usual Daily Oral Dose (mg) Over Age 65	Frequency
Phenothiazines						
Chlorpromazine	Thorazine	100	200-600	25-100	50-200	bid*
Thioridazine	Mellaril	100	200-600	N/A	50-200	bid
Mesoridazine	Serentil	50	150	25-175	25-100	bid
Trifluoperazine	Stelazine	5	5-10	1-2	2-10	qd+
Fluphenazine Hcl	Permitil, Prolixin	1	2.5-10	2-5	1-3	qd
Perphenazine	Trilafon	9	16-64	5-10	4-16	bid
Thioxanthenes						
Chlorprothixene	Taractan	40	75-200	75-200	25-75	bid
Thiothixene	Navane	4	6-30	4	2-10	bid
Butyrophenone						
Haloperidol	Haldol	1	2-12	2-5	0.5-5	bid
Dibenzoxazepine						
Loxapine	Loxitane	10	20	12.5-50	5-10	bid

*Twice a day
+Once daily

Continued

Table 13-1

Selected Antipsychotic Drugs—cont'd

Class/Generic Name	Trade Name	Dose Equivalent (mg)	Usual Daily Oral Adult Dose (mg)	Single Parenteral Adult Dose (mg)	Usual Daily Oral Dose (mg) Over Age 65	Frequency
Indole derivative Molindone	Moban	5	15-60	N/A	5-15	bid
Diphenylbutylpiperidine Pimozide	Orap	4	2-10		200	bid
Dibenzodiazepine Clozapine	Clozaril	400	200-900	N/A	200	bid
Benzisoxazole Risperidone	Risperdal	3	1-6	N/A	0.5-1	bid
Thienobenzodiazepine Olanzepine	Zyprexa	10	5-20	N/A	5-10	qd

Table 13-2

Abnormal Involuntary Movement Scale (AIMS)

Patient's name _____   Rater _____   Date _____

Instructions: Read the examination procedure (opposite page) before rating.

Movement ratings: Rate highest severity observed. Rate movements that occur upon activation one less than those observed spontaneously.

Facial and Oral Movements					
1. Muscles of facial expressions: include movements of forehead, eyebrows, periorbital area, cheeks. Note frowning, blinking, smiling, and grimacing. Circle one	0 None	1 Minimal, may be extreme normal	2 Mild	3 Moderate	4 Severe
2. Lips and perioral area: include puckering, pouting, and smacking.	0	1	2	3	4
3. Jaw: include biting, clenching, chewing, mouth opening, and lateral movement.	0	1	2	3	4
4. Tongue: rate only increase in movement both in and out of mouth, not inability to sustain movement.	0	1	2	3	4

Extremity Movements					
5. Upper (arms, wrists, hands, fingers): include choreic movements (rapid, objectively purposeless, irregular, spontaneous) and athetoid movements (slow, irregular, complex, serpentine). Do not include tremor (repetitive, regular, rhythmic).	0	1	2	3	4
6. Lower (legs, knees, ankles, toes): include lateral knee movement, foot tapping, heel dropping, foot squirming, and inversion and eversion of the foot.	0	1	2	3	4

Form for scoring the Abnormal Involuntary Movement Scale. (From Department of Health and Human Services, National Institutes of Mental Health, Washington, DC.)

Continued

Table 13-2

Abnormal Involuntary Movement Scale (AIMS)—cont'd

		0	1	2	3	4
Trunk Movements	7. Neck, shoulder, hips: include rocking, twisting, squirming, and pelvic gyrations.	0	1	2	3	4
Global Judgments	8. Severity of abnormal movements.	0 None, normal	1 Minimal	2 Mild	3 Moderate	4 Severe
	9. Incapacitation due to abnormal movements: Rate as in item 8.	0	1	2	3	4
	10. Patient's awareness of abnormal movements. Rate only patient's report.	0 No awareness	1 Aware, no distress	2 Aware, mild distress	3 Aware, moderate distress	4 Aware, severe distress
Dental Status	11. Current problems with teeth and/or dentures?	0 No	1 Yes			
	12. Does patient usually wear dentures?	0 No	1 Yes			

The following side effects have been noted for antipsychotic drugs:

- Anticholinergic effects, including dry mouth, constipation, impairment of erectile functioning, urinary delay or obstruction, tachycardia, impaired sweating, and delusions.
- Antiadrenergic effects, particularly orthostatic hypotension.
- Extrapyramidal effects, consisting of dystonia, parkinsonian symptoms and signs (rigidity, tremor, shuffling gait, rolling of finger), akathisia, akinesia, and, most serious, tardive dyskinesia are sometimes noted. Akathisia is particularly troublesome. It is manifested by restlessness, muscle cramps, jitteriness, pacing, and "inner anxiety." Frequently, patients who develop akathisia will be unwilling to continue taking the drug.
- Other less common but serious side effects that may occur are agranulocytosis, epileptic seizures, cholestatic jaundice, photosensitivity, alterations in cardiac conduction, and neuroleptic malignant syndrome.

Clozapine, risperidone, and olanzepine are far less likely to produce extrapyramidal side effects in the elderly population. Clozapine is unfortunately associated with blood dyscrasias, and patients taking it must have weekly blood draws to check their white blood count. However, Risperidone and olanzepine do not require this. All three drugs produce sedation and weight gain, and can also affect the prolactin levels, causing lactation. Clozapine is particularly likely to produce orthostatic hypotension.

Some noncompliant patients with a demonstrated need for a neuroleptic drug may require intramuscular depot medication. The most commonly used ones are haloperidol decanoate (given monthly) and fluphenazine decanoate (given every 14 days).

ANXIOLYTICS AND HYPNOTICS

The benzodiazepines have almost entirely replaced barbiturates and meprobamate in the treatment of anxiety and insomnia. Other drugs used for these purposes include antihistamines (particularly hydroxyzine) and beta-blockers (propranolol).

Buspirone is particularly well tolerated in the anxious, elderly patient with dementia but, like all anxiolytic agents, it is not as effective in controlling agitation as the neuroleptics.

Benzodiazepines are generally divided into three groups: short-acting, intermediate-acting, and long-acting. The long-acting examples (diazepam, chlordiazepoxide, and flurazepam) accumulate in elderly individuals and increase the risk of toxicity. Drugs that are more rapidly eliminated, such as alprazolam, lorazepam, and triazolam are preferable.

Clonazepam is a unique member of this class because it stimulates serotonin production and has value in the management of aggression. This drug appears to be useful for patients who display hyperactivity, insomnia, social intrusiveness, and impulsivity. My experience suggests that clonazepam is also useful in conjunction with a low-dose neuroleptic such as haloperidol. The side effects of benzodiazepines include sedation, worsening of cognitive impairment, transient global amnesia, ataxia, falls, and paradoxical worsening of symptoms.

Injuries due to falls are the leading cause of injury-related deaths in those over 75 and are the most common reason for injury-related admissions to hospital in this age group. Benzodiazepine use is an important iatrogenic risk factor in both the community and institutions. Ten percent of men and 20% of women over the age of 65 use benzodiazepines daily, either for control of anxiety or for sleep.

Propranolol has been described as decreasing aggression in individuals with dementia, but it may need to be taken for several weeks before any effect is noted. The potential side effects of propranolol include hypotension, depression, sleep disturbance, and worsening of both chronic obstructive airway disease and heart failure. This drug may also mask the signs of hypoglycemia.

ANTIDEPRESSANTS

The relationship between dementia and depression is a complex one. Short-lived dysphoria may occur as a reaction to loss of cognitive abilities, and major depressive disorders of late onset may be superimposed on Alzheimer's disease. Antidepressant drugs may be useful in either situation. The choice of antidepressant depends on four considerations:

- Previous treatment for depression. What drug, if any, was useful?
- Drug management of other family members. If a first-degree relative was responsive to a particular antidepressant, it is a good idea to try the same drug for this patient.
- Other medications that the patient may be taking, including over-the-counter drugs. Because patients often do not remember their medications, it is helpful to have them bring drugs in a bag and ask a relative who knows the patient to accompany him.
- Possible need for psychiatric counseling. Treatment-resistant depression may require referral to a psychiatrist, particularly one familiar with psychopharmacology.

Antidepressants are of the following types: tricyclics (TCAs), tetracyclics, triazolopyridines, lithium, monoamine oxidase inhibitors (MAOIs), stimulants, serotonin reuptake inhibitors, and drugs that primarily influence norepinephrine and dopamine, such as bupropion (Table 13-3).

Tricyclic and tetracyclic antidepressants are effective and useful but they vary in their side effect profiles. Particularly troublesome for older individuals are the anticholinergic actions (see discussion of antipsychotics). All these drugs have a propensity to cause orthostatic hypotension, although imipramine, amitriptyline, and doxepin are more likely to cause this problem than nortriptyline. Orthostasis is particularly troublesome in older individuals because of the risk of falls. In younger patients, the medication is often given at bedtime, but in the elderly, divided doses are preferred because of the risk of nocturnal (*hora somni* [hs]) loading and an associated fall when the patient arises at night to use the bathroom or answer the telephone.

Cardiac conduction can be affected by antidepressants, inducing irregularities in the cardiac rhythm. Skin rash, liver toxicity, tinnitus, and myoclonus are other side effects that also occur.

Table 13-3

Antidepressants: Dose Ranges and Frequency

Class	Drug Name	Dose Range (mg/day)	Frequency
Tricyclics	Imipramine	25-300	hs*
	Desipramine	10-300	hs
	Amitriptyline	25-300	hs
	Nortriptyline	10-150	hs
	Doxepin	10-300	hs
Tetracyclines	Maprotiline	25-150	hs
MAOIs	Phenelzine	15-90	bid+
Triazolopyridine	Trazodone	50-600	tid++
Stimulants	Dextroamphetamine	25-30	bid (not at bedtime)
	Methylphenidate	5-40	bid (not at bedtime)
Serotonin Reuptake Inhibitors	Fluoxetine	10-60	qd+++
	Sertraline	50-600	qd
	Paroxetine	10-60	qd
	Fluoxamine	50-200	bid
Chloropropiophenones	Bupropion (SR)	150-300	bid
Phenylpiperazine	Nefazodone	100-300	bid
alpha-2 antagonist	Mirtazapine	15-45	qd
NE & 5HT Reuptake inhibitor	Venlafaxine	500-300	bid

*At bedtime.
+Twice a day.
++Three times a day.
+++Every day.

Plasma levels of these drugs are useful when noncompliance is suspected, when no response is elicited with a therapeutic dose, or when a change in efficacy occurs after a switch to a generic brand.

Low starting doses are recommended in the elderly. Increases in dosage should continue until improvement is noted or until side effects become intolerable. Duration of treatment is often longer for older patients. After the age of 50 years a typical depressive cycle lasts for 3 to 5 years, compared to 9 to 18 months in younger patients. MAOIs are not recommended in the depressed patient with dementia. The use of these agents is complicated by dietary and medication restrictions that are easily forgotten.

Trazodone is a useful drug in the elderly depressed patient. Although it is relatively free from anticholinergic side effects, it does produce sedation, hypotension, and dizziness.

Stimulants are rarely prescribed to any patient except children with attention deficit disorder and individuals with narcolepsy. These agents are associated with abuse and dependency. However, stimulants may be the only antidepressant drugs that work in a depressed person with dementia, particularly one who has another complicating medical illness such as stroke or congestive heart failure.

Although it is advisable to administer the last dose of the day of a stimulant no later than 4 PM (because of the drug's tendency to produce insomnia), stimulants are remarkably free of side effects in the elderly.

Lithium is used in the treatment of bipolar disorder, but it has also been used in the elderly to enhance the action of antidepressants and to manage agitation. Since lithium is excreted via the kidneys and renal clearance is typically reduced in older individuals, great care must be exercised both before and during treatment. Side effects include a fine tremor, nausea, headache, lassitude, and polyuria.

The selective serotonin reuptake inhibitors (SSRIs) include fluoxetine, paroxetine, sertraline, and fluoxamine, although the latter was introduced primarily to treat obsessive-compulsive disorders. The SSRIs have a very favorable side effect profile in the elderly. Not only are they minimally anticholinergic, but they also are noncardiotoxic and do not produce orthostatic hypotension. They can produce nausea, insomnia, and sometimes diarrhea early in treatment. A more serious side effect is autonomic hyperactivity, often described by the patient as "nervous inside." Some authors have referred to this as "internal akathisia."

Many physicians currently use these agents as the antidepressant of first choice. Although fluoxetine comes in a standard 20-mg capsule form, it is also available in a liquid form, which allows lower doses to be prescribed. Fluoxetine, sertraline, and paroxetine are more expensive than generic tricyclics or trazodene.

The SSRIs are highly protein bound and therefore may affect the toxicity of other protein-bound drugs. Particularly serious are those with a narrow therapeutic window such as digoxin, coumadin, and dilantin. Another cause for concern with SSRIs is their action on the cytochrome P450 system in the liver. This is the major pathway for the human body to metabolize many drugs in the liver.

No SSRI should be administered without due consideration of drug/drug interaction. An important but incomplete list of drugs interacting with SSRIs include:
• Antipsychotics
• Beta-blockers
• Benzodiazepines
• Calcium channel blockers
• Erythromycin
• Lidocaine
• Quinidine
• Tricyclic antidepressants

The SSRIs are also associated with a high percentage of cases of sexual dysfunction, erectile problems in males, and anorgasmia in both men and women. In patients with subcortical dementia, SSRIs have been associated with apathy.

Bupropion is a safe and effective antidepressant without the drug/drug interactions of the SSRIs. This agent appears to have a relatively selective action on dopamine reuptake. Bupropion has few anticholinergic actions, induces little or no sedation, and is noncardiotoxic. It is the one antidepressant least likely to produce erectile dysfunction in males and anorgasmia in females that is currently available in the United States. Most important, it is safe for use in elderly patients with dementia.

Venlafaxine which inhibits the reuptake of both serotonin and norepinephrine, is probably not a drug of first choice for the treatment of depression in the elderly. It produces more nausea than the SSRIs and is more likely to cause hypertension. It also produces drug/drug interactions.

Nefazodone is chemically related to trazodone, affects the serotonin system but has less likelihood of producing sexual side effects than the SSRIs. Mirtazapine is an alpha-2 antagonist. It is very sedating and produces weight gain.

GENERAL CONSIDERATIONS

Compliance and drug-taking behavior are often ignored by health care professionals. Yet the following important principles of psychopharmacology need to be considered:

- New drugs are more expensive than established ones.
- Prescriptions for large amounts of antidepressants are dangerous because of the risk of overdose if the patient feels suicidal.
- Older individuals, especially those who are 75 years and older, are often taking multiple drugs, some of which may have been purchased as over-the-counter medications.
- Older patients are more affected by troublesome side effects than younger, more resilient individuals.
- It is usually best to "start low and go slow," that is, to begin with a small dose of the psychoactive medication and gradually increase the dose to achieve the desired therapeutic effect.
- Coordination of the various specialists involved in the care of the patient is essential, and the CNA is in a unique position to perform this role.

SUMMARY

To achieve the best results from psychoactive drugs in the treatment of psychiatric complications of dementia, special attention must be given to careful review. Relatives and patients always have questions, and an atmosphere must be created that encourages the development of a rapport that fosters an understanding of the disease and the drugs being used for treatment, including the side effects and potential benefits of these agents.

BIBLIOGRAPHY

Banazak DA: Difficult dementia: Six steps to control problem behaviors, *Geriatrics* 51(2):36-42, 1996.

Carter C, Swift RM, Turnbull JM: When are long-term anxiolytics warranted? *Patient Care* (March):155-177, 1996.

Cummings, JL, Ross R, Absher J et al: Depressive symptoms in Alzheimer disease: Assessment and determinants, *Alzheimer Dis Assoc Disord* 9(2):87-93, 1995.

Harvey RJ: Review: Delusions in dementia, *Age Ageing* 25:405-408, 1996.

Neutel CI, Hirdes JP, Maxwell CJ et al: New evidence on benzodiazepine use and falls: the time factor, *Age Ageing* 25:273-278, 1996.

Rapp MS, Flint AJ, Herrman N et al: Behavioral disturbances in the demented elderly: phenomenology, pharmacotherapy and behavioral management, *Can J Psychiat* (Nov)37:651-657, 1992.

Turnbull JM: Tips on prescribing psychotropic drugs, *Fam Pract Recert* (April) 18(4):54-72, 1996.

Specific Drug Therapy

Sharon Wyatt Moore

*It is impossible to cure all patients; that would
be an achievement surpassing in difficulty even
the forecasting of future developments.*

—Hippocrates

INTRODUCTION

Prior to the 1970s, approved treatment options were unavailable for the memory problems associated with dementia. Although few such drugs are commercially available at this time, many areas of research appear promising for new drug development. Extensive efforts are underway to understand the mechanisms of nervous system pathology of patients with Alzheimer's disease, and such insights are critical to develop effective treatments. It is now clear that there is not one specific defect in the disease, but several processes or pathways are affected. Certainly, the progress researchers have made in the last 20 years gives families hope for future breakthroughs to ease the suffering now endured. New efforts are also underway to determine whether some medications may help prevent Alzheimer's disease.

This chapter will attempt to provide the reader with an overview of the major medications previously used, currently used, and now under study for the treatment of this disease. None have the prospect of curing Alzheimer's disease, but some patients may experience beneficial effects or delayed worsening. Because all medications have possible side effects, the physician must weigh the risks and benefits with each medication decision.

—▸ With any treatment measure, it is especially important for the physician to exclude delirium, psychosis, and potentially reversible causes of dementia before starting therapy.

HYDERGINE

Hydergine (generic name, ergoloid mesylates) is a combination of four derivatives of ergotoxine and was the first medication approved by the United

States Food and Drug Administration (FDA) for *"senile mental decline."* The package insert for this medication now states it is indicated for *"an idiopathic decline in mental capacity,"* and those who respond tend to have *"some ill-defined process related to aging or . . . some underlying dementing condition (i.e., primary progressive dementia, Alzheimer's dementia, senile onset, multi-infarct dementia)."*

The mechanism of its actions are complex and poorly understood. Although use of Hydergine dates back to the 1940s for a variety of conditions, interest in the drug peaked with reported improvements in confusion. The majority of the studies in patients with decreased cognition were then performed in the 1970s and 1980s. These early studies had relatively small numbers of subjects, less refined diagnostic criteria, and simpler statistical techniques than current methodology. Yet, few results were seen in patients with Alzheimer's disease. Although the effects of Hydergine were recently reassessed with a new metaanalysis, the results remained similar. The authors concluded that future studies with longer follow-up times and higher dosages of the drug than currently approved in the United States would be necessary for adequate drug assessment, but others consider ergot mesylates to have limited value.

CHOLINERGIC STRATEGIES

The first major research area specifically in Alzheimer's disease therapy concerned neurotransmitters. Neurotransmitters are the chemical messengers between nerve cells in the brain and other parts of the nervous system. Most of the attention has focused on acetylcholine, a neurotransmitter that is decreased early in the disease in parts of the brain of Alzheimer's disease patients. Choline acetyltransferase (ChAT) is the key enzyme in the production of acetylcholine and is reduced in the cerebral cortex of Alzheimer's disease patients. Furthermore, the reduced ChAT levels correlate with the density of neuritic plaques, which contain the amyloid protein.

Four main approaches with drug therapy have involved attempts to increase the acetylcholine in the brain:
1. Increasing the building blocks from which acetylcholine is made (precursors) within the presynaptic neuron
2. Increasing the release of acetylcholine from the presynaptic neuron
3. Inhibiting acetylcholinesterase, the enzyme that breaks down the acetylcholine, so that the acetylcholine remains in the synapse for a longer time to carry messages between nerve cells
4. Directly stimulating cholinergic receptors to increase the action of acetylcholine by using acetylcholine-like compounds called agonists

Acetylcholine Precursors

Early studies, mostly with small numbers of Alzheimer's disease patients, assessed whether the building blocks of acetylcholine, choline, and phosphatidyl choline (lecithin), improved cognition. The majority of these studies did not report any significant improvement.

Acetylcholine Releasers

Although these compounds help increase the presynaptic release of acetylcholine, the first agent studied, 4-aminopyridine, demonstrated mixed results. The second drug, Dup 996 (also known as linopiridine or AVIVA), continues to be studied. In addition to increasing acetylcholine release, it also increases dopamine and serotonin, other neurotransmitters affected by Alzheimer's disease, but Dup 996 is associated with side effects on the liver and seizures.

Cholinesterase Inhibitors

Tacrine (Cognex). In 1993, tacrine became the first agent approved in the United States specifically for the treatment of mild to moderate Alzheimer's disease. It works by slowing the breakdown of the acetylcholine molecule by the acetylcholinesterase enzyme, thereby prolonging the action of the acetylcholine. An early report in 1986 demonstrated marked improvement in cognitive defects in 14 of 17 patients with Alzheimer's disease treated with tacrine, which then stimulated multicenter studies with various doses. Initially, the maximum daily dosage assessed was 80 mg/day given for periods up to 12 weeks, but later studies evaluated dosages up to 160 mg/day for longer periods. Cognition and global improvements were observed to be dose-dependent.

Several points about the use of tacrine are important for the caregiver and patient to understand. Not everyone can or should take tacrine. Tacrine is not recommended in patients with a history of allergic reaction to tacrine or related drugs; liver disease such as cirrhosis, hepatitis, hepatoma; significantly abnormal liver function tests; jaundice; prior stroke, hydrocephalus, subdural hematoma, or brain tumor. Risks should be carefully assessed in patients with other medical problems such as asthma, kidney disease, low blood pressure, slow heart rate, a heart condition known as sick sinus syndrome, seizure disorder, and prior upper gastrointestinal bleeding. It can also stimulate acid secretion in the stomach, potentially worsening peptic ulcer disease, and can increase levels of theophylline, a medicine used to aid breathing. Tacrine should not be administered to patients taking drugs with significant anticholinergic effects.

Of those who do take tacrine, the initial dosage is small, 10 mg four times a day. Dosage may be increased at 6-week intervals to 20 mg, 30 mg, then 40 mg four times a day, if tolerated. It therefore takes a minimum of 4 1/2 months to reach the most effective dose, if no significant problems arise.

Patients must have regular blood tests. When starting tacrine, patients must have weekly blood tests to check liver function for at least 18 weeks. Frequency of blood tests may then be decreased to every 3 months, but it is increased to weekly again for 6 weeks each time the dosage is increased. Additional tests are needed if liver function tests become abnormal or if the patient resumes tacrine after stopping it for 4 weeks or longer. Some of the other possible side effects include nausea, vomiting, diarrhea, heartburn, and decreased appetite, which have caused up to 10% to 20% of patients to stop the medication.

At best, only about a third of patients who take tacrine will show improvement. Sometimes the patient's response is to stay the same, rather than get worse. It is possible that patients taking tacrine at 80 mg/day or more who discontinue the drug abruptly may experience a sudden worsening of their condition.

During clinical trials, increased liver function tests (Alanine transferase [ALT], specifically) occurred in about half of patients. About one-fourth of patients developed an ALT greater than 3 times the upper limit of normal, requiring a reduction of dosage. If ALT becomes greater than 5 times the upper limit of normal, tacrine is stopped. Once the drug is stopped, liver function abnormalities should resolve with time. In certain circumstances, the drug may be reintroduced later, but careful monitoring is necessary.

Costs of the drug itself, blood testing, and follow-up office visits amount to approximately $2500 to $3000 per year.

Donepezil (Aricept). In November 1996 the FDA approved a second acetylcholinesterase inhibitor for patients with mild to moderate Alzheimer's disease, donepezil (previously known as E2020). The main advantages of this medication are the absence of liver toxicity in clinical trials, need for fewer blood tests since frequent monitoring of liver function tests is not required, a relatively high degree of selectivity for the nerve tissue enzyme that breaks down acetylcholine, and the once daily dosage schedule. These differences originate from its belonging to a different group of anticholinesterase, the piperidines rather than the acridines, and its longer duration of action.

The starting dosage for donezepil is 5 mg, and it takes about 15 days to reach a steady level of medication in the body. While donezepil can be taken with or without food, it is recommended that it be taken just before bedtime. Studies indicate that some patients may tend to experience greater benefit with a 10-mg dose, but the dose should not be increased before 4 to 6 weeks on the 5-mg dose.

In results to date, donezepil has demonstrated efficacy in three main clinical trials: An initial 14-week dose-finding study with 141 patients demonstrated a 50% reduction in the percentage of patients exhibiting clinical decline with a 5-mg dosage of donepezil (11% of patients) compared with a placebo (20% of patients).

Over 900 patients were then enrolled in 2 randomized, double-blind studies lasting 15 weeks (ARICEPT[TM] package insert) and 30 weeks, in which donezepil again yielded improvements in cognition and functioning relative to placebo. One open-label extension of treatment report (without a placebo control group) indicates that the cognitive improvement with donezepil may persist at least two years, but further studies are needed to substantiate this.

The main side effects of donezepil occur in a small percentage of patients and include nausea, diarrhea, insomnia, vomiting, muscle cramps, fatigue, and anorexia. Like tacrine, caution should be used in patients with asthma, kidney disease, low blood pressure, slow heart rate, a heart condition known as sick sinus syndrome, seizure disorder, and prior upper gastrointestinal bleeding. The drug is also expected to stimulate acid secretion in the stomach, potentially worsening peptic ulcer disease, and should not be administered to patients taking drugs with significant anticholinergic effects. Unlike tacrine, significant drug interactions with theophylline have not been reported. No drug interactions have been reported with cimetidine, warfarin, or digoxin.

At this point, no direct comparison studies are available between tacrine and donepezil. Both drugs are considered to help some symptoms of Alzheimer's disease in some patients, but there is no evidence that either agent is able to alter the course of the underlying disease.

Other cholinesterase inhibitors. Several other drugs with anticholinesterase activity remain under study. Velnacrine is identical to the body's main metabolic product of tacrine. Short-term studies have demonstrated that higher dosages (up to 225 mg/day) have modest but significant benefits in cognitive behavior and memory for patients with Alzheimer's disease. As with tacrine, the main side effects are abnormal liver function tests and diarrhea.

A sustained-release formulation of physostigmine has been developed. Although physostigmine was the initial cholinesterase inhibitor studied, drawbacks included the need for intravenous administration, an individualized dosage for optimal intracerebral concentration, and lack of effect with advanced dementia. The newer sustained-release physostigmine can be given orally and has a longer duration of action.

Other second-generation cholinesterase inhibitors under study include galanthamine and related compounds, heptyl-physostigmine, metrifonate, and ENA-713. Metrifonate is considered a pro-drug that is transformed into a relatively nonselective cholinesterase inhibitor. In early studies it exerted beneficial effects on cognition at medium to high doses and was not associated with significant liver function abnormalities. ENA-713 (also known as Exelon) belongs to the carbamate class and is a relatively selective inhibitor of cortical and hippocampal acetylcholinesterase. A 26-week multicenter study of ENA-713 yielded encouraging results with doses of 6 to 12 mg/day.

Cholinergic Agonists

The muscarinic type of acetylcholine (cholinergic) receptors in the brain have important functions in learning and memory. Although the postsynaptic receptors are relatively unaffected in Alzheimer's disease, the presynaptic receptors that regulate acetylcholine release are decreased. By giving a cholinergic agonist, the acetylcholine activity theoretically increases. The first cholinergic agonists studied in Alzheimer's disease were bethanechol, oxotremorine, pilocarpine, RS-86, and arecholine. Bethanechol produced small benefits but had to be given into the ventricle of the brain, and the risks of administration outweighed the benefits. Use of arecholine was limited by the need for frequent intravenous (IV) administration, while results with oxotremorine and pilocarpine were not encouraging. RS-86 had mixed results but significant side effects. Other newer cholinergic agonists are being studied and are hoped to have less toxicity and more selective actions.

DOPAMINERGIC AND ANTIOXIDANT STRATEGIES

Other neurotransmitters reportedly decreased in Alzheimer's disease patients include serotonin, norepinephrine, and dopamine, while alterations in somatostatin, corticotropin-releasing factor, and gamma aminobutyric acid (GABA) may also play important roles. Dopamine has been extensively studied, and a traditional medication for Parkinson's disease, L-deprenyl (also known as selegiline), has been tried in patients with Alzheimer's disease. Parkinson's disease is caused by a deficiency of dopamine resulting from a loss of the nerve cells that produce it. L-deprenyl is believed to work by increasing central dopamine, but it may also contribute to preservation of surviving neurons from neurotoxins that use oxidative/free radical mechanisms.

The largest study with L-deprenyl is from the National Institute of Aging's Alzheimer's Disease Cooperative Study trial, which began in 1992. This study has enrolled 342 patients with mild to moderate Alzheimer's disease and has compared whether L-deprenyl and vitamin E (an antioxidant) can slow progression of the disease. Data is now being analyzed. However, interest in antioxidants for treatment of Alzheimer's disease is growing. Researchers at the Salk Institute found that in cell culture the neurotoxicity of β-amyloid may result from its effects on nerve cells to increase hydrogen peroxide production. Hydrogen peroxide then releases free radicals, which can damage cell components. Antioxidants, such as vitamin E, could block the toxic effects of β-amyloid. Two other compounds that are similar to L-deprenyl are also being studied in other trials with Alzheimer's disease and Parkinson's disease patients: lazabemide (RO10-6327) and MDL 72,974A.

NMDA AND AMPA RECEPTOR-RELATED STRATEGIES

Glutamate is another major neurotransmitter in the central nervous system with important roles in learning and memory. It acts on four post-synaptic receptors, two of which are called N-methyl-D-aspartate (NMDA) and alpha-amino-3-hydroxy-5-methyl-4-isoxazolepropionic acid (AMPA) receptors. Glutamate as well as abnormal accumulations of β-amyloid are now believed to contribute to the degeneration of nerve cells in patients with Alzheimer's disease. When glutamate exerts neurotoxic effects by activating these post-synaptic receptors, it is called excitotoxicity. An increase in intracellular calcium is involved in these events. In cell cultures glutamate can induce neurofibrillary tangles, and β-amyloid or its precursor protein can increase the excitotoxic effects of glutamate or NMDA.

NMDA Receptor Strategies

Early research efforts indicated that the density of the NMDA receptor decreases in the cortical and hippocampal regions of the brain with aging and as a result of Alzheimer's disease. Some researchers hypothesized that in response to the reduced receptor density with aging, the receptor function increases.

NMDA agonists. Initial treatment strategies in treating Alzheimer's disease involved the use of agonists at the NMDA receptors (compounds that bind to the receptor and cause it to function). Although the compound L-glutamate showed some positive effects on memory and learning in animal models, it was not studied further due to neurotoxic effects. After observation of these adverse effects, very few studies with NMDA itself or other NMDA agonists were pursued.

Glycine agonists. There are several sites on the NMDA receptor where chemicals can bind and modify the action of the receptor. The glycine-B receptor is adjacent to the NMDA receptor and can indirectly activate it. Recent studies with d-cycloserine, a partial glycine agonist, have had mixed results: 108 patients with mild to moderate Alzheimer's disease received d-cycloserine or a placebo for ten weeks, and those who received the intermediate dosage of medication demonstrated significant improvements on memory testing. An earlier study with larger numbers of patients in a 26-week treatment period also demonstrated improvements on one section of a memory test with the same dosage of d-cycloserine. However, there were no other significant differences from the placebo group. Neither were any effects observed when cycloserine was administered to 40 patients for 6 months. Another agent, milacemide, is called a pro-drug because it is converted to glycinamide and glycine once it crosses the blood-brain barrier. Although it improved memory in animal studies, a large multicenter trial with Alzheimer's disease patients did not demonstrate any significant benefit.

NMDA receptor antagonists. Also in early stages of study are NMDA receptor antagonists, such as memantine. In animal models this compound appears to improve cognition, but its mechanism of action remains incompletely understood. Clinical trials in patients with Parkinson's disease have demonstrated some positive results, and other NMDA receptor antagonist compounds are being investigated.

AMPA receptor strategies. Another type of glutamate receptor is the AMPA receptor. Ampakines, chemicals that increase signal transmission through the AMPA receptor, are also projected to be possible treatments for patients with Alzheimer's disease. Ampakine CX-516, discovered in 1991 by Dr. Gary Lynch and coworkers at the University of California, Irvine, was tested in animals in 1993. Trials with healthy adults started in 1994 and have thus far shown encouraging improvements in memory, particularly with older subjects. Additional trials are scheduled to begin in 1997 under the direction of the National Institute of Health.

NOOTROPICS

This category of medications is chemically related to γ-aminobutyric acid (GABA), but apparently they do not exert GABA-like effects. Their mechanism of action remains poorly understood but was originally thought to involve effects on energy metabolism. Then research indicated other possible mechanisms of the nootropics: stimulation of central cholinergic activity, enhancement of NMDA receptor density in aging, and steroid sensitivity of the memory-enhancing effects. The issue is complicated by observations that different medications have different results in studies.

Within the group of nootropics are piracetam, oxiracetam, pramiractam, and aniracetam. Although results from animal studies initially appeared promising, few significant results have been seen in several studies with these medications in Alzheimer's disease.

NEUROTROPHIC FACTORS

Neurotrophic factors such as nerve growth factor (NGF), brain-derived neurotrophic factor (BDNF), and neurotrophin-3 (NT-3) are believed to be important in nerve cell maintenance and repair. Recent work has suggested that increased levels of NGF are present in the brains of patients with Alzheimer's disease, except in the region of the basal nucleus of Meynert. It is possible that these increased levels of cerebral NGF may be secondary to degenerative changes in the basal forebrain cholinergic system.

Researchers hypothesized that increased availability of these neurotrophic factors might be beneficial to Alzheimer's disease patients to potentially slow or counteract cholinergic degeneration. However, NGF does not cross the blood-brain barrier and would have to be administered directly into the brain or attached to a carrier molecule that could cross the blood-brain barrier.

Two alternatives have been suggested:

1. A compound known as K-252, which can stimulate the neurotrophin NT-3 outside the body in cell systems, has also been discovered.
2. Cells genetically engineered to produce NGF have been implanted into specific brain areas of rats.

The National Institute of Aging has actively supported this innovative preclinical work through their Drug Discovery Groups for Alzheimer's Disease, but further trials must be performed to determine if these compounds would be useful in patients.

GANGLIOSIDES

While these compounds are found naturally in cell membranes, the highest concentrations are in the brain, especially in the connections between nerve cells. Ganglioside content is significantly decreased in the brains of patients with Alzheimer's disease, and ganglioside GM1 has been proposed as a therapeutic agent in the disease. This agent reportedly increases nerve cell responsiveness to neurotrophic factors and helps nerves rebuild and replace lost nerve endings. Early studies with intramuscular or intravenously injected ganglioside GM1 revealed that very little of the drug penetrates the blood-brain barrier. The drug was then administered in five Alzheimer's disease patients by a reservoir and tubing connected directly into the lateral ventricle of the brain. The disease process was halted in all five patients after one year of treatment. Subsequently, the drug was found to have higher serum concentrations by subcutaneous administration but longer elimination times after intramuscular injection. In a short, double-blind trial with 12 patients with probable Alzheimer's disease who received 6 weeks of placebo and 6 weeks of intramuscular ganglioside GM1, cognitive improvement was not seen. Further studies are needed to determine the utility of this agent.

NONSTEROIDAL ANTIINFLAMMATORY DRUGS (NSAIDS)

Initial interest in these medications began after observations that fewer patients with arthritis, particularly rheumatoid arthritis, had Alzheimer's disease. Then epidemiologic studies discovered a similar inverse association of Alzheimer's disease with steroids and antiinflammatory treatments including steroids and NSAIDs. NSAIDs include such medications as indomethacin, ibuprofen, naproxen, aspirin, and several others available only by prescription. The degree of Alzheimer's disease risk reduction with NSAIDs has varied from 50% to 75% in the studies, although results with aspirin have been less consistent.

The proposed mechanism by which these drugs work involves an inflammatory process occurring in the brain of patients with Alzheimer's disease. Part of the normal immune system involves a pathway of factors called complement. When the body recognizes a danger, the complement factors are activated to protect the body. Researchers have recognized that some of the materials associated with senile plaques, such as β-amyloid protein, can bind complement factors and start the inflammatory response. NSAIDs and steroids act by decreasing the inflammatory response. Of note, a recent report indicates that extended use of H2 (histamine 2)-blocking drugs (such as cimetidine, ranitidine, famotidine, nizatidine) may also delay the onset of Alzheimer's disease, independent of NSAIDs, as histamine potentiates the inflammatory events.

Two published studies have described treatment of Alzheimer's disease with these medications. A preliminary report with indomethacin lasting 6 months and a newer report with daily NSAIDs or aspirin lasting 12 months indicated that patients taking these medications had less cognitive decline during the study period. Currently, the National Institute of Aging's Alzheimer's Disease Cooperative Study is studying the steroid prednisone in 150 patients with mild to moderate Alzheimer's disease to determine if this drug can slow the course of the disease. Although more potent than NSAIDs, it is also associated with more potential side effects, and the study should yield important information about the risks versus benefits of using steroids in treating Alzheimer's disease.

At this point, further studies are definitely needed before these medications could be recommended. Patients and subjects at risk for Alzheimer's disease should not start these medications without other indications and then only after discussion with a physician because of the potential for side effects and interactions with other drugs.

CALCIUM CHANNEL BLOCKERS

Researchers now have a heightened awareness of calcium's role in neurodegenerative diseases. Research has found that nerve cells from aged rats have approximately three times as many channels to allow calcium into the cells as those from young rats, and the calcium ion channel density appeared to be associated with poorer results on learning tasks. They hypothesized that calcium channel density may be related to an increased vulnerability to neurotoxic damage. A few years ago, intracellular free calcium was thought to play a role in nerve cell damage in Alzheimer's disease because of its activation of some destructive enzymes, and calcium channel blocking drugs began to be tested in patients.

Nimodipine

Although the drug nimodipine is a calcium channel blocker similar to those used to treat hypertension, it has a greater effect on cerebral arteries than on other arteries. It is currently approved for use in the United States for preventing ischemic deficits in patients with subarachnoid hemorrhage from ruptured congenital cerebral aneurysms. These beneficial effects on cerebral blood flow, together with the calcium channel blocking properties, led to its marketing in Europe as a cognitive enhancer. Clinical trials have reported beneficial effects in patients with dementia treated with nimodipine over a 10- to 12-week period and when compared with Hydergine and placebo. However, further studies are needed to determine its utility in treating Alzheimer's disease.

OTHER APPROACHES

Acetyl-L-Carnitine (ALCAR)

ALCAR is the acetyl ester of L-carnitine and has a structure very similar to acetylcholine. It reportedly has several effects relevant to neuronal metabolism. It functions as an intracellular carrier of acetyl groups for the synthesis of acetylcholine, increases the activity of choline acetyltransferase and the high-affinity uptake of choline, protects nerve cells against oxidative injuries, helps stabilize neuronal membranes, and helps aging nerve cells retain nerve growth factor binding properties. Its actions on a short-term basis, however, are probably not directly through classical neurotransmitter systems. Clinical trials have suggested ALCAR may slow the rate of deterioration in Alzheimer's disease patients, but studies are ongoing.

Angiotensin Converting Enzyme (ACE) Inhibitors

The role of these medications, such as captopril and ceranapril (SQ 29,852), remains uncertain in dementia. Some animal studies have suggested that ACE inhibitors improve memory, and increased ACE activity has been observed in some parts of the brain of Alzheimer's disease patients. Captopril and ceranapril have also been reported in animal studies to protect the cerebral cortical microcirculation against acute hypotension, but further studies are needed to clarify this issue.

Estrogen

Estrogen is proposed to have several effects on decreasing the risk of Alzheimer's disease:

1. It may promote survival and growth of cholinergic nerve cells through actions on nerve growth factor.
2. It may alter the processing of amyloid precursor protein, causing less deposition of β-amyloid and a reduction in senile plaques.
3. While β-amyloid may cause constriction of blood vessels, estrogen may increase cerebral blood flow by stimulation of the blood vessel dilator endothelial derived relaxing factor, and inhibit the blood vessel constrictor endothelin.

Two main studies have reported that women treated with estrogen had significantly less AD. The latter researchers commented that estrogen did not prevent AD, but those who took it had later onset of the disease. Of 1124 elderly women in the study, the incidence of Alzheimer's disease was 16.3% in those not taking estrogen and only 5.8% in those receiving it. Three other studies failed to find a significant relationship between estrogen usage and risk of Alzheimer's, but each of these studies had limitations.

An ongoing study called the Women's Health Initiative Memory Study (WHI-MS) of Estrogen and Alzheimer's disease will enroll over 8,000 women at least 65 years of age, evaluate the effectiveness of estrogen in delaying the onset of Alzheimer's disease, and follow subjects at least 6 years.

A few very small studies have been published that describe beneficial effects of estrogen in the treatment of Alzheimer's disease. In addition, the tacrine clinical trial data was reanalyzed for improvement in women receiving both estrogen and tacrine. There appeared to be a synergistic interaction between the two drugs. However, at this point available information is inadequate to conjecture that estrogen could prevent or treat Alzheimer's disease, and further studies are needed.

DRUG DEVELOPMENT

The drug development process may appear slow and difficult, but it contains many precautions to prevent unsafe medications from being tested in humans. After discovery of a potential drug, it must go through rigorous studies in the laboratory and in animals (preclinical studies) for a period of 1 to 6 years. If it needs to be chemically changed to increase effectiveness, further preclinical testing is required. Then if the drug appears to have some effectiveness in a disease and a reasonable safety profile, the pharmaceutical company developing the agent files an Investigational New Drug (IND) application with the FDA. Clinical trials may begin 30 days later if the FDA does not object.

The clinical trials are divided into three phases:

- Phase I studies involve 20 to 100 healthy subjects and aim to learn about dosage levels; absorption, break down, and elimination in the body; and further safety information.
- Phase II studies are larger, including 100 to 300 individuals with the disease under study. Additional safety information and preliminary efficacy data are gathered.
- Phase III studies, requiring an additional 2 to 4 years, include between 1000 and 3000 patients with the disease under study to ensure adequate information is collected to judge safety and efficacy.

If problems are detected at any point in the development process, the studies may be stopped, but if the drug appears promising, the pharmaceutical company will file a New Drug Application (NDA) with the FDA. The NDA is a very detailed report including all the information learned about the drug in the studies, which the FDA will study and eventually grant approval for marketing if the drug is determined to be safe and effective. The pharmaceutical company must continue to monitor safety information on every reported adverse experience after marketing because rare adverse effects (such as occurring 1 per 100,000 or less) may only be detected when large numbers of patients receive the drug.

SUMMARY

A wide variety of agents are now under study for the treatment and even prevention of Alzheimer's disease. It must be emphasized that while some of these agents are commercially available for other uses, only tacrine and donepezil are approved by the Food and Drug Administration for use in treating Alzheimer's disease. Much work remains to be performed to determine if the benefits of each of the other drugs will outweigh the risks, and under what circumstances the drugs should be used, if at all. At this point, some of the agents have only been studied in animals, while others have been studied in healthy adults. The results may differ significantly from those in patients with Alzheimer's disease, and may differ further depending on the progression of the disease and degree of concurrent illnesses. Therefore, findings with each drug mentioned in this chapter must be considered in light of its stage in the drug development process. Finally, a person should not begin any of these agents without careful discussion with his or her physician, as some agents may have harmful interactions with other drugs and underlying diseases.

With serious and life-threatening diseases, such as Alzheimer's disease, several steps are underway to speed up the drug development process. The FDA has allowed some Phase II studies to be combined with Phase III studies. In addition, collaboration between government, academic researchers, pharmaceutical companies, and biotechnology firms is helping to hasten the development of possible new treatments. The Alzheimers's Association has prepared drug fact sheets for Alzheimer's disease patients who are interested in participating in clinical trials with a new medication, and these are available from either the local chapter or the national office. In the coming years, hope is alive and well that new treatments and even prevention efforts will become available for Alzheimer's disease.

BIBLIOGRAPHY

Aisen PS, Davis KL: Inflammatory mechanisms in Alzheimer's disease: implications for therapy, *Am J Psychiatry* 151:1105-1113, 1994.

Alzheimer's Association: Advances in Alzheimer research. From test tube to treatment: the rigorous road of drug testing, *Alzheimer's Association National Newsletter* 16 (3):1A-4A, 1996.

Antuono PG: Effectiveness and safety of velnacrine for the treatment of Alzheimer's disease: a double-blind, placebo-controlled study, *Arch Intern Med* 155:1766-1772, 1995.

Barrett-Connor E, Kritz-Silverstein D: Estrogen replacement therapy and cognitive function in older women, *JAMA* 260:2637-2641, 1993.

Birge SJ: Is there a role for estrogen replacement therapy in the prevention and treatment of dementia? *J Am Geriatr Soc* 44:865-870, 1996.

Bores GM, Huger FP, Petko W et al: Pharmacologic evaluation of novel Alzheimer's disease therapeutics: acetylcholinesterase inhibitors related to galanthamine, *J Pharmacol Exp Ther* 277:728-738, 1996.

Breitner JC, Gau BA, Welsh KA et al: Inverse association of anti-inflammatory treatments and Alzheimer's disease: initial results of a co-twin control study, *Neurology* 44:227-232, 1994.

Breitner JC, Welsh KA, Helms MJ et al: Delayed onset of Alzheimer's disease with nonsteroidal anti-inflammatory and histamine H2 blocking drugs, *Neurobiol Aging* 16:523-530, 1995.

Brenner DE, Kukull WA, Stergachis A et al: Postmenopausal estrogen replacement therapy and the risk of Alzheimer's disease: a population-based case-control study, *Am J Epidemiol* 140:262-267, 1994.

Bruno G, Scaccianoce S, Bonamini M et al: Acetyl-L-carnitine in Alzheimer's disease: a short-term study on CSF neurotransmitters and neuropeptides, *Alzheimer Dis Assoc Disord* 9:128-131, 1995.

Buckholtz NS: Alzheimer's disease drug development and testing at the National Institute on Aging, *Psychopharm Bull* 30:15-17, 1994.

Cohen SA, Müller WE: Age-related alterations of NMDA-receptor properties in the mouse forebrain: partial restoration by chronic phosphatidyl-serine treatment, *Brain Res* 548:174-180, 1992.

Crutcher KA, Scott SA, Liang S et al: Detection of NGF-like activity in human brain tissue: increased levels in Alzheimer's disease, *J Neurosci* 13:2540-2550, 1993.

Davis KL, Powchik P: Tacrine, *Lancet* 345:625-630, 1995.

Doraiswamy PM: Current cholinergic therapy for symptoms of Alzheimer's disease, *Primary Psychiatr* 3:56-68, 1996.

Dysken MW, Mendels J, LeWitt P et al: Milacemide: A placebo-controlled study in senile dementia of the Alzheimer type, *J Am Geriatr Soc* 40:503-506, 1992.

Fakouhi TD, Jhee SS, Sramek J et al: Evaluation of cycloserine in the treatment of Alzheimer's disease, *J Geriatr Psychiatry Neurol* 8:226-230, 1995.

Fillit H, Weinreb H, Cholst I: Observations in a preliminary open trial of estradiol therapy for senile dementia (Alzheimer's type), *Psychoneuroendocrinology* 2:337-345, 1986.

Flicker C, Ferris SH, Kalkstein D et al: A double-blind, placebo-controlled crossover study of ganglioside GM1 treatment for Alzheimer's disease, *Am J Psychiatry* 151:126-129, 1994.

Gage FH, Fisher LJ: Genetically modified cells for intracellular transplantation, *Basic Clin Aspects Neurosci* 5:51-51, 1993.

Graves AB, White E, Koepsell TD et al: A case-control study of Alzheimer's disease, *Ann Neurol* 28:766-774, 1990.

Gray CW, Patel AJ: Neurodegeneration mediated by glutamate and beta-amyloid peptide: a comparison and possible interaction, *Brain Res* 691:169-179, 1995.

Green RC, Goldstein FC, Auchus AP et al: Treatment trial of oxiracetam in Alzheimer's disease, *Arch Neurol* 49:1135-1136, 1992.

Harbaugh RE, Reeder TM, Senter HJ et al: Intracerebroventricular bethanecol chloride infusion in Alzheimer's disease: results of a collaborative, double-blind study, *J Neurosurg* 71:481-486, 1989.

Hellweg R, Jockers-Scherübl M: Neurotrophic factors in memory disorders, *Life Sci* 55:216-2169, 1994.

Henderson VW, Paganini-Hill A, Emanuel CK et al: Estrogen replacement therapy in older women: comparisons between Alzheimer's disease cases and nondemented control subjects, *Arch Neurol* 51:896-900, 1994.

Hollister L, Gruber N: Drug treatment of Alzheimer's disease. Effects on care giver burden and patient quality of life, *Drugs Aging* 8:47-55, 1996.

Honjo H, Ogino Y, Naitoh K et al: In vivo effects by estrone sulfate in the central nervous system—senile dementia (Alzheimer's type), *J Steroid Biochem* 34:521-525, 1989.

Jaffe AB, Toran-Allerand CD, Greengard P et al: Estrogen regulates metabolism of Alzheimer's amyloid beta precursor protein, *J Biol Chem* 269:13065-13068, 1994.

Kanowski S, Fischof P, Hiersemenzel R et al: Wirksamkeitsnachweis von nootropika am beispiel von Nimodipin - ein beitrag zur entwicklung geeigneter klinischer prufmodelle, *Zeitscrift fur Gerontopsychologie und Psychiatrie* 1:35-44, 1988.

Knapp MJ, Knopman DS, Solomon PR et al: A 30-week randomized controlled trial of high-dose tacrine in patients with Alzheimer's disease, *JAMA* 271:985-991, 1994.

Knusel B, Hefti F: K-252 compounds: Modulators of neurotrophin signal transduction, *J Neurochem* 59:1987-1996, 1992.

Kuller LH: Hormone replacement therapy and its potential relationship to dementia, *J Am Geriatr Soc* 44:878-880, 1996.

McGeer PL, McGeer EG: Anti-inflammatory drugs in the fight against Alzheimer's disease, *Ann NY Acad Sci* 777:213-220, 1996.

McGeer PL, Schulzer M, McGeer EG: Arthritis and anti-inflammatory agents as possible protective factors for Alzheimer's disease: a review of 17 epidemiologic studies: *Neurology* 47:425-432, 1996.

Marx J: Searching for drugs that combat Alzheimer's, *Science* 273:50-53, 1996.

Mattson MP, Barger SW, Cheng B et al: beta-amyloid precursor protein metabolites and loss of neuronal Ca^{2+} homeostasis in Alzheimer's disease, *Trends Neurosci* 16:409-414, 1993.

Mohr E, Knott V, Sampson M et al: Cognitive and quantified electroencephalographic correlates of cycloserine treatment in Alzheimer's disease, *Clin Neuropharmacol* 18:28-38, 1995.

Mondadori C: In search of the mechanism of action of the nootropics: new insights and potential clinical implications, *Life Sci* 55:2171-2178, 1994.

Moore NC, Gershon S: The brain-renin-angiotensin system and behavior, *Dementia* 1/4:225-236, 1990.

Müller WE, Mutschler E, Riederer P: Noncompetitive NMDA receptor antagonists with fast open-channel blocking kinetics and strong voltage-dependency as potential therapeutic agents for Alzheimer's dementia, *Pharmacopsychiatry* 28:113-124, 1995.

Müller WE, Scheuer K, Stoll S: Glutaminergic treatment strategies for age-related memory disorders, *Life Sci* 55:2147-2153, 1994.

Ohkura T, Isse K, Akazawa K et al: Evaluation of estrogen treatment in female patients with dementia of the Alzheimer's type, *Endocrine J* 41:361-371, 1994.

Ohkura T, Isse K, Akazawa K et al: Long-term estrogen replacement therapy in female patients with dementia of the Alzheimer's type: seven case reports, *Dementia* 6:99-107, 1995.

Paganini-Hill A, Henderson VW: Estrogen deficiency and risk of Alzheimer's disease in women, *Am J Epidemiol* 104:256-261, 1994.

Parnetti L: Clinical pharmacokinetics of drugs for Alzheimer's disease, *Clin Pharmacokinet* 29:110-129, 1995.

Polderman KH, Coen D, Stehouwer A et al: Influence of sex hormones on plasma endothelin levels, *Ann Intern Med* 118:429-432, 1993.

Rich JB, Rasmusson DX, Folstein MF et al: Nonsteroidal anti-inflammatory drugs in Alzheimer's disease, *Neurology* 45:51-55, 1995.

Rogers J, Kirby LC, Hempelman SR et al: Clinical trial of indomethacin in Alzheimer's disease, *Neurology* 43:1609-1611, 1993.

Rogers SL, Doody R, Mohs R et al: E2020 produces both clinical global and cognitive test improvement in patients with mild to moderately severe Alzheimer's disease (AD): results of a 30-week phase III trial, *Neurology* 46:A217, 1996.

Rogers SL, Perdomo C, Friedhoff LT: Clinical benefits are maintained during long-term treatment of Alzheimer's disease with the acetylcholinesterase inhibitor, E2020, *Eur Neuropsychopharmacol* 5:386, 1995.

Rogers SL, Friedhoff LT, the Donepezil Study Group. The efficacy and safety of donepezil in patients with Alzheimer's disease: results of a US multicentre, randomized, double-blind, placebo-controlled trial, *Dementia* 7:293-303, 1996.

Sadoshima S, Nagao T, Ibayashi S et al: Inhibition of angiotensin-converting enzyme modulates the autoregulation of regional cerebral blood flow in hypertensive rats, *Hypertension* 23:781-785, 1994.

Sano M, Bell K, Cote L et al: Double-blind parallel design pilot study of acetyl levocarnitine in patients with Alzheimer's disease, *Arch Neurol* 49:1137-1141, 1992.

Schneider LS, Farlow MK, Henderson VW et al: Estrogen replacement therapy may enhance response to tacrine in women with Alzheimer's disease, *Neurology* 45(Suppl):A288, 1995.

Schneider LS, Farlow MR, Henderson VW et al: Effects of estrogen replacement therapy on response to tacrine in patients with Alzheimer's disease, *Neurology* 46:1580-1584, 1996.

Schneider LS, Olin JT: Overview of clinical trials of Hydergine in dementia, *Arch Neurol* 51:787-798, 1994.

Schneider LS, Tariot PN: Emerging drugs for Alzheimer's disease: mechanisms of action and prospects for cognitive enhancing medications, *Med Clin North Am* 78:911-934, 1994.

Schwartz BL, Hashtroudi S, Herting RL et al: d-Cycloserine enhances implicit memory in Alzheimer patients, *Neurology* 46:420-424, 1996.

Scott SA, Mufson EJ, Weingartner JA et al: Nerve growth factor in Alzheimer's disease: increased levels throughout the brain coupled with declines in nucleus basalis, *J Neurosci* 15:6213-6221, 1995.

Simpkins JW, Singh M, Bishop J: The potential role for estrogen replacement therapy in the treatment of the cognitive decline and neurodegeneration associated with Alzheimer's disease, *Neurobiol Aging* 15(Suppl 2):S195-S197, 1994.

Spagnoli A, Lucca U, Menace G et al: Long-term acetyl-L-carnitine treatment in Alzheimer's disease, *Neurology* 41:1726-1732, 1991.

Sramek JJ, Anand R, Wardle TS et al: Safety/tolerability trial of SDZ ENA 713 in patients with probable Alzheimer's disease, *Life Sci* 58:1201-1207, 1996.

Summers WK, Majovski LV, Marsh GM et al: Oral tetra-hydro-amino-acridine in long-term treatment of senile dementia, Alzheimer's type, *N Engl J Med* 315:1241-1245, 1986.

Svennerholm L: Gangliosides—a new therapeutic agent against stroke and Alzheimer's disease, *Life Sci* 55:2125-2134, 1994.

Tam SW, Zaczek R: Linopiridine. A depolarization-activated releaser or transmitters for treatment of dementia, *Adv Exp Med Biol* 363:47-56, 1995.

Tang M-X, Jacobs D, Stern Y et al: Effect of estrogen during menopause on risk and age at onset of Alzheimer's disease, *Lancet* 348:429-432, 1996.

Tariot PN, Schneider LS, Patel SV et al: Alzheimer's disease and (−)-deprenyl: rationales and findings. In Szeleny I, editor: *Inhibitors of monoamine oxidase B: pharmacology and clinical use in neurodegenerative disorders,* Basel, 1993, Birkhauser Verlag AG, pp: 301-307.

Thibault O, Landfield PW: Increase in single L-type calcium channels in hippocampal neurons during aging, *Science* 272:1017-1020, 1996.

Thomas RJ: Excitatory amino acids in health and disease, *J Am Geriatr Soc* 43:1279-1289, 1995.

Tollefson GD: Short term effects of the calcium channel blocker nimodipine (Bay-e 9736) in the management of primary degenerative dementia, *Biol Psychiatry* 27:1133-1142, 1990.

Toran-Allerand CD, Miranda RC, Bentham WD et al: Estrogen receptors colocalize with low affinity nerve growth factor receptors in cholinergic neurons of the basal forebrain, *Proc Natl Acad Sci USA* 89:4668-4672, 1992.

Van Buren G, Yang D, Clark KE: Estrogen-induced uterine vasodilatation is antagonized by L-nitroarginine methylester, an inhibitor of nitric oxide synthesis, *Am J Obstet Gynecol* 16:828-833, 1992.

Vernon MW, Sorkin EM: Piracetam: An overview of its pharmacological properties and a review of its therapeutic use in senile cognitive disorders, *Drugs Aging* 1:17-35, 1991.

Watkins PB, Zimmerman HJ, Knapp MJ et al: Hepatotoxic effects of tacrine administration in patients with Alzheimer's disease, *JAMA* 271:992-998, 1994.

Woo JK, Lantz MS: Alzheimer's disease: how to give and monitor tacrine therapy, *Geriatrics* 50:50-53, 1995.

Urinary and Fecal Incontinence

Ronald C Hamdy
Larry B Hudgins

*They say man has succeeded where the animals
fail because of the clever use of his hands, yet
when compared to the hands, the sphincter ani
is far superior. If you place into your cupped
hands a mixture of fluid, solid and gas and then
through an opening at the bottom, try to let only
the gas escape, you will fail. Yet the sphincter ani
can do it. The sphincter apparently can differentiate between solid, fluid and gas. It apparently can
tell whether its owner is alone or with someone,
whether standing up or sitting down, whether his
owner has his pants on or off. No other muscle in
the body is such a protector of the dignity of
man, yet so ready to come to his relief. A muscle
like this is worth protecting.*

—Walter C. Bornemeier

Urinary incontinence is the inappropriate and involuntary passage of urine. Its
exact prevalence is difficult to establish because it can occur in varying degrees
and the patient may deny having the problem. Its prevalence is particularly
difficult to determine in patients with Alzheimer's disease.

Although the underlying dementia may be responsible for some of the
incontinence, other conditions that are treatable and reversible are often present.
Thus the caregiver has the initial burden of recognizing incontinence and
arranging for further evaluation of the patient. Urinary incontinence is an issue
of quality of life that should be neither ignored nor denied.

RELUCTANCE TO ADMIT INCONTINENCE

In the early stages of Alzheimer's disease, when the patient still has insight into
his condition, he may try to conceal his incontinence so as not to draw the

attention of his cohabitants and social contacts. The patient recognizes he has a problem with his mental state, which he may find difficult to cope with and may try to hide from his immediate social contacts. Rather than admitting the additional problem of urinary incontinence and seeking medical advice, the patient often resorts to concealing it. He may hide soiled clothes or wear towels in his underwear. Often the patient feels ashamed of having lost control over his bodily functions and may be embarrassed to mention the problem. Finally, the patient may be afraid that he will be forced to accept institutional care and give up his possessions and independence. In fact, urinary incontinence often is the factor that convinces relatives and caregivers that institutionalization is necessary.

> Urinary incontinence is often the main reason for admission to a nursing home.

Frequently, urinary incontinence seen in the early stages of Alzheimer's disease is not related to the disease itself but is caused by an unrelated condition that often can be easily treated. Unfortunately, the patient often feels that the urinary incontinence represents another step in his gradual and relentless deterioration and loss of control over his mind and body. This attitude usually leads to profound depression punctuated by bouts of irritability when the patient becomes angry with himself and fails to understand what is happening to him.

In late stages of Alzheimer's disease, urinary incontinence often is the result of the underlying condition and the global reduction in the number of cerebral cortical neurons (nerve cells). Because of this reduction in neurons, no inhibitory impulses are sent out from the micturition center in the brain to the urinary bladder. Alternatively, the patient may urinate in inappropriate places because he is unaware of his environment and is disoriented. At this stage, the patient may also become incontinent of feces.

DISCUSSING INCONTINENCE

The treating physician and other caregivers must be alert to the problem of urinary incontinence and need to be prepared to discuss it openly with the patient before its impact undermines the patient's self-confidence, worsens his general condition, and disrupts his precarious equilibrium with his environment. The caregivers must stress that urinary incontinence is not necessarily related to Alzheimer's disease and that it may be possible to correct it. Unfortunately, a conspiracy of silence often develops when the patient, the relatives, and the caregivers know that the patient is incontinent and yet pretend not to have noticed it.

> Urinary incontinence is a quality of life issue that should neither be denied nor ignored.

It is remarkable how often the patient's relatives try to conceal the problem. When questioned, they may deny that their relative is incontinent until the situation becomes intolerable, in which case often little can be done apart from seeking institutional care. This situation is unfortunate because, even in late cases, a reversible cause for urinary incontinence sometimes can be found and treated.

COMMON TYPES OF URINARY INCONTINENCE

A number of classifications for urinary incontinence have been proposed. However, patients often have more than one type simultaneously. The various types are not mutually exclusive; in fact, one type often potentiates another.

Types of Urinary Incontinence

- Stress incontinence
- Urge incontinence
- Overflow incontinence
- Functional incontinence
    Often more than one type of incontinence exists at the same time.

STRESS INCONTINENCE

Stress incontinence characteristically occurs when the patient stands up, coughs, laughs, or sneezes. The patient usually is dry in between these episodes and at night. Stress incontinence is caused by weakness of the urinary sphincter and/or perineal muscles, which allows small quantities of urine to be passed when the intraabdominal pressure is suddenly increased, and exceeds the pressure of the internal sphincter, as occurs during sneezing, laughing, and coughing.

Stress incontinence also may result from anatomical changes that interfere with the urethrovesical angle (the angle between the urinary bladder and urethra). In women, the change may be a result of several pregnancies and childbirth or surgical interventions. In addition, estrogen deficiency in postmenopausal women often leads to urethral inflammation, which is associated with senile vaginitis that may further aggravate stress incontinence. In these instances the diagnosis can be suspected by the appearance of the vagina and can be confirmed by microscopic examination of a mucosal smear, demonstrating findings of estrogen deficiency.

Characteristics of Stress Incontinence

- Urine is lost when abdominal pressure is increased.
- Small quantities of urine are lost during each episode.
- Patients are dry in between episodes and at night.
    Stress incontinence often is aggravated by diseases that cause muscle weakness or interfere with the patient's mobility, such as Parkinson's disease, strokes, or osteoarthritis. In these circumstances the patient may need to strain or heave himself as he struggles to get up from his chair. Such straining increases the intraabdominal pressure, which is transmitted to the urinary bladder. If this pressure exceeds that of the urinary sphincters, urinary incontinence results. A similar situation may arise when a patient tries to get up from a very low chair. Stress incontinence is more common in women and usually responds well to pelvic floor and perineal muscle exercises (Kegel exercises), provided the patient is able to comprehend and perform these exercises on a regular basis.

URGE INCONTINENCE

Urge incontinence, or detrusor instability, results when uninhibited contractions of the detrusor muscle (the muscle layer lining the urinary bladder) are strong enough to overcome the pressure of the internal urethral sphincter. This type of urinary incontinence, also known as unstable bladder, spastic bladder, or uninhibited bladder, is the most common kind occurring in old age. It is characterized by the almost continuous passage of small quantities of urine, with the patient being wet most of the time, day and night. The patient may feel the desire to micturate but be unable to postpone the act.

In late stages of Alzheimer's disease, detrusor instability is also caused by decreased cortical inhibition because the number or the integrity of the neurons in the micturition center of the brain is affected, in which case uninhibited contractions of the bladder occur before it reaches its full capacity. Stress incontinence often potentiates detrusor instability.

Detrusor instability also may be caused by local or pelvic processes, including inflammation, infection, prostatic hypertrophy, neoplasms, fecal impaction, uterine or bladder prolapse, and foreign bodies such as calculi in the urinary bladder.

Characteristics of Urge Incontinence

• Almost continuous passage of small quantities of urine.
• Patient is incontinent most of the time and at night.

When urinary tract infections are responsible for this type of urinary incontinence, the incontinence usually is associated with a certain amount of dysuria (pain or burning sensation while passing urine). It must be emphasized, however, that although acute bladder infection often is responsible for incontinence, chronic infection does not always lead to urinary incontinence.

OVERFLOW INCONTINENCE

As with other types of urinary incontinence, overflow incontinence occurs when the pressure inside the bladder exceeds that of the internal urinary sphincter. Unlike all other causes of urinary incontinence, however, overflow incontinence is caused by an actual obstruction to the flow of urine through the urethra. As a result of this obstruction, urine is retained in the bladder, which progressively increases in size. The pressure in the bladder also increases until it exceeds the pressure obstructing the flow of urine, at which point urine is discharged from the bladder until the pressure in the bladder falls below that of the obstructing lesion. Characteristically, patients with overflow incontinence have grossly distended bladders that can be palpated clinically, and the urine flow rate is significantly reduced, often amounting to no more than a dribble.

Characteristics of Overflow Incontinence

• Patient passes small quantities of urine.
• Urine flow is decreased.
• Bladder is grossly distended.

One of the main problems associated with overflow incontinence is incomplete emptying of the bladder. A residual volume of urine frequently is present, even at the end of a bout of incontinence (therefore the bladder is palpable). This residual urine invites bladder infections, which may spread to the kidneys via the ureters.

Many causes may be responsible for urinary obstruction and overflow incontinence, including fecal impaction, pelvic tumors, urethral stricture, bladder neoplasms, and calculi. In men, one of the most common causes of obstruction to the flow of urine is prostatic hypertrophy. In women, uterine or bladder prolapse may be responsible. The obstructing lesion may distort the urethra enough to cause an angulation that obstructs the flow of urine, thus interfering with micturition. Often when these patients try to micturate but cannot, they strain and increase the intra-abdominal pressure, which is transmitted not only to the intravesical pressure but also to the base of the bladder and the structures surrounding the urethra. As a result of this increased pressure, the angulation of the urethra becomes more pronounced and further increases the obstruction and difficulty in initiating micturition.

Then another problem develops. As the intra-abdominal pressure increases during straining, the venous return from the abdomen to the heart is reduced; this causes pelvic congestion and may further increase the volume of the obstructing lesion or the already distended prostate and complicate the initiation of micturition. The solution to this problem is a simple exercise that consists of taking deep breaths to decrease the pressure in the thoracic cavity and to increase the flow of blood from the abdomen and pelvic cavity to the heart. This action reduces the intraabdominal and intrapelvic congestion (including that of the pelvic structures and urethra), thus lessening the obstruction to the flow of urine and allowing micturition to take place.

Drug-Induced Urinary Retention and Overflow Incontinence

Occasionally, urinary retention and overflow incontinence are precipitated by medications, which include over-the-counter or prescribed antihistamines, sedatives, and other psychoactive drugs with anticholinergic properties. Many hypotensive medications affect continence via smooth muscle relaxation. This relaxation causes a dysfunctional bladder that allows urinary overfill.

Certain drugs that cause constipation, such as narcotics, antidiarrheals antidepressants and antihypertensive drugs, may lead to fecal impaction. In severe cases the fecal masses in the rectum may distort the urethra, alter the angle between the urethra and the urinary bladder, and cause urine retention and eventually overflow incontinence.

FUNCTIONAL INCONTINENCE

Functional incontinence is caused by factors outside the urinary bladder and its nervous connections, which remain intact. The patient is incontinent of urine because he is unable to postpone the act of micturition until a suitable place for voiding is reached. In other words, the patient feels the desire to micturate, may start taking appropriate steps to go to the toilet, but does not have enough time to

---

● Information the Physician Needs to Know:

- Is it genuine or "apparent" incontinence?
- Is it recent or long-standing?
- Is the patient urinary incontinent all the time, or is it episodic?
- What medication is the patient taking?
- Is the incontinence related to any physical activity?
- Any associated symptoms?
- Does the patient feel the urge to pass urine?
- Can the patient walk easily?

---

reach the toilet before micturition takes place. Stress incontinence often potentiates this type of urinary incontinence.

Characteristics of Functional Incontinence

- Patient feels the urge to pass urine.
- Patient is unable to reach a suitable voiding place in time.
- Patient is dry in between episodes of incontinence.

Incontinence and Curtailed Patient Mobility

Functional incontinence commonly results when a patient becomes less mobile. For instance, patients with severe osteoarthritis, Parkinson's disease, strokes, or any other condition that limits their physical capabilities may suffer from functional incontinence. In these situations it is often useful to advise patients to anticipate when the urinary bladder is likely to be filled and to attempt to empty it at regular intervals of 2 to 3 or 4 hours rather than waiting to feel the urge to micturate.

Incontinence and Inability to Locate Toilet

Patients with Alzheimer's disease are prone to develop functional incontinence because they cannot find their way to the toilet. They may become incontinent because the toilet is located too far from their bedroom or sitting area. The maximum distance between toilet and room or sitting area should be approximately 100 feet.

Similarly, if the way to the toilet is not clearly illuminated, or if there are many obstacles on the way to the toilet, the patient may not be able to reach the toilet before his bladder empties. Since a patient with Alzheimer's disease is likely to forget the way to the toilet, it is important to make sure that the patient has easy access to the toilet, that he knows the way there, and that the way is well marked with signs. Easy access is particularly important in institutions where a patient may wake up at night wanting to void his bladder but is confused and cannot recognize the way to the toilet. This situation is especially likely to occur during the first few days after admission to a nursing home or other similar institution.

If a patient with Alzheimer's disease cannot remember to empty his bladder at regular intervals, the caregiver may need to offer reminders. Alternatively, an alarm clock may be used to remind the patient to go to the toilet at certain intervals. In residential institutions a bladder-emptying schedule individualized for each patient may be helpful.

Incontinence and Physical Restraints

Functional incontinence may result from the use of physical restraints, which frequently are applied to patients who tend to wander, fall repeatedly, or become aggressive, such as those who have Alzheimer's disease. Even though patients in restraints may feel the urge to micturate, they cannot free themselves to reach the toilet in time. The development of urinary incontinence in such patients often is a serious setback and may considerably increase their degree of frustration, irritability, and even violence. Such behaviors serve to reassure the caregivers that using restraints was justified, and thus a vicious cycle is begun. Often the rate of deterioration is dramatically increased when sedatives are also prescribed to "quiet" the patient. As a result, the patient's condition declines rapidly, and the complications of being bedridden quickly appear. Caregivers who use restraints must make sure that the patients empty their bladders at regular intervals to avoid the problem of functional incontinence.

Incontinence and Inability to Communicate

Patients with anomia, aphasia, or other speech problems common to individuals with Alzheimer's disease may not be able to notify the caregivers appropriately of their desire to micturate. For this reason caregivers who care for such patients must develop a set of vocabulary signals or a ritual by which the patient notifies them of the desire to micturate. Body language is important to watch with Alzheimer's disease patients as restlessness, pulling at clothes, undressing, and other similar actions may indicate the need to urinate, and "accidents" can be prevented. If such communication is not possible, regular toileting should be instituted. This subject is discussed in greater detail in Chapter 16.

Drug-Induced Functional Incontinence

Functional incontinence can also be precipitated by drugs. Loop diuretic drugs (e.g., furosemide, bumetanide, and ethacrynic acid), which suddenly increase the volume of urine severalfold, may lead to functional incontinence, especially if the patient does not expect this result after taking the tablets. By suddenly increasing the volume of the bladder, loop diuretic drugs also may lead to pelvic congestion. In some instances, particularly in men with prostatic hypertrophy, this increased volume may lead to obstruction of the flow of urine and eventually to overflow incontinence.

Characteristically, incontinence induced by loop diuretic drugs develops shortly after these tablets have been taken. Patients, along with their relatives or the nursing staff, should be warned about the sudden increase in volume of urine that is likely to occur after this medication is taken. Also, patients taking loop diuretic drugs must be kept near a toilet, must know their way to the toilet, or must be taken to the toilet at regular intervals. Similarly, these patients should not be encouraged to go on outings or for walks within a few hours of taking the diuretic drug without making sure that they have ready access to a toilet.

> A bout of urinary incontinence, even an isolated one, can be so humiliating for the patient that it completely undermines self confidence and significantly accelerates the rate of decline.

Functional incontinence may occur during deep sleep and sometimes is induced by potent hypnotic drugs, when the patient's sleep is so deep that even though impulses are reaching the micturition center in the brain, they do not elicit any response from the other areas of the brain. Since no inhibitory impulses reach the sacral plexus, micturition takes place. In addition, alcohol use in the elderly should not be forgotten because of its potential for inducing polyuria, urinary frequency, urinary urgency, sedation, delirium, and immobility.

INFORMATION FOR THE PHYSICIAN

Although the patient's physician diagnoses the cause of the urinary incontinence, this task can be eased considerably if the right information is provided. The caregiver therefore plays an active and important role in diagnosing and managing the patient who has urinary incontinence.

Genuine Versus "Apparent" Urinary Incontinence

Even before referring the patient to a physician, the caregiver should attempt to determine whether the patient has genuine urinary incontinence or whether the leakage of urine was accidental, for example, having spilled from the urinal bottle or bedpan, as often happens with patients who are bedridden or confined to bed by either physical restraints or guard rails.

Characteristics of Incontinence

Recent versus long-standing incontinence. Once it has been established that the patient is genuinely incontinent of urine, the caregiver should determine whether the incontinence is of recent onset or has been a long-standing problem. Incontinence of recent onset has a better prognosis since it is usually the result of some reversible disease.

Is the patient incontinent of urine all the time? Attempts should be made to find out whether the patient is incontinent of urine all the time or if the incontinence tends to occur at specific times of the day or is related to taking certain drugs. Urinary incontinence that is worse late in the morning could be caused by a loop diuretic taken earlier in the morning. On the other hand, incontinence that is worse at night could be related to hypnotic preparations, which may profoundly inhibit the higher cortical (brain) functions. This condition is particularly likely if the patient is taking large doses of hypnotic drugs.

What medication is the patient taking? Since there are other possibilities for drug-induced urinary incontinence, it is essential to know all the medications that the patient is taking and whether they were prescribed by a physician or bought over the counter. Certain over-the-counter drugs intended to assist in weight loss may contain diuretic preparations. Other drugs prescribed for allergies or the common cold induce sedation or produce anticholinergic side effects that may lead to urine retention and eventually to overflow incontinence.

Elderly patients and those with Alzheimer's disease may take or may be given medications that were prescribed for their friends, neighbors, or relatives. The caregiver should inquire in detail about all medications that the patient is taking. The management of drug-induced urinary incontinence is fairly simple and consists of discontinuing the offending drug or substituting a less offensive one. Nevertheless, it is important to consult the patient's physician before discontinuing any prescribed medication, even if the drug is believed to be responsible for the urinary incontinence.

Are there any factors that precipitate incontinence? Next, the caregiver must determine whether the urinary incontinence is related to any of the patient's activities, such as standing up, coughing, laughing, or sneezing. If the patient tends to be incontinent while doing any of these activities, the diagnosis is probably stress incontinence. As noted earlier, this type of incontinence often responds to pelvic floor and perineal muscle exercise.

Are there any associated symptoms? If the patient is not incontinent all the time, it is helpful to know how many times he needs to micturate, the amount of urine passed, and whether there is any associated urgency, dysuria (pain on urination), scalding, difficulty in starting micturition, or dribbling. Urgency, dysuria, or scalding suggests a lower urinary tract infection. Difficulty in initiating micturition or dribbling suggests prostatic hypertrophy. Finally, the patient should be asked about bladder sensation and whether the act of micturition can be voluntarily initiated and interrupted.

How mobile is the patient? If the physician is given all this information before seeing the patient, the task of diagnosing the condition will be much easier and the diagnosis itself will more likely be accurate. The physician should be told about the patient's mobility and physical capabilities. Patients with disorders that interfere with their mobility are more likely to have urinary incontinence (functional incontinence) than are fully mobile patients. Obesity may be a factor in aggravating urinary incontinence by weakening the pelvic floor muscles.

Clinical Examination

Although the clinical history is frequently enough to suggest the type of urinary incontinence and its underlying cause, a thorough physical examination is also necessary. The examination should include a rectal examination and, in women, a vaginal examination. In stress incontinence, urine leakage can be assessed when the bladder is full and by asking the patient to strain. Feeling a distended, enlarged bladder after the patient has voided suggests bladder outlet obstruction or a weak bladder muscle. Pelvic examination is done to identify inflammation of the urethra or vagina, pelvic muscle laxity, and pelvic masses. Rectal examination should also help to identify perianal fissure, anal sphincter muscle tone, prostate size, and nodules.

Laboratory Investigations

After the physical examination, laboratory studies may be indicated, including a urinalysis, urine culture, blood chemistry profile, and sometimes x-ray imaging of the urinary tract. Fiberoptic cystoscopy with a direct view into the bladder is also sometimes necessary to check for the anatomy of possible lower urinary tract obstruction and to note intrinsic bladder lesions, inflammation, or tumor. Urodynamic studies may also be indicated, especially if it is suspected that there is more than one cause for the incontinence.

FECAL INCONTINENCE

Fecal incontinence is the involuntary passage of stools. Established fecal incontinence is both socially isolating and a common cause of institutionalization of the patient with dementia. Like urinary incontinence, fecal incontinence is commonly denied by the patient and sometimes underreported by the family caregivers. Both situations are unfortunate because the majority of affected patients can be helped.

COMMON CAUSES OF FECAL INCONTINENCE

Fecal Impaction

Fecal impaction is the most common cause of fecal incontinence in the elderly.

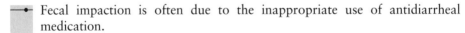 Fecal impaction is often due to the inappropriate use of antidiarrheal medication.

Injudicious use of antidiarrheal agents often precipitates fecal incontinence. These drugs are commonly overused by elderly patients and their caregivers. Initially, these compounds may be taken because of a bout of diarrhea or loose stools. If the patient continues to take the agent after the diarrhea has been controlled, constipation may result. In severe cases, fecal masses may become impacted in the rectum and later in the descending colon. Water is gradually absorbed from these fecal masses, which become hardened (fecoliths). In turn, these masses irritate the mucosal lining of the descending colon and rectum, increasing the production of mucus. This occurrence may be interpreted by the patient as another bout of diarrhea, and she may take more constipating agents. As time goes by, the fecal masses may reach the proximal part of the descending colon, where the fecal matter is semisolid. At this stage the fecal material bypasses the fecoliths and may reach the rectum. The patient may not be able to control its evacuation and may think that she is having another bout of diarrhea. As a result, constipating agents may be taken, thus completing the vicious cycle and worsening the condition.

Many elderly patients are highly conscious of their bowel habits and think that they should have a bowel movement daily. They report feeling terrible if they are not "regular." Therefore laxative use and abuse are rampant among the elderly. However, since daily use limits the effectiveness of the laxative as a cathartic, it allows constipation to persist.

Medications

Medications frequently taken by the elderly, either prescription or over-the-counter drugs, are always suspect in contributing to constipation. Iron supplements, for example, can cause intestinal irritation and have been reported to aggravate constipation. Diuretics, given for hypertension, congestive heart failure, or edematous states, by inducing urinary potassium loss and dehydration, may reduce stool hydration and adversely affect colon motility. Similarly, calcium channel blocking agents relax smooth muscle in the bowel wall, thus impairing gut propulsion. Sedatives prolong immobility and slow gut activity but may also affect sphincter control. Codeine and other narcotic analgesics can cause constipation and are occasionally used for severe diarrhea. Aluminum-containing antacids are also frequent offenders. Clonidine may cause constipation by affecting autonomic neuromuscular bowel control. However, this drug has been used successfully in controlling neuropathic diarrhea in patients with diabetes.

Neurogenic Factors

Fecal incontinence may be caused by neurological disorders such as strokes, spinal cord disease, and autonomic neuropathy resulting from diabetes mellitus. Patients with neurogenic fecal incontinence are not incontinent of stools all the time, as is the case with patients whose incontinence results from impaction. Instead, such patients tend to be incontinent once or twice daily, usually following the intake of food when the gastrocolic reflex is stimulated and the stools are usually well formed. This association between intake of food, gastrocolic reflex, and incontinence can be used successfully in the management of such incontinence.

A rectal glycerine suppository may be given on wakening or prior to breakfast. A bedside commode chair is advisable for less mobile patients who are confined to bed. Velcro clothes fasteners are also helpful aids for patients who lack normal dexterity and cannot undress easily. Some patients with Alzheimer's disease may not appreciate the need to postpone the desire to defecate until reaching an appropriate setting. In addition, some patients may not be able to distinguish flatus from feces.

Gastrointestinal Conditions

Severe diarrhea of any cause may lead to incontinence, particularly if the patient's mobility is reduced. Diarrhea may result from a variety of conditions, ranging from acute infections of the bowel to neoplastic lesions. Acute infections may be the result of food poisoning, which is particularly likely to occur in patients who live alone and are provided with previously cooked food, whether through a senior citizens program or prepared by relatives. Instead of consuming such food promptly, they commonly store it, often unhygienically, and reheat it later to a temperature that is insufficient to kill possible pathogens. The introduction of the microwave oven, with its tendency to heat foods unevenly, may worsen the situation by promoting a false sense of security. Other gastrointestinal causes of fecal incontinence are the same as those in patients who do not have dementia and include irritable bowel syndrome, ulcerative colitis, diverticulitis, neoplastic tumors of the colon and rectum, and the pseudomembranous colitis that often complicates antibiotic therapy.

Abnormalities in thyroid functions can affect bowel function. Hyperthyroidism may be a cause of chronic diarrhea, and hypothyroidism may lead to chronic constipation.

CLINICAL EVALUATION

Recently discovered or prolonged and sustained fecal incontinence mandates a search for reversible and treatable disorders. Caregivers should be able to note the frequency and consistency of the stools and any associated symptoms, including abdominal or rectal pain, bleeding, abdominal cramps, or abdominal distention or bloating. Pertinent questions to be answered include the following:

1. Are there any new focal signs of weakness that suggest recent stroke?
2. Is the patient physically able to get to the toilet, or is he limited by arthritis, muscle weakness, or poor eyesight?
3. What medication does the patient routinely take (both prescribed and over-the-counter drugs)?
4. Is the patient's physical environment "user friendly"? In other words, is it free of obstacles in the patient's path? Does it afford good lighting and bed rails? Is clothing easy to unfasten?
5. Can the patient remember the way to the toilet?
6. Has the patient had noticeable or documented weight loss?

Having obtained this history, a complete physical examination should be done. A neurological evaluation is needed to determine the patient's mental status, mobility, and motor strength. The abdominal examination should focus on any abdominal distention, activity of bowel sounds, enlarged organs or masses, or tenderness in palpation. Digital rectal examination helps to define anal sphincter tone, masses, or impaction. A stool specimen should be obtained to check for occult blood. A "high" impaction may be present but not detectable on rectal examination. A plain film of the abdomen may be necessary to evaluate this possibility. Other investigations may be indicated to diagnose uncommon causes of incontinence.

SUMMARY

Urinary and fecal incontinence have profound implications on the quality of life of both patient and caregiver. Neither type of incontinence is a diagnosis per se and appropriate evaluation is needed. In many instances neither condition is directly related to Alzheimer's disease and may stem from causes that can be treated successfully. A positive attitude toward the management of incontinence and an attempt to identify the underlying cause or precipitating factors is needed. Even if the incontinence cannot be corrected, a number of aids can be used to make the management of incontinent patients easier and to lighten the burden on the caregivers. These aids are discussed in detail in Chapter 16. The management of fecal incontinence is discussed in Chapter 18.

BIBLIOGRAPHY

Barrett JA: Colorectal disorders in elderly people, *Br Med J* 305:764-766, 1992.

Chutka DS, Fleming KC, Evans MP et al: Urinary incontinence in the elderly population, *Mayo Clin Proc* 71(1):93-101, 1996.

Clinical Practice Guideline. Urinary incontinence in adults. US Department of Health and Human Services, Public Health Service, Agency for Health Care Policy and Research, 1992.

Diokno A, Yuhico M, Jr: Preference, compliance and initial outcome of therapeutic options chosen by female patients with urinary incontinence, *J Urol* 154(5): 1727-1731, 1995.

Fanti JA et al: Efficacy of bladder training in older women with urinary incontinence, *JAMA* 265:609, 1991.

Maloney C: Evaluation and treatment of urinary incontinence: a primary care approach, *Nurse Pract* 20(2):74-75, 1995.

O'Brien J: Evaluating primary care interventions for incontinence, *Nurs Stand* 10(23):40-43, 1996.

Osterberg A, Graf W, Karlom U et al: Evaluation of a questionnaire in the assessment of patients with fecal incontinence and constipation, *Scand J Gastroenterol* 31(6):575-580, 1996.

Ouslander JG, Schnelle JF: Incontinence in the nursing home, *Ann Intern Med* 122(6):438-449, 1995.

Rao SS: Functional colonic and anorectal disorders. Determining and overcoming causes of constipation and fecal incontinence, *Postgrad Med* 98(5):115-119, 124-126, 1995.

Resnick NM: Urinary incontinence in older adults, *Hosp Pract* 27(10):139-184, 1992.

Romanzi LJ, Heritz DM, Blaivas JG: Preliminary assessment of the incontinent woman, *Urol Clin North Am* 22(3):513-520, 1995.

Romero Y, Evans JM, Fleming KC et al: Constipation and fecal incontinence in the elderly population, *Mayo Clin Proc* 71(1):81-92, 1996.

Sandvik H, Hunskaar S, Vanvik A et al: Diagnostic classification of female urinary incontinence: an epidemiological survey corrected for validity, *J Clin Epidemiol* 48(3):339-343, 1995.

Skelly J, Flint AJ: Urinary incontinence associated with dementia, *J Am Geriatr Soc* 43(3):286-294, 1995.

Szonyi G, Collas DM, Ding Y et al: Oxybutynin with bladder retraining for detrusor instability in elderly people: a randomized controlled trial, *Age Ageing* 24(4):287-291, 1995.

Versi E, Orrego G, Hardy E et al: Evaluation of the home pad test in the investigation of female urinary incontinence, *Br J Obstet Gynaecol* 103(2):162-167, 1996.

Yim PS, Peterson AS: Urinary incontinence. Basic types and their management in older patients, *Postgrad Med* 99(5):137-140, 143-144, 149-150, 1996.

Management of Urinary Incontinence

Mary M Lancaster

Take time to deliberate,
but when the time for action arrives,
stop thinking and go in.

—Andrew Jackson

Urinary incontinence is a disturbing and often distressing problem for both patients and caregivers. Its management can be costly and time consuming. The onset can result in the placement of the affected person in a long-term care facility. When magnified by the decreased mental ability of patients with dementia, the management can become a seemingly insurmountable task. Strategies currently exist that can help lessen the strain on patients and caregivers.

Urinary incontinence is a problem all too often left untreated out of embarrassment or lack of knowledge of available treatment options. However, its treatment and management are receiving greater attention from health care personnel and the general public than in the past. In March 1996 the Agency for Health Care Policy and Research (AHCPR) issued an updated Clinical Practice Guideline entitled "Urinary Incontinence in Adults: Acute and Chronic Management." This publication goes beyond the original guidelines published in 1992 to include management strategies for persons with chronic incontinence. Groups such as Help for Incontinent People (HIP) and the International Continence Society are making strides in assisting caregivers in the public and health care domains to be knowledgeable of treatment and management options.

GENERAL GUIDELINES

When the patient has had a complete evaluation of the incontinence, as discussed in Chapter 15, and no "reversible" cause is identified, finding the most appropriate form of management is the first step. The management strategy

213

chosen should be the least invasive and with the fewest potential adverse complications. Additional criteria that caregivers should keep in mind are the patient's physical and mental capabilities and quality of life issues. Maintaining the patient's self-esteem and independence are a primary goal. The easiest method of managing incontinence for the caregiver may not always be the safest, the best for the patient, or the most cost effective.

SPECIAL CONSIDERATIONS FOR PATIENTS WITH ALZHEIMER'S DISEASE

For the management of urinary incontinence in patients with Alzheimer's disease, caregivers must consider the nature of the disease when selecting management strategies. Successfully reversing or achieving complete independent management of urinary incontinence requires an intact central nervous system. Because patients with Alzheimer's disease are continually undergoing degenerative changes in the brain, they may no longer "feel" or "recognize" the need to void, may be unable to communicate the need to void, may be immobile or restrained, may not be able to control the urge to void, may not recognize the appropriate time or place to void, and/or may not be able to remember a toileting schedule. Successful management of incontinence becomes dependent on a caregiver who is attentive, available, and creative. This adds to the physical and psychosocial strain caregivers experience as they care for patients with Alzheimer's disease. Several factors affect the management of urinary incontinence in patients with Alzheimer's disease.

PATIENT FACTORS AFFECTING URINARY INCONTINENCE

Mobility

In many older adults, especially those afflicted with Alzheimer's disease, impaired mobility, slow gait, or the use of restraints may lead to incontinence. Simply being able to reach the bathroom in time becomes a real challenge. Caregivers often unknowingly contribute to incontinence by restricting a patient's movement with restraints, geri-chairs, side rails, and table tops. Even for a cognitively intact older person, the above barriers to continence can be difficult to overcome.

Manual Dexterity

Since manual dexterity may be impaired in older persons, from arthritis, Alzheimer's disease, or stroke, such steps as unzipping pants or removing hosiery may interfere with the patient's ability to stay dry. There are many ways to be creative with clothing to make it easier to remove and thus keep the patient cleaner and dryer. Velcro strips can be used to replace snaps, buttons, and zippers. Clothing with an elastic waistband can be more quickly and easily removed. Undergarments are available with flap openings that eliminate the need to "pull down" or remove the undergarment. Wrap-around skirts and dresses are convenient and inexpensive. These steps can help maintain the patient's self-esteem and independence. However, since not all "accidents" can be prevented, the use of durable wash-and-wear clothing is recommended.

Patients with Alzheimer's disease often are unable to perform a certain task because they can no longer remember how to get started in the task or the correct sequence of events in a task.

This may be the reason the patient goes to the bathroom, but stands at the toilet not knowing exactly what to do. Simply helping the patient with the first step or two of the task will be enough to jog the memory and the patient will be able to complete the task. This is termed "task breakdown" or "sequencing." It can be done through verbal instruction, demonstration, or hands-on initiation of the first steps. Some patients may need assistance each step of the way. Although it may seem easier and quicker to pull down the patient's pants and seat him or her on the commode, this does not help to promote the patient's self-esteem and independence. By assisting the patient only when needed, self-esteem is promoted and independence is prolonged. Once caregivers begin taking over tasks for the patient, the ability to perform those tasks will be lost forever.

Flexibility

Since older adults have less flexible hip and knee joints, going to the bathroom can be difficult and uncomfortable. Simply sitting down on the toilet and getting up from it can be problematic. Elevated seats that increase the height of the toilet seat are available and make going to the bathroom easier and less painful. In addition, some toilet seats are padded to promote comfort while sitting on the commode. Handrails can be installed for added support and safety when sitting down and getting up. If the patient has trouble maintaining an upright position or has a tendency to fall to the side, chair arms that can be placed around the toilet to provide an additional degree of safety are also available. Nursing homes and other long-term care facilities are required by licensing agencies to have these types of supports and protective/assistive devices installed in the bathroom facilities (Box 16-1).

DEVICES AND AIDS TO ASSIST IN MANAGEMENT OF URINARY INCONTINENCE

Many devices and aids are available to assist caregivers in managing incontinence. However, some of the products discussed in this chapter may not be covered by health insurance policies, Medicare, or Medicaid. Insurance policies should be checked carefully to determine whether or not incontinence management is a covered service. Because these products can be expensive, an adequate workup to rule out reversible causes of the incontinence is strongly recommended.

Commode Chairs

Commode chairs can accommodate the needs of patients who are relatively mobile. The commode chair can be placed in the area the patient spends most of the day. There are several different types of commode chairs, and selection should be based

---

● **Box 16-1**
Strategies to Reduce Urinary Incontinence:

• Get medical workup to rule out correctable problem.
• Assess and observe voiding pattern.
• Set up regular schedule for voiding.
• Provide verbal/visual cues.
• Do not scold or lecture if accidents occur.
• Offer praise for using toilet and staying dry.
• Place clear signs or pictures to label bathroom.
• Portable commodes.
• Highrise toilet seat/grab bars.
• Simplify clothing.
• Proper lighting.
• Provide privacy and do not rush.
• Coach person while on toilet.
• Diuretics during daytime, if incontinence is mostly nocturnal.

---

on the individual needs and capabilities of the patient and the caregiver. Most chairs have wheels that allow easy movement from place to place and brakes to allow safe transfer to the chair. Caregivers should always check to make sure that any commode chair with wheels also has wheel locks/brakes and that the locks are on whenever the patient is in the chair. Some have pans that slide underneath the seat and can be easily removed for cleaning. This type of chair can also be rolled directly over the existing toilet, allowing the patient to use the bathroom facilities. Some commode chairs are upholstered and have lids and can double as regular cushioned chairs.

Urinals and Bedpans

For patients who have a significant degree of immobility, or for those who spend a great deal of time in wheelchairs, hand-held urinals for both men and women are available from medical equipment suppliers, pharmacies, and department stores. Caregivers are most likely to be familiar with urinals designed for male patients, but not with those for female patients.

There are various types of urinals, but they are all generally made of plastic and have a wide opening and a collection device. The collection device may be molded directly with the urinal or there may be tubing from the urinal to the collection device. In general, most urinals hold at least 1000 ml. For female patients, it is easiest to use this type of device in a sitting position. If this type of equipment is not available, a plastic milk jug can be adapted as a male urinal and a plastic bowl can be used as a female urinal. As these devices are sometimes awkward to use, patients who use urinals should be checked regularly to make sure that spillage has not occurred.

A bedpan may occasionally be needed for a patient who for whatever reason cannot use other types of equipment. Problems associated with the bedpan include difficulty in voiding in a lying position, the difficulty in cleaning the patient after the bedpan has been used, and the possibility of spillage in the bed. However, most importantly, the bedpan is awkward and quite uncomfortable if used for any length of time. Most bedpans are made of plastic, which has a tendency to stick to the bare skin. Applying some powder over the edges of the bedpan can help to prevent this from occurring. When a bedpan is used, caregivers must be attentive to removing it as soon as the patient is finished. Patients must be cleansed well after using the bedpan. Such cleansing is usually best accomplished by turning the patient on his or her side.

Absorbent and Protective Products

The use of absorbent and protective products is recommended while patients are undergoing evaluation of urinary incontinence, and for patients with chronic, long-term incontinence. Jeter and associates have provided guidelines for the selection of products for managing urinary incontinence. According to them, the ideal product should do the following:
1. Contain urine completely and prevent leakage onto clothing, bedding, and furniture.
2. Be comfortable to wear, and protect vulnerable skin from maceration, chafing, and pressure ulcers.
3. Be easy to use.
4. Disguise or control odor.
5. Be inconspicuous under clothing, without bulk or noise.
6. Be easy to dispose of or clean.
7. Be reasonably priced and readily available.

Absorbent products are designed only to help manage incontinence, not treat it. These products either directly contain the urine or serve as a barrier that protects clothing, bedding, and furniture. Absorbent and protective products come in many styles and shapes, may be washable or disposable, and have various names. They have become extremely popular over the past few years and have been marketed as the "answer" to adult incontinence problems. The increased availability and marketing of these products contributes to the problem of persons not seeking professional help for their incontinence.

Although many of the products work in essentially the same manner, serious considerations are involved in choosing the most appropriate product. The availability of laundry facilities, the cost of the various products, and the degree of absorbency should be considered. Useful and conclusive data are lacking comparing reusable products with disposable products. The degree of absorbency and the ease of use may vary greatly. If the patient voids large quantities of urine, the volume of urine the product will effectively contain should be of primary concern. On the other hand, if the patient's problem is occasional dribbling, a pad that is more comfortable and less bulky may be considered. Regardless of the type chosen, absorbent products have made life easier and more dignified for many older adults. Because these products can be concealed under clothing, the person can often return to a more active and social life.

Shields or Guards

One form of absorbent product is pant liners, also referred to as shields and guards. These are pads that the patient wears inside an undergarment. Some of them come with a light stretchy undergarment with a pouch into which the pad can be placed. Others are full-length pads held in place by a waist strap. These products differ greatly in the amount of urine that can be contained, but most have a waterproof outer lining that protects clothing. When soiled, the pad can be removed and replaced with a clean, dry one. The undergarment is washable and reusable.

Adult guards and shields that come with an undergarment typically come in sizes according to waist measurements, thus offering a good fit. Some have elastic waistbands that allow the garment to be easily pulled up while others have Velcro closures, snaps, or buttons. These products are less bulky than adult diapers and are more suitable for patients who are still socially active. Because the slip-in guard pads are not as absorbent as the shields, the guards work best with patients who void small amounts or have a dribbling problem. These products usually have a stay-dry lining next to the patient's skin, which offers protection from skin irritation, rashes, and excoriation.

Protective Underpads

Protective underpads come in both reusable (washable) and disposable forms. The major purpose of this type of product is to protect linens and furniture from becoming soiled with urine or feces. Several different sizes are available, depending upon the size of the area to be protected. When used to protect bed linens, the pad should cover an area that stretches from approximately midback to midthigh and extends beyond the sides of the patient. Such coverage will promote protection when the patient turns and moves around in bed. A much smaller area can be covered when the patient is sitting in a chair since less movement will take place.

At a minimum, the protective underpad should have a thin layer of absorbent material backed by a waterproof cover. Because an underpad is usually less absorbent than a diaper, it may need to be used in conjunction with one of the other management strategies discussed above. Caution and care must be used with the protective underpad because they tend to become rolled or wadded underneath the patient during movement. This can result in undue pressure on certain areas of the body, and if the pressure is not relieved, can eventually lead to skin breakdown.

Adult Diapers

One of the most readily recognized products on the market today is the adult diaper (briefs). Basically fashioned after diapers used for infants, adult diapers are good for people who are incontinent of both bowel and bladder. This product usually comes in sizes (S,M,L) and is fastened with adhesive strips. Adult diapers have been improved greatly by incorporating comfort measures and "accident prevention."

Most adult diaper garments have elastic waistbands and leg bands to help prevent leakage, and many have stay-dry liners. Adult diapers can be used with ambulatory or nonambulatory patients. Although one of the bulkiest types of absorbent products, adult diapers can be worn underneath loose outer clothing. They can also be easily applied to bedridden patients.

Most adult diapers have absorbent inner layers covered by a waterproof outer layer. Frequently the layer closest to the skin will pull the urine away from it toward the outer layer, thereby preventing moisture from remaining in constant contact with the skin. Newer products have a substance in the inner layers that forms a gel as it draws the urine. Patients who use adult diapers must be checked regularly for soiling, the diaper must be changed regularly, and skin care provided as needed.

Underpads should be straightened and all wrinkles removed on a regular basis; a clean, dry pad should be applied whenever soiling has occurred.

CATHETER DEVICES

If the patient's incontinence is not controlled by any of the treatments discussed previously, there are drainage and collection (catheter) systems that can facilitate management. Catheter systems are closed tube devices by which the patient's urine passes into a catheter and flows through drainage tubing into a collection reservoir. These devices can be either internal or external. According to the 1996 AHCPR guideline, catheter systems should be used judiciously and only when other methods of management have failed.

Internal Catheters

Internal catheters are commonly called indwelling or Foley catheters. These systems consist of a silicone, latex, or Teflon tube (catheter) that is passed through the urethra into the bladder (Figure 16-1). The catheter remains in place by means of

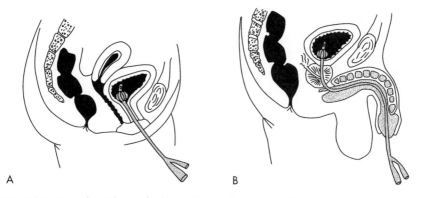

A   B

Figure 16-1, A   The Foley catheter in the female bladder. The inflated balloon at the top prevents the catheter from slipping out of the urethra. **B,** A Foley catheter with the balloon inflated in the male bladder. (From Sorrentino SA et al: *Mosby's textbook for long-term care assistants,* ed 2, St Louis, 1994, Mosby.)

an inflatable balloon. The end of the catheter (outside the body) is connected to a larger and longer piece of plastic tubing, which in turn drains into a bag. The urine is emptied directly and continuously from the bladder and flows to the collection bag. Because this device is inside the body, the risk of infection is very high. In fact, most persons with internal catheters develop bacteriuria (bacteria in the urine) within 2 to 4 weeks after catheter insertion. Therefore, internal catheters are not recommended for the treatment and management of urinary incontinence except in very specific instances. These instances are: for urinary obstruction when other interventions are not feasible, for selected terminally ill patients, for short-term treatment of pressure ulcers in incontinent patients, for severely impaired patients in whom alternative measures are not an option, and/or for patients who live alone and a caregiver cannot provide other supportive measures. Every effort should be made to find a noninvasive method to manage the urinary incontinence.

Problems associated with indwelling catheters are infection, trauma to the urethra or bladder, loss of bladder tone, obstruction secondary to occlusion, leakage, bladder spasms, and accidental removal. Extreme care must be exercised to reduce the occurrence of any of the above complications. Patients who require long-term indwelling catheters may need to have the catheter changed. There is currently no data available to support an optimal frequency of catheter changes. Usual community practice is to change the catheter every 30 days, however some patients may need their catheter changed more frequently. A good rule of thumb is to change the catheter whenever encrustation forms, blockage develops, or urinary tract infection occurs. Sterile technique must be followed for insertion of an indwelling catheter by a caregiver. Additionally, the drainage/collection bag should always be kept lower than the level of the patient's bladder to prevent urine from flowing backward into it.

The area where the catheter enters the body should be cleansed at least daily. This can be accomplished during the bath, as long as a clean washcloth and soap and water are used. The catheter should be taped to the inner thigh of the patient to prevent pulling. The patient's urine should be monitored for signs of infection, including odor, cloudiness, and the presence of mucus or blood. Such monitoring is important because acute infection in the older adult often occurs atypically, with little or delayed physical symptoms. Caregivers should be alert to evidence of pain, tenderness in the abdomen or back, fever, increasing restlessness, pulling at the catheter, increasing lethargy, or confusion. Any patient with an indwelling catheter should be encouraged to drink plenty of fluids. Fruit juices that are acidic are also recommended to help make the urine a less desirable medium for bacterial growth. Cranberry juice is frequently the preferred choice.

External Catheters

The external catheter provides a safer alternative to the indwelling catheter, yet it too is associated with urinary tract infections. These devices are recommended for patients who adequately empty the bladder, who have intact skin, and for whom other interventions have failed or are not appropriate. For men, the condom catheter is the most frequently used drainage and collection device. This device is usually a thin latex or silicone condom that fits over the penis and connects to a drainage tube and bag. The condom should have some sort of firm molding at the connecting end to prevent the condom from twisting closed and preventing drainage of the urine. An external catheter is usually held in place by an elastic adhesive strip that fits either between the penile skin and the condom or directly over the top of the condom. Some companies make an external catheter that has an adhesive inner surface that adheres to the penile skin. If an external catheter with an adhesive strip is being used, it must be wrapped snugly around the penis to hold the catheter in place. However, extreme care must be taken not to make the adhesive strip too tight because doing so can result in impaired blood circulation to the penis. If swelling or a change in skin color is noted, the adhesive strip is too tight and must be removed immediately. Care must also be taken to avoid taping the pubic hair with the adhesive because doing so can cause great discomfort when the catheter is removed.

External catheters should be removed at least daily. The skin should be washed with warm, soapy water; rinsed thoroughly; and dried well before a clean catheter is applied. Some patients may demonstrate an allergy to the latex condom; if a reaction occurs, another brand should be tried. In addition, some patients, regardless of proper hygiene, will develop skin irritation underneath the catheter. Such irritation can be healed quickly by discontinuing use of the external catheter for a few days and relying on another form of management. There are now skin barrier wipes available that can be applied to the penile skin prior to applying the condom catheter, which help prevent skin irritation.

A few external drainage devices are available for female patients. However, the female anatomy poses difficulty in using these products successfully. The female incontinence system usually consists of a pliable, funnel-shaped device that fits snugly over the vulva and is held in place by pressure, straps, or adhesive. Some of these systems also use an undergarment that is worn to hold the funnel in place. Much more work needs to be done in designing an external collection system for women that is easily applied, comfortable, and effective. As with men, the female collection device should be removed and changed (or cleansed) daily and good perineal care provided.

Drainage bags or reservoirs for both indwelling and external catheters come in two basic forms: a leg bag and a chair/bed bag. The leg bag is a much smaller unit that holds less urine. The bag is strapped to the leg, which allows it to be concealed underneath clothing and enables the patient to engage in social activities without embarrassment or the need to carry around a larger bag. Leg bags are ideal for short trips, parties, or shopping. If the bag requires emptying while the patient is away from home, the urine can be easily drained into any toilet.

The larger bedside bag or chair bag is used mainly when the patient is at home, in the hospital, or away for long periods. Because these bags hold larger amounts of urine, they require emptying less frequently and are ideal for nighttime urine collection. The larger bag usually is marked in graduated increments, which is useful when monitoring the patient's total output. Care must be taken to avoid turning the patient on the tubing, which can result in increased pressure and skin damage. The tubing should be kept free of any kinks and the drainage bag must always be kept lower than the level of the patient's bladder. The tubing should be coiled on the bed to promote drainage and anchored to the sheet to prevent pulling on the catheter.

WHAT CAN THE CAREGIVER DO?

Access to Facilities

The best strategy for maintaining access to toileting for mobile patients is to remove any type of physical barrier that hinders freedom to go to the bathroom. If this is not a possibility, then the caregiver must be sure to assess the patient's need to void frequently. Making toilet facilities easily accessible and available is also very important. A situation in which the person must climb stairs to reach an upstairs bathroom invites "accidents" as well as falls when impaired mobility or urge incontinence is a factor.

The pathway to the bathroom needs to be uncluttered, well marked, and well lit. For patients who cannot remember where the bathroom is located, signs and drawings can be used in hallways and on doors to help them find the correct place to void. Leaving a light on at night in the bathroom may help draw the patient's attention to the bathroom when awakened at night.

When getting to the bathroom constitutes a major problem, other methods may be more appropriate. If the patient is fairly mobile, portable commode chairs can be used. Medical equipment suppliers usually rent or sell these chairs. Another source to check is with the area Alzheimer's Association and support groups for access to equipment.

Behavioral Techniques

The use of behavioral techniques is the first-line strategy for treating/managing urinary incontinence. The advantages of behavioral techniques are that there are no reported side effects and their use does not limit future treatment options. All behavioral techniques involve the patient and caregivers, and the use of positive reinforcement for effort and progress. These techniques are designed to decrease the frequency of incontinent episodes and fall into two main categories: caregiver-dependent techniques and active rehabilitation and education techniques. Due to the nature of Alzheimer's disease and the progressive memory impairment experienced by the patient, the active rehabilitation and education techniques generally do not prove useful.

Behavioral techniques for treatment of urinary incontinence:
- Toileting assistance (scheduled toileting, habit training, prompted voiding)
- Bladder training
- Pelvic muscle rehabilitation

Included in the toileting assistance techniques are routine/scheduled toileting, habit training, and prompted voiding. Routine or scheduled toileting is caregiver dependent and is recommended for those patients who cannot participate in independent toileting. A fixed schedule of toileting (every 2–4 hours) is established and the caregiver takes the patient to the bathroom according to the schedule, around the clock. This technique is used to keep the patient dry and avoid accidental voiding. Because no effort is made to have the patient change his voiding behavior, this method is most useful for patients with advanced Alzheimer's disease.

Habit training. Habit training is similar to scheduled toileting but the schedule is set according to the patient's voiding habit. A baseline assessment must be carried out prior to implementation of habit training in order to establish the patient's voiding pattern. The caregivers then take the patient to the bathroom during the times of greatest voiding frequency (e.g., upon arising in the morning, after breakfast, before bed, etc.). In order to establish the patient's voiding pattern, the caregiver must:
1. Observe patient to find what times he/she urinates.
2. Take patient to bathroom at those times everyday.
3. Praise patient for being dry and using toilet.

Prompted voiding. Prompted voiding carries the above techniques a step further. With this method, the patient plays a significant part by recognizing the need to void, asking for assistance, or by responding when prompted to void. This technique is most useful for patients in the early stages of the disease. Prompted voiding uses monitoring, prompting, and praising:
• Monitoring—patient is checked by caregiver on a regular basis and asked to report verbally if wet or dry.
• Prompting—patient is prompted to try and use the toilet.
• Praising—patient is praised for maintaining continence and for trying to use toilet.

Bladder training/retraining programs combine education, scheduled voiding with delay of voiding, and positive reinforcement in order to have voiding occur more on a set timetable rather than as a result of the urge to void. Cooperation and limited understanding on the patient's part are required in bladder training. Because of the steps involved, bladder training is used primarily for urge and mixed incontinence and can be useful for only a small number of patients with Alzheimer's disease or other dementias. The initial schedule is set between 2 and 3 hours and does not occur during sleep. Gradually, the interval between voiding is lengthened, and the patient actively attempts to delay voiding until the next set time.

The success of routine/scheduled toileting, habit training, and prompted voiding in reducing incontinent episodes lies with the caregivers. Those caregivers who are not educated in the proper technique and/or fail to adhere to the intervention decrease the effectiveness of these management strategies. Caregivers need to understand that these techniques are not designed to achieve total continence, only to reduce the frequency of incontinence. This understanding will help keep them from becoming disappointed and disheartened when an accidental voiding occurs.

Fluid and Dietary Management

Overall fluid intake should not be restricted in an effort to reduce incontinence. Older persons are already at risk for dehydration and further reducing fluid intake

---

─● Key Points in the Management of Urinary Incontinence:

1. Attend to patient as soon as possible.
2. Do not rush the patient.
3. Provide enough time to empty bladder.
4. Provide privacy.
5. Do not scold patient if accidents occur.

---

can have serious consequences. Fluid intake should be encouraged and should consist of a variety of fluids, including plain water. Caffeine products such as coffee, tea, colas, and chocolate should be avoided, particularly by those persons with urge incontinence and urinary frequency. If the patient is taking a medication to help eliminate fluid from the body, caregivers should talk with their doctor regarding how much fluid the patient can have and about avoiding giving the fluid medication at nighttime.

Constipation is a common problem in older adults and for those with chronic urinary incontinence. Measures to establish a normal bowel pattern should accompany those to reduce urinary incontinence. By eliminating bowel impaction, the pressure on the bladder and urethra is reduced. This can only help the patient who is experiencing problems with urinary continence. Adequate fluid intake, dietary fiber, and exercise are important components of a bowel program. Laxatives and stool softeners are not recommended for the management of bowel function and the prevention of constipation.

Skin Care

Regardless of the strategies and products selected to aid in the management of incontinence, particular and regular attention must be paid to providing good hygiene and skin care. Urinary incontinence is one of the major factors underlying the development of skin irritation and breakdown. Prolonged contact with moisture and urine lessens the skin's ability to remain intact. Skin breakdown can lead to increased length of hospital stays, increased cost of care, increased risk for infection, and can be extremely painful for the patient.

If an absorbent or protective product is being used, it should be changed whenever it becomes saturated, and the patient's skin should be cleansed with a mild soap and warm water, rinsed thoroughly to remove the soap, and dried. There are specially designed spray washes available that help to cleanse the patient's skin, yet are gentle and control odor. The patient should be checked about every 2 hours to see if care is needed. The perineal area needs to be assessed frequently for signs of rash or irritation.

Newly developed skin care products are on the market that can be used to help prevent and treat rashes and irritation. Barrier products are applied directly to clean, dry skin and act as a layer between the patient's skin and the urine.

Some of these products contain alcohol and are not recommended for use on excoriated, weepy skin due to burning. However, there are some brands now available that do not burn and are very helpful in healing open skin. Whenever a rash or irritation occurs, it may be helpful to choose another form of management for a few days. Often just cleansing the skin and exposing the area to air can help it heal. If the rash or irritation persists, a health care professional should be consulted. Occasionally, patients may be allergic or sensitive to materials used in some products. If this occurs, another brand or one that is hypoallergenic can be tried.

SUMMARY

Urinary incontinence is a treatable and manageable problem faced by millions of people. Care of patients with chronic urinary incontinence must include a combination of behavioral interventions, environmental interventions, fluid and dietary considerations, and the use of the most skin friendly products possible. Urinary incontinence need not control the life of the patient or the caregiver. When the physician, patient, family, and nursing personnel work together, a successful and amenable management plan can be developed. This unified approach leads to fewer worries, eases the burden of caregiving, and allows a more normal and enjoyable life.

BIBLIOGRAPHY

Agency for Health Care Policy and Research. Urinary incontinence in adults: acute and chronic management. Clinical practice guidelines AHCPR Pub No 96-0682. Rockville (MD): 1996, US Department of Health and Human Services, Public Health Service.

Brink C: Absorbent pads, garments and management strategies, *J Am Geriatr Soc* 38:363-373, 1990.

Brooks MJ: Assessment and nursing management of homebound clients with urinary incontinence, *Home Health Nurse* 13(5):11-16, 1995.

Catazaro J: Managing incontinence: an update, *RN* 59(10):38-46, 1996.

Godec CJ: Timed voiding: a useful tool in the treatment of urinary incontinence, *Urology* 23(1):97-100, 1994.

Hu TW, Kaltreider DL: The cost-effectiveness of disposable versus reusable diapers, *J Gerontol Nurs* 16(2):19-24, 1990.

Hutchinson S, Leger-Krall S, Wilson HS: Toileting: a biobehavioral challenge in Alzheimer's dementia care, *J Gerontol Nurs* 22(10):18-27, 1996.

Jeter KF: The use of incontinence products. In Jeter KF, Faller N, Norton C, editors: *Nursing for continence*, Philadelphia, 1990, WB Saunders.

Long ML: *Managing urinary incontinence*. In Chenitz WC, Stone JT, Salisbury SA, editors: *Clinical gerontological nursing: a guide to advanced practice*, Philadelphia, 1991, WB Saunders.

McCormick KA, Burgia LD, Engel BT et al: Urinary incontinence: an augmented prompted void approach, *J Gerontol Nurs* 18(3):3-10, 1992.

McDowell BJ, Engberg S, Weber F et al: Successful treatment using behavioral interventions of urinary incontinence in homebound older adults, *Geriatr Nurs* 15(6):303-307, 1994.

Ouslander JG, Schnelle J, Uman GC et al: Predictors of successful prompted voiding among incontinent nursing home residents, *JAMA* 273:1366-1370, 1995.

Penn C, Lekan-Rutledge D, Joers AM et al: Assessment of urinary incontinence, *J Gerontol Nurs* 22(1):8-19, 1996.

Rousseau P: Urinary collection devices in geriatric incontinence, *J Enterostom Therapy* 18(1):26-31, 1991.

Skelly J, Flint AJ: Urinary incontinence associated with dementia, *J Am Geriatr Soc* 43:286-294, 1995.

Smith D: Continence restoration in the homebound patient, *Nurs Clin North Am* 23:207-217, 1988.

Thomas A, Morse J: Managing urinary incontinence with self-care practices, *J Gerontol Nurs* 17(6):9-14, 1991.

Wanich C, Reilly N: Incontinence care products: non-surgical management of urinary incontinence, *Ostomy Wound Manage* 34(3):45-51, 1991.

Warkentin R: Implementation of a urinary continence program, *J Gerontol Nurs* 18(1):31-36, 1992.

Warren JW: Urine-collection devices for use in adults with urinary incontinence, *J Am Geriatr Soc* 38:364-367, 1990.

Wyman J, Elswick RK Jr, Ory MG et al: Influence of functional, urological, and environmental characteristics on urinary incontinence in community-dwelling older women, *Nurs Res* 42(5):270-5, 1993.

Agencies

National Association for Continence (NAFC)
P.O. Box 8310
Spartanburg, SC 29305-8310
1-800-BLADDER
1-864-579-7900 for South Carolina

Wound, Ostomy and Continence Nurses Society (WOCN)
2755 Bristol Street
Suite 110
Costa Mesa, CA 92626
1-714-476-0268

Safety and Accident Prevention

Mary M Lancaster

Accidents will occur in the best-regulated families, . . .
. . . they may be expected with confidence, and must be borne with philosophy.

—Charles Dickens (David Copperfield)

Patients who have Alzheimer's disease are prone to a number of accidents and injuries. In the earlier stages of the disease the majority of accidents and safety concerns stem from the progressive cognitive deterioration (loss of memory and judgment) of the patient. These include safety issues such as driving, poisonings, and fires. However, as the disease progresses and begins to take its toll on the physical functioning of the patient, other safety issues become apparent (falls, restraints, etc.) The safety of the patient and others is of paramount concern.

DRIVING A CAR

Traffic accidents often are one of the earliest signs that alert caregivers to the fact that something is wrong with the person's mental functioning. Common driving problems include becoming lost and failing to stop at traffic lights, stop signs, or yield signs. Persons with Alzheimer's disease may forget the meaning of road signs, may confuse the meaning of red and green traffic lights, may incorrectly gauge the distance between vehicles, or simply may forget which way to go. Any one of these mistakes can cause a serious accident.

Individuals who are in the early stage of Alzheimer's disease also find it difficult to integrate and understand the meaning of several stimuli received simultaneously. As a result, they are easily distracted, which is often a cause of traffic accidents. For instance, the person may be distracted by road construction and may not notice that a traffic light has changed to red, that they are about to crash into a nearby car, or that they may run off the road.

As discussed in Chapters 7 and 8, a patient who is in early stages of Alzheimer's disease may appear normal or just "eccentric" (at least to people who are strangers), although definite impairment of memory and other cognitive functions is present. Because of this apparent normalcy, the decision about whether to stop the person from driving is always a difficult one, especially since driving may represent the individual's only means of independence. Sometimes a spouse may be unable to drive and relies on the patient with Alzheimer's disease for transportation.

Many persons with Alzheimer's disease are able to drive themselves to the local shopping center or to the home of a relative or friend. They do so almost automatically. Nevertheless, because these individuals have definite mental impairment and their reaction time is slower than normal, they are a hazard to other drivers, to pedestrians, and to themselves. Persuading a person with Alzheimer's disease that he or she should not drive a car can be difficult.

> For many adults, men in particular, the loss of the car represents a serious insult to their independence.

Simply explaining to the person that driving is not safe may not work. The caregivers should attempt to provide the person with as many specific details about her driving habits as possible. Caregivers should help the person to find alternative forms of transportation. Having the physician tell the patient that she can no longer drive may also be effective. Most states require physicians to notify the Department of Transportation when they determine that someone is no longer capable of driving. Taking the person in for license retesting may be another avenue of persuading the person to stop driving. However, when verbal interventions fail in getting the person to give up the car keys, it may become necessary to hide the keys. As a last resort, the car can be sold or the engine can be altered so that it will not start (e.g., by disconnecting the distributor).

BECOMING LOST

Persons with Alzheimer's disease frequently lose their way. Since they cannot integrate various stimuli and orient themselves, they are often unable to retrace their steps. In many instances individuals with Alzheimer's disease have taken a bus, a car, or the train and later have been found wandering miles from home. Patients in the early stage of Alzheimer's disease generally have a specific purpose or destination in mind when they leave home (e.g., shopping or visiting). However, once away from the familiar surroundings of their home, they no longer recognize the way to the store or to their friend's home and they become lost. Because of this tendency to become lost, such persons run the risk of being mugged, becoming victims of other forms of violence, or being exposed to extreme weather.

The problem of becoming lost that occurs in the early stage of Alzheimer's disease differs from that of wandering, seen in the later stages of the disease.

> Persons with Alzheimer's disease appear to have a deep-rooted need to keep moving, a phenomenon that seems even more pronounced in the middle stages of the disease.

This problem raises the issue of how to constrain the person. Deciding whether to prevent the patient from leaving the house presents another difficult matter, since this measure often increases agitation and irritability, and damages self-esteem and independence. All patients with Alzheimer's disease should wear some sort of identification bracelet that provides a phone number that can be called in the event the patient becomes lost. (This is discussed in greater detail later in this chapter.) Finally, caregivers should try to accompany the patient on outings as much as possible. This helps to preserve freedom to move about and continue in activities while providing for the patient's safety.

POOR JUDGMENT AND GULLIBILITY

Persons with Alzheimer's disease may not be fully aware of the risks they take or the consequences of their actions. Their ability to weigh risks and benefits or to accurately determine the steps and "equipment" necessary to complete a task are impaired. For example, a person may not remember to make sure that traffic is clear before crossing the street and consequently can be hit by a car. Similarly, at home a person may use a poorly balanced ladder to try to reach an object on a high shelf.

Because most persons in the early stages of the disease are still relatively independent and able to communicate, it is not unusual for unscrupulous people to take advantage of their impaired mental functioning. The affected person may be approached by someone who persuades him or her to part with his or her money or property, and complex legal problems may ensue. If the person's judgment is considered to be poor, power of attorney probably should be granted to a more capable person or guardianship should be sought from the courts. Protecting the person's money is a major concern to caregivers. Small amounts of money can be left with the person to make him or her feel as if some control still exists, while the majority of money (or checks) is deposited into an account that the person cannot access. This way the person's bills can be paid out of the major account by someone who can protect the person's interest. It is also important to remember that individuals with Alzheimer's disease may invite strangers into the home, who may abuse them or steal from them.

FIRE AND ELECTRICAL SAFETY

Persons with Alzheimer's disease are at high risk for personal injuries and for causing injuries to others through improper or inappropriate use of household equipment and devices. The person's poor memory, curiosity, and poor coordination and judgment are responsible for most of these injuries. For example, after deciding to cook a meal, the person may turn on the gas but forget to light it, or may forget about the food placed on the stove to cook. These actions are particularly hazardous for the person who is still living alone. For these individuals, the gas to the stove can be disconnected and a caregiver can bring hot meals into the home.

Persons with Alzheimer's disease inadvertently pose frequent fire hazards because they often do not appreciate the significance of many of their actions, and they are easily distracted. Electrical appliances, stoves, heaters, and smoking materials pose particular dangers. Frequently, the person may turn on one of these appliances and leave it unattended. Changing or removing control knobs from stoves and heaters can help to prevent accidents. Gas stoves are especially hazardous because if the gas is turned on but not lit, gas poisoning or an explosion can result. Electrical outlets should be covered when they are not in use. This can be accomplished by using the childproof covers available at most department stores. Fuse boxes and circuit boards should also be secured to prevent the person from tampering with the power supply.

> The person who smokes should always be supervised while smoking and the smoking materials secured when not in use.

The home environment should be checked for matches and lighters. Smoke alarms in several strategic locations are essential.

Another major component of safety is fire safety in the institutional setting. All the precautions regarding fire hazards that were previously cited should also be considered in a fire safety program in an institutional setting. When the institution houses patients with Alzheimer's disease, particular attention should be paid to the need for an efficient evacuation plan. This plan should require as little assistance for the patients as possible. Each employee should be able to automatically initiate the plan. Practice sessions are required, which should include handling the patients in a "fire scenario" so the employees know how the patients react to relocation. The confusion and curious nature of many patients with Alzheimer's disease may also lead to patient-initiated false fire alarms. This problem usually can be addressed by having a two-step process for initiating fire alarms, one that is too complicated to be mastered by a patient with dementia.

HEAT AND COLD INJURIES

Injuries resulting from heat and cold include burns, hyperthermia, and hypothermia. The effects of aging and Alzheimer's disease on sensory perception and interpretation places these patients at risk for such injuries.

Bathing can be risky for Alzheimer's disease patients. They may suffer scalds/burns from bath water that is too hot or expose themselves to hypothermia from water that is too cold. Caregivers should test the bath water for the patient prior to bathing. Regulators can be placed on the water heater and set to a temperature that will prevent the water from being too hot (no greater than 115 degrees.) Often, persons with Alzheimer's disease are easily distracted while preparing to bathe. As a result, the faucet may be left on and the person may not realize the water is overflowing the tub. Additionally, hot water bottles and heating pads should never be used unsupervised as the patient may not sense when damage is being done to the affected body part.

Similarly, affected persons may forget to (or be unable to) turn on the heat. This can result in hypothermia, particularly during the winter months. They may not realize that although the heat is on, the house will not become warm if the windows are open. Conversely, persons with Alzheimer's disease may turn the heat up too high, creating an environment conducive to hyperthermia. Thermostats should be secured with covers that will prevent the patient from turning the heat on and off. If fans are used in the environment, they should have a protective guard to prevent the patient from placing fingers into the fan blades. Because of impaired memory and judgment, Alzheimer's patients may dress inappropriately for the environmental temperature. These persons tend to layer clothing, which can result in hyperthermia during the summer, or they go outside inappropriately dressed in the winter, which can result in hypothermia. Careful supervision is required for most patients with Alzheimer's disease to help prevent injuries from heat and cold.

FALLS

Falls commonly occur in older persons, but those with Alzheimer's disease are at even greater risk. On average, approximately half of the falls among older persons are secondary to an intrinsic problem such as orthostatic hypotension, arrhythmias, Parkinson's disease, neuropathies, epilepsy, and medications the patient may be taking. The other half are caused by environmental factors such as poor lighting, loose carpeting, or cluttered surroundings. Persons who have trouble perceiving their surroundings because of diminished vision or hearing also are more likely to fall.

Persons with Alzheimer's disease often take unnecessary risks. For example, the person may place a chair atop a table and attempt to climb on both to reach an item on a high shelf, and the results are often disastrous. Similarly, the person may decide to paint a room, repair a window, or clean out the gutters and in doing so may take risks that increase chances of falling.

The person with Alzheimer's disease reacts more slowly than normal, which makes it difficult to regain balance if he or she starts to fall. This slow reaction time is one reason that it is so important to ensure that the person's surroundings are free of any potential hazards that might cause falls. Such hazards include poorly placed electrical wires, uneven floors, and throw rugs. Friends and family members who visit the affected person should be reminded not to rearrange furniture or place things on the floor. They need to understand that the person cannot easily adapt to changes in his environment and that he performs best in familiar surroundings. When furniture or household items are moved, the person may bump into them and fall.

Throw rugs are very dangerous to elderly people, especially persons with Alzheimer's disease. Loose rugs are hazardous because the person may catch his foot underneath the edge, trip, and fall, and possibly suffer a broken hip. All rugs should be made slip proof for everyone's safety. Certain throw rugs or decorative rugs may have been in place for many years and therefore may have great sentimental value to the family. In addition, they may help with the person's orientation by keeping the surroundings familiar. Such rugs should be given nonslip backing, or the edges should be secured to the floor with nails or double-sided adhesive tape. Bulky rugs should be replaced by thinner ones that are not so high off the floor.

Removing obstacles from the common path of traffic throughout the house is important. On furnitures, any sharp edges or corners should be padded. All traffic areas, pathways, and rooms commonly used should be well lit. Bedrooms, bathrooms, hallways, and stairwells also require good lighting. Highly polished floors and direct sunlight in rooms should be avoided since both produce glare, which presents a difficulty for older people. Glare can be reduced by using low-luster polishes on floors, by placing sheer curtains over windows, and by using indirect lighting.

Persons with Alzheimer's disease may not be able to gauge the height of steps, curbs, and door thresholds accurately, a situation that often leads to falls. The edges of steps can be highlighted in a bright color to help draw attention to the steps. As an alternative, barriers can be used to block stairways; however, the barriers should be high enough that the person will not try to walk over them. Doors leading to basements should be kept locked.

As the dementia of Alzheimer's disease progresses, the person may develop an ataxic gait and may be at even greater risk of falling, even in a safety-conscious environment. Although little can be done to affect the processes underlying these changes, there are many other factors that increase the risk of falls for patients with Alzheimer's disease. Controlling these risk factors provides a major opportunity for reducing the injuries associated with falling.

One of the major activities of caregivers should be assessment of the effect of medications on the risk that a patient will fall. Since antipsychotics, antidepressants, sedatives/hypnotics, vasodilators, and diuretics are particularly associated with increased risk of falls, they should be used in the smallest doses that will achieve the desired effects.

Caregivers should consistently assess the resident's stability during standing, ability to change positions safely, and balance and coordination. All these skills may deteriorate in the patient with advancing dementia. Sometimes assistive devices such as walkers or wheelchairs can be used by the patient to provide support during ambulation. Because of the patient's poor memory and impaired learning, he or she cannot be relied on to use these devices each time he is walking or to use them correctly. Offering general activities to maintain strength, ensuring that sensory deficits are corrected with eyeglasses and hearing aids, and constantly assessing for environmental risks may be all that can be done practically to prevent falls.

In the past, physical restraints were often used to prevent falls. However, it is becoming increasingly obvious that the negative effects of this practice, such as increased agitation and deterioration in overall physical and mental condition, make this an option of last resort in the management of patients at risk of falling. The use of restraints is discussed in greater detail later in this chapter.

POISONING AND PICA

Accidents with common household cleaners, caustic agents, and poisons are more likely to happen to persons who have Alzheimer's disease than to unaffected individuals. The affected person's inability to read or recognize labels, forgetfulness, and inquisitive nature are responsible for many of the accidental poisonings and ingestions that occur. Many substances are ingested because the person no longer recognizes or understands the appropriate used of the substance. Therefore all potentially hazardous materials and substances should be kept secured.

In cases of food poisoning, the person's diminished senses of smell and taste may prevent him or her from noticing a strong smell or "off" taste in spoiled food. Thus he or she may not be able to recognize food that has gone bad. Similarly, the person may forget to properly prepare food or to return it promptly to the refrigerator after cooking or eating.

Pica, the craving for or eating of unusual foods or substances, is a trait that is not uncommon among persons with Alzheimer's disease. The person with Alzheimer's disease can have a very curious nature and, just like a child, may use her mouth to investigate both liquids and solids. Therefore all cleaning products, medications, and other poisonous substances must be kept safely locked in a cabinet. The person may no longer recognize which things are appropriate to eat and may pick up items such as soap, cigarette butts, and flowers and put them in the mouth. Products such as mouthwash, toothpaste, and liquid detergent also should be kept out of sight; although not actually poisonous, they can make a person very ill if taken in large amounts. Many household plants have poisonous leaves, flowers, or berries and should be removed from the environment.

MEDICATIONS

Persons with Alzheimer's disease are likely to take the wrong medicines, the correct medicine at the wrong time, or too much of any medication.

● **Case Study—The Patient Who Mixed Up His Medication**
One patient known to us who was in stage 2 of Alzheimer's disease took his sleeping medication first thing in the morning and his diuretic the last thing before going to bed. Consequently, he tended to be lethargic and sleepy most of the day, and incontinent and fully awake at night. It was generally assumed that these two conditions were the result of his Alzheimer's disease but, in fact, the problems were caused by the inappropriately taken medication.

An individual with Alzheimer's disease must not have uncontrolled access to medications. The patient may take a sleeping tablet, then forget that it was taken, and a few minutes later take another one. This sequence may be repeated several times until the patient has taken an overdose of a hypnotic medication. A number of devices can be used to prevent the person from taking more medication than is required. For instance, all the day's medication can be placed in a small compartment of a special container while the main compartment, which contains the rest of the medication, remains inaccessible. A note can be left in the container saying that, since no tablets are left, the medication for the day has been taken and the person should not try to take any more. This reminder may prevent the patient from becoming agitated at not being able to take additional medication.

The same risk of overdose applies to a person who is in pain, has analgesic preparations at hand, and tries to relieve the pain. Because the person's memory is poor, he or she may forget having taken an analgesic tablet and therefore may take too much of this medication. Overdosage of many preparations, such as hypotensive medications and medications that act on the heart, may be associated with serious side effects. Therefore no medication should be left lying around. As much as possible, the person should be given his medication on a day-to-day basis.

The caregiver should take charge of all the person's medication and administer it as prescribed. The caregiver must be instructed about how and when to give the medication and should know the common side effects. In this way the caregiver will be prepared and able to consult with the physician if any side effects should occur and to keep the patient safe from unintentional overdose.

WANDERING

Wandering is a problem many caregivers must face with persons who have Alzheimer's disease. Nursing homes with special units for these individuals have an advantage because they usually have an area that is locked for safety yet allows the person to move about freely. Although the person should be granted as much independence as possible, the prevention of accidents caused by wandering outside the house must be considered when it is no longer safe for the person to be out alone.

Doors leading to the outside should be kept locked. Often, simply changing to a new type of lock that the person is not familiar with can solve the problem (Figure 17-1). If this step does not work, deadbolt locks or locks having a number sequence keypad can be installed. Regular door handles can be replaced with childproof models that require a combination of actions to turn the handle. The person with Alzheimer's disease probably will not be able to figure out the sequence necessary to open the door. Doors may be concealed with drapes, pull-down shades, or portable decorative screens. However, one of the dangers of changing doors and locks is fire. In each town the local fire marshal often will have specific suggestions to deal with this problem.

Alarm systems on doors also can be helpful. These systems allow the door to be opened but signal that the person is going outside. Sometimes the alarm itself is enough to scare the person so that he will close the door and stay inside. In another type of alarm system the patient wears a wristband that triggers either an alarm or door-locking mechanism as the patient comes close to a sensor. Many types of alarm systems are available, and they vary on sophistication and cost. Families can shop around to find the system best suited to the living arrangement and the budget. Many nursing homes use alarm systems on the outside doors of buildings.

If the person with Alzheimer's disease is still able to go outside, fencing around the yard can serve as added protection. This arrangement allows the person to get some fresh air and to exercise in an enclosed, safe area. The yard should be kept clear of branches or other objects that might cause harm. In addition, the person should have adequate identification on her body, such as a medic-alert bracelet or a locket that provides the name and phone number of the individual to be contacted if the person becomes lost.

Law enforcement officers recommend that I.D. bracelets not give the person's name and address, due to the risk of exploitation by unscrupulous people. The family should have a recent photograph of the person that can be given to the

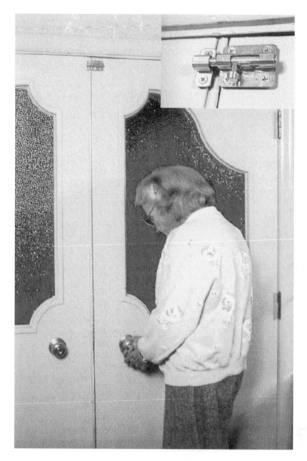

Figure 17-1 A slide lock is placed at the top of the door. The person tries to open the lock on the knob. (From Sorrentino SA et al: *Mosby's textbook for long-term care assistants,* ed 2, St Louis, 1994, Mosby.)

neighbors or the police if a search should become necessary. Neighbors and friends should be told of the person's condition so that they can notify the caregiver if they see the person wandering outside. The phone numbers of the police department and the neighbors should be kept readily accessible. Caregivers should be encouraged to contact the local chapter of the Alzheimer's Association in their area to see if the chapter offers a "wanderer's program." The "Safe Return" program sponsored by many community Alzheimer's Association chapters registers the person with Alzheimer's disease with the local chapter, local police, and 911. Then, in the event that the person wanders away from home, one phone call will activate search procedures. The Alzheimer's Association has been instrumental in providing education and training to local police agencies on how to assist the lost or wandering Alzheimer's disease patient and the caregivers. This is further discussed in Chapter 27.

Some persons will not go outside unless they are wearing their favorite jacket or shoes or carrying their purse or wallet. This practice is probably a lifelong habit that the person with Alzheimer's disease has maintained. Putting these articles out of sight until they are needed can help prevent the person from wanting to go outside.

In the institutional setting wandering becomes a safety issue when the resident is able to wander into a section of the facility that is unsafe for him or for other residents, or to leave the facility altogether. Many institutions now have mechanisms to alert staff when a resident wanders beyond safe limits. Such devices allow a staff member to locate the resident, accompany him briefly, and then redirect him to a safe area. Wandering behavior often can be contained by having cues that anchor the resident to a safe area, such as the presence of familiar or pleasing items.

In some instances, residents must be placed in special care areas where wandering can be restricted. Such restriction can be achieved through the use of extensive monitoring systems or by locking doors to prevent exit. These units should be designed to maximize the resident's freedom to move about and should include access to indoor and outdoor recreational activities (Figure 17-2).

Some wandering can be contained by manipulating the environment to make it seem more restrictive than it actually is. Complicated opening mechanisms on exit doors are often enough to frustrate the patient with cognitive impairments. This illusion of containment also can be fostered by including noxious stimuli, such as rough walls or disorienting designs near exits. Some facilities have found that using a dark grid area on the floor has helped to prevent patients from moving into unsafe

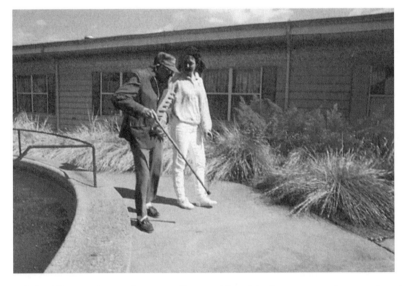

Figure 17-2   The nursing assistant walks outside with the person who wanders. He is guided back into the facility. (From Sorrentino SA et al: *Mosby's textbook for long-term care assistants*, ed 2, St Louis, 1994, Mosby.)

or restricted areas. Another common problem is wandering into other patients' rooms. Simply placing some ribbon or police tape across the doorway is enough to keep the person out of the room.

In spite of the institution's efforts to deal with the wanderer, occasionally a resident will wander away from a facility. The facility should have a clearly defined procedure for searching for missing residents and for notifying appropriate authorities and family members. The use of identification bracelets and the presence of a current photograph can be lifesaving in such situations.

Guns

In the US, in contrast to other societies, guns are common in many households. Obviously they should be secure or removed in the presence of a person with dementia.

CONSIDERATIONS IN LATER DISEASE STAGES

In the later stages, the person with Alzheimer's disease has physical disabilities in addition to mental impairment. Because of failing physical status, the person with late-stage Alzheimer's disease is much more likely to be confined to a chair or bed. In some ways this confinement reduces the risk for many of the accidents previously described; however, different concerns for overall safety arise. This person is at greater risk for falling (if still ambulatory), for becoming incontinent of urine, for developing decubitus ulcers, and for becoming dehydrated (see Chapter 6).

In addition to failing physical status, the person's mental abilities decline. As the patient's degree of confusion increases, she may wander more frequently or may become agitated or combative toward caregivers or others in her environment. This combination of mental and physical decline frequently results in placement of the person in a hospital or nursing home. Safety in these institutions is complicated by the presence of a number of residents with similar behaviors and by the necessity for staff to closely monitor the idiosyncrasies of these individuals.

Environmental Safety

Environmental safety encompasses a program for the evaluation of all aspects of the environment in regard to the safety of patients and caregivers. One of the major safety risks posed by the person with severe dementia is the tendency to place objects in her mouth. This tendency may be caused by confusion over whether or not the item is food, or it may represent a need for oral stimulation. Whatever the reason for this action, any item that could be swallowed or aspirated must be placed out of the resident's reach. Caregivers must be particularly careful to alert family and other visitors to this risk and must inspect all personal items given to the patient. Institutions should have policies concerning the identification and storage of unsafe items and the supervision of residents during potentially risky activities. This safety measure includes monitoring the use of medical devices and appliances and even monitoring routine activities of daily living such as bathing or shaving.

Safety during mealtime is another concern, particularly in the later stages of the disease, and is discussed in Chapter 19.

Use of Restraints

Physical restraints or restraint achieved by means of drugs can be used to ensure the patient's safety. The primary objective in using restraints is to protect the person from self-injury (falling) or inflicting injury on others. Because the use of restraints conflicts with the overall treatment goal of maintaining independence and can result in serious complications, all alternative measures for safety should be exhausted before restraints are prescribed (see Box 17-1 on p. 239 for some alternatives to restraint.) Restraints never should be seen as the first or the definitive solution to a safety or behavior problem. They also should not be used solely for the convenience of the caregivers.

In an institutional setting it must be remembered that a physician must order any restraint and the order must be time-limited. The need for restraint must be clearly documented in the medical record.

Whenever a restraint is used, the goal is to eliminate it as soon as possible. Restraints violate the patient's rights, restrict the patient's movement, and deny him or her independence and a sense of freedom.

A common unwanted side effect of restraints, especially when used with persons with Alzheimer's disease, is aggressive and agitated behavior. Often the person does not comprehend the reason for the restraint and begins to fight it. The patient may think that he or she is being tied down or punished. Conversely, some individuals may exhibit regressive behavior and retreat further into isolation by not interacting. In either situation the person's confusion, isolation, and dependence will probably increase. If this situation occurs, engaging the person in some activity and using therapeutic touch can help to decrease the agitation by distracting his or her attention from the restraints. Restraint-free periods should be attempted on a regular basis to provide an opportunity for exercise and to assess the need for continuing the restraint.

Many types of restraints are available, such as vest restraints, wrist and ankle restraints, bar restraints, and belt restraints. Each type has advantages and disadvantages that should be considered when selecting the one most appropriate for the person's needs.

Vest restraints are used frequently because they allow free movement of the arms and legs while supporting the upper body. This type of restraint is particularly useful for persons who tend to lean forward and are at risk of falling out of a wheelchair. Vest restraints also can be effective for persons who try to climb out of bed.

Disadvantages of the vest restraint are: the person can slide down and wiggle out of the vest, these can restrict normal respiration if it becomes lodged around the chest, and accidental death cases have been reported when the vest became lodged around the patient's neck, causing strangulation. Vest restraints always must be applied properly and according to the manufacturer's specifications to help prevent

---

● Box 17-1
Alternative to Restraints

1. Use of diversional activities: music, exercise, art, books, videos, etc.
2. Use positioning aids such as foam pillows, wedges, cushions, arm boards.
3. Use proper footwear—shoes can be worn in bed.
4. Hang up visual reminders such as stop signs, do not enter signs, ribbons across doors.
5. Ensure protection for fallers: helmet, knee and elbow pads, hip pads.
6. Use low beds, which are commercially available.
7. Place pads on floor next to bed.
8. Place mattress on floor.
9. Involve in task of the day (sweeping, cleaning, dusting, folding clothes).
10. Use sensory aids such as eyeglasses and hearing aids.
11. Reduce medications that can cause drowsiness and confusion.
12. Educate patient and family on use of call bell.
13. Check every 2 hours for need to void and for hunger, thirst.
14. Elicit volunteer support to engage and observe patients.
15. Implement a buddy system.
16. Keep necessary items within reach.
17. Use velcro seat belts.
18. Use rocking chairs.
19. Use a calm, gentle approach—engage person in social conversation.
20. Use massage, therapeutic touch.
21. Use a nonthreatening manner—try not to tell person "what they can't do."
22. Pad corners of furniture.
23. Have nonslip backing on rugs.
24. Enhance family involvement with patient.
25. Ensure thorough assessment of possible causes for behavior.
26. Use prosthetic devices such as wheelchairs, walkers, canes.
27. Locate patient near central nursing station.
28. Install alarm systems for doorways, exits, and beds/chairs.
29. Place bed rails in down position.
30. Decrease overstimulation by lower lighting, soft music, quiet area.

---

respiratory distress or strangulation. This includes securing the long straps to a stable object (such as the bed frame) and using quick-release knots.

Many persons can get out of a restraint even if it has been correctly applied. By no means should the restraint be considered a sure safeguard against falls and accidents. The person in restraint should be checked frequently to ensure that the restraint remains in place and that circulation and respirations are not restricted. The person's needs for toileting, food, fluid, and activity also must be assessed and met by releasing the restraints every 2 or 3 hours. In the institutional setting, all checks on the restrained patient should be recorded in the nursing notes or on a flowsheet. In addition, there must be documentation in the nurse's notes regarding the person's response to the restraint and the assessment performed for continued justification for the restraint.

A restraint always must be secured to a stable object. Restraints used for persons confined to bed should be secured to the bed frame, not to the side-rail. The person should be able to roll from side to side in a vest restraint. Restraints for a person in a wheelchair should never be fastened to a movable part of the chair. Belt restraints can be securely fastened underneath the seat of the wheelchair. This type of restraint is best used with cooperative persons who need reminding only to call for assistance when they want to get up.

Side rails are a form of restraint that helps to remind the individual to stay in bed. Because judgment and reasoning are impaired, patients with Alzheimer's disease frequently do not understand the need for side rails and will try to climb over them. When rails are used, the bed should always be in the low position. If the person should decide to climb over the side rails and the bed is in the high position, the added distance that the person will fall can significantly increase injury. Most individuals who climb over side rails or fall from bed report that they were trying to get to the bathroom. Therefore it is vitally important for caregivers to attend to the person's elimination needs frequently.

Arm, leg, or wrist restraints are used less frequently than other methods. They should be used only when the person's agitation is severe and this method is the only way to keep the person from harming self or others. This type of restraint should be used only for short periods because it completely restricts movement of the extremity. Sedatives are frequently used in combination with arm, leg, or wrist restraints. If the person requires this type of combination restraint, he must be assessed at regular intervals, and this assessment must be documented. Hand mittens, which allow free movement, can be used instead of wrist restraints for persons who try to remove their intravenous lines or feeding tubes. The ankle or wrist restraint must be removed frequently, and the extremity must be massaged and placed through range-of-motion exercises. The area where the restraint is applied must be assessed for tissue injury.

The use of restraints is a controversial issue. Each state and local institution must have a policy outlining the requirements and procedures for using physical restraints. In addition, each situation must be analyzed individually. New regulations and guidelines are being enforced that mandate that restraints, in any form, be used only when absolutely necessary and then only under a physician's order and for a limited time period. Caregivers must be aware that the use of restraints adversely affects behavior and outcomes. The person's safety and well-being must be weighed against the risks and side effects of restraints, and the goal of using restraints for the least amount of time possible must always be kept in mind.

Families are becoming more involved in decisions related to restraints. Family conferences are the ideal setting for discussing the pros and cons of restraint, explaining why temporary restraint may be needed, and assessing the family's beliefs and attitudes about the use of restraints. If a family is opposed to the use of restraint for maintaining the person's safety, this decision should be entered in the record during the family conference and all in attendance should sign the note (including family members). For a more in-depth discussion on the regulations governing restraint use and the care of persons in restraint, the reader is directed to the Bibliography section.

SUMMARY

Safety and accident prevention for persons with Alzheimer's disease pose many difficulties for caregivers. Being aware of potential hazards and realizing that the affected person can no longer be responsible for his own safety is the first step in preventing accidents. Providing a safe environment, either at home or in the institution, can help lessen the strain on caregivers. Considerable patience and creativity are required to make an environment safe yet stimulating for persons with Alzheimer's disease.

BIBLIOGRAPHY

Bradley L, Siddique CM, Dutton B: Reducing the use of physical restraints in long-term care facilities, *J Gerontol Nurs* 21(9):211-34, 1995.

Capezuti E, Evans L, Strumpf N et al: Physical restraint use and falls in nursing home residents, *JAGS* 44(6):627-633, 1996.

Cohen C, Neufeld R, Dunbar J et al: Old problem, different approach: alternatives to physical restraints, *J Gerontol Nurs* 22(2):23-29, 1996.

Chenitz WC, Kussman H, Stone JT: Preventing falls. In Chenitz WC, Stone JT, Salisbury SA, editors: *Clinical gerontological nursing: a guide to advanced practice*, Philadelphia, 1991, WB Saunders.

Eigsti D, Vrooman N: Releasing restraints in the nursing home, *J Gerontol Nurs* 18(1):21-23, 1992.

Freedman ML, Freedman DL: Should Alzheimer's disease patients be allowed to drive? A medical, legal, and ethical dilemma, *JAGS* 44(7):876-877, 1996.

Hensel T: OBRA Regulations, *Topics in Geriatric Rehab* 11(I):39-45, 1995.

Johansson K, Bronge L, Lundberg C et al: Can a physician recognize an older driver with increased crash potential? *JAGS* 44(10):1198-1202, 1996.

Johnson D: Restraint-free care: a look back, *Nurs Homes* 44(7):26, 1995.

Josephson K, Fabacher D, Rubenstein L: Home safety and fall prevention, *Clin Geriatr Med* 7:707-731, 1991.

Kaszniak AW, Keyl PM, Albert MS: Dementia and the older driver, *Hum Factors* 33:527-537, 1991.

Lach HW, Reed AT, Smith LJ, et al: Alzheimer's disease: assessing safety problems in the home, *Geriatr Nurs* 16(4):160-164, 1995.

Matteson MA, Linton A: Wandering behavior in institutional persons with dementia, *J Gerontol Nurs* 22(9):39, 1996.

Matthiesen V, Lamb KV, McCann J et al: Hospital nurses' views about physical restraint use with older patients, *J Gerontol Nurs* 22(6):8-16, 1996.

Namazi KH, Rosner TT, Calkins MP: Visual barriers to prevent ambulatory Alzheimer's patients from exiting through emergency doors, *Gerontologist* 29:699-702, 1989.

Neufeld RR, White H, Foley W et al: Can physically restrained nursing home residents be untied safely? Intervention and evaluation design, *JAGS* 43(11): 1264-1268, 1995.

Oleske DM, Wilson RS, Bernard BA et al: Epidemiology of injury in people with Alzheimer's disease, *JAGS* 43(7):741-746, 1995.

Robinson A, Spencer B, White L: *Understanding difficult behaviors: some practical suggestions for coping with Alzheimer's disease and related illnesses,* Geriatric Education Center of Michigan, 1988.

Schnelle JF, MacRae PG, Giacobassi K et al: Exercise with physically restrained nursing home residents: maximizing benefits of restraint reduction, *JAGS* 44(5):507-512, 1996.

Silliman, RA: Injury prevention in Alzheimer's disease patients: possibility or pipe dream? *JAGS* 43(7):831-833, 1995.

Strumpf NE, Evans LK, Schwartz D: Physical restraint of the elderly. In Chenitz WC, Stone JT, Salisbury SA, editors: *Clinical gerontological nursing: a guide to advanced practice,* Philadelphia, 1991, WB Saunders.

Tibbitts GM: Patients who fall: how to predict and prevent injuries, *Geriatrics* 51(9):24-31, 1996.

Daily Care and Management

Mary M Lancaster

Nothing in life is to be feared, it is only to be understood.

—Marie Curie

As the course of Alzheimer's disease progresses, patients begin to demonstrate a lack of attention to personal hygiene and grooming. This development may be caused by changes in memory that interfere with the patient's ability to perform tasks that require sequential steps or by simply ignoring the need for personal hygiene. Whatever the cause may be, patients with Alzheimer's disease soon experience problems with bathing, changing clothes, eating, and using the bathroom. To caregivers, these tasks seem quite simple, but to those whose memory is impaired, the tasks of daily living can be frustrating, confusing, and overwhelming.

Caregivers need to continually assess the patient's skill in performing activities of daily living (ADLs) since this skill level can change on a daily basis. Expecting the patient to perform an activity that he or she cannot do will lead to frustration for the caregiver and the patient. Catastrophic reactions occur when the patient becomes overwhelmed and frustrated by expectations. Caregivers must be attuned to the patient's general hygienic needs and to their specific areas of impairment in order to promote good personal hygiene, independent functioning, and strong self-esteem.

Maintaining set routines for all ADLs also helps to keep the patient functioning independently. For instance, every morning upon arising from bed, the patient should go through the same activities in the same sequence and at approximately the same time. The patient may use the bathroom, eat breakfast, take a bath, dress, and then brush his or her teeth. This routine should be followed every day. When routines and schedules are disrupted or changed, the patient finds the situation confusing and frustrating. A catastrophic reaction may occur that could be avoided by planning for hygienic needs in a way that is compatible with the patient's needs.

243

TASK BREAKDOWN

ADLs such as bathing, eating, and toileting are actually quite complicated tasks that are comprised of a series of sequential steps. Forgetting any one of the steps of an activity can block the patient's ability to perform the task. For example, brushing teeth requires the patient to recognize all the equipment needed (toothbrush, toothpaste, sink) and to remember how to use each piece of equipment. In addition, the patient needs to remember to find the equipment, put the toothpaste on the toothbrush, brush his teeth, and rinse his mouth. Early in the disease, providing assistance with the one step that is forgotten may be all that is needed for the patient to finish the task. Eventually, the entire activity will need to be performed for the patient.

Task breakdown (breaking down an activity into its simplest steps) is a very useful tool in keeping the patient with Alzheimer's disease functioning on her own. The caregiver needs to be present to coach the patient through the task rather than completing the task for her. When the patient is allowed to actually perform the activity, she will retain the ability longer.

—• Completing tasks for the patient is not always the best approach.

Providing cues such as labeling, breaking tasks down into very simple steps, giving verbal reminders and prompts, and offering demonstrations are all useful in keeping the patient functioning. As the patient's capabilities continue to decline, increased verbal and visual assistance will become necessary. For the patient with Alzheimer's disease, once a skill is lost it is virtually impossible to regain. Daily care for terminal or end-stage Alzheimer's disease is discussed in Chapter 20.

Regardless of the daily task involved, the technique of task breakdown can be applied to assist the patient in maintaining independent or minimally assisted functioning for as long as possible. The following sections describe routine practices that are essential to the daily care of the patient with Alzheimer's disease.

Oral Care and Hygiene

Care of the mouth is one area of daily hygiene that is most often neglected when patients no longer perform the task independently. However, it is vitally important that oral care be provided. Improper or inadequate oral care can result in serious problems with both teeth and gums, and can lead to systemic infection. When neglected, the gums can quickly become irritated and inflamed, resulting in pain, bleeding, and exposure of the root of the tooth, which can provide an excellent site for infection. In addition, improperly cleansing of the oral cavity causes bad breath, which can decrease the person's comfort level and self-esteem.

Periodic examinations by a dentist or dental hygienist should be continued as long as possible. Some dentists will make trips to the home or nursing home if the patient is unable to come to the office. Edentulous patients should have a yearly oral examination and those patients with natural teeth should be checked twice each year. All patients entering a long-term care facility should have a comprehensive oral assessment by a dentist or health care professional to provide a baseline for treatment and management.

Patients with natural teeth. If the patient has his natural teeth, attention must be given to proper brushing at least once or twice a day. All tooth surfaces must be brushed to remove food particles and plaque. The gum line needs to be gently brushed to stimulate circulation and remove imbedded food. If the patient is performing the activity, caregivers may need to provide assistance. Check the patient's mouth to make sure he or she is adequately cleansing his teeth, gums, and tongue. Inspect frequently for signs of gum inflammation, swelling, and tenderness.

Adaptive equipment, such as long toothbrushes, suction toothbrushes, and toothbrushes with large handles, is available to make oral care easier. Ingestible toothpaste can be used for the patient who tends to swallow after brushing instead of spitting. When the patient cannot brush her own teeth, the caregiver must assume this task. Props designed to keep the patient's mouth open are available from medical equipment suppliers. These make getting into the mouth to provide adequate care much easier. Dental hygienists are a resource caregivers can use when needing some assistance or instruction on proper oral care.

Edentulous patients. The patient who no longer has any natural teeth still requires daily oral care. It is a myth that patients who are edentulous do not require oral care. All the soft tissues of the mouth should be cleansed at least once a day. A soft toothbrush, sponge, or moist gauze wrapped around a toothbrush can be used to clean the edentulous patient's mouth.

Patients with dentures. If the patient wears dentures, particular attention must be given to oral care. The dentures should be removed at least once a day and scrubbed with a soft brush and cleanser. This practice helps to remove the food particles that adhere to the dentures. The top and bottom of each denture should also be cleansed to remove any trapped food, mucus, and adhesive. Ideally, the patient's dentures should be removed each evening, cleansed, and stored in a denture cup filled with water until the next morning. Just before the dentures are to be placed in the patient's mouth, they should be rinsed.

Dentures can improve the patient's chewing ability, looks, and speech. The patient should be assisted in inserting his dentures each morning. Certain problems unique to denture wearers need to be noted. If the patient has lost a significant amount of weight, which is common in Alzheimer's disease, the dentures may become very loose and actually inhibit chewing and speech. If the dentures do not stay in place, a dentist should be consulted. "Wobbly" dentures and ones that are left in place for long periods can be sources of soft tissue irritation. Large ulcerations can develop and interfere with eating and speaking. They can also cause significant pain. The accompanying case history illustrates the impact of inadequate denture care on health and functioning.

Case Study—Inadequate Denture Care

Mrs. W. is a 72-year-old woman who has been residing in a nursing home for the last 4 years. She was diagnosed as having probable Alzheimer's disease 3 years ago. Her daughter comes to visit every day at supper time to encourage her to eat. For the past several weeks Mrs. W. has become more agitated and irritable and has been losing weight. She has also been noted rubbing her face. Because of this agitation, Mrs. W. has been given increasing doses of a tranquilizer. She now sits slumped over in her chair, and her speech is slurred. Mrs. W.'s daughter is quite concerned about her mother's rapid deterioration and her grimacing during eating. As a last resort, she consults her own dentist and asks him to see her mother.

The dentist arrives and finds Mrs. W. in her usual position, slumped in her chair. He inspects Mrs. W.'s mouth and sees that she has all her natural lower teeth, but has an upper denture. The lower teeth are in good shape, except that they need brushing. The dentist asks Mrs. W. if she is having any problems. Mrs. W. pulls at her upper denture and shakes her head. After removing the upper denture, the dentist finds a large ulcer on the hard palate covered with a thick layer of mucus and food. After cleansing the area, the dentist is relieved to note that the ulcer is superficial. He recommends that the denture be left out for one week, after which it is to be used only when eating. He also leaves instructions for cleansing of the denture and Mrs. W.'s mouth (hard palate in particular) after each meal.

Two weeks later, the dentist comes to see how Mrs. W. is progressing. He is amazed to find a woman who is sitting up, communicating, and eating very well. The staff report that the dose of the tranquilizer has been greatly reduced and that Mrs. W. has gained 3 pounds.

BATHING

As Alzheimer's disease progresses, the patient may begin to resist bathing. There are numerous possible causes for this resistance toward bathing. Some causes are fear, lack of privacy, the overwhelming aspect of the mechanics of bathing, changes in hot/cold sensations, embarrassment, and depression. The patient may associate a shower with being out in the rain, may fear what will happen if undressed, may no longer recognize the person who is helping her, or may have forgotten how to turn on the water. Caregivers need to investigate the possible cause of the patient's reluctance so that appropriate corrective action can be taken.

Bathing Routines

The caregiver needs to evaluate the best time of day for bathing. This decision should take into consideration the patient's past routine. Some persons bathe in the

---

—● Possible Causes for Difficulty in Bathing

- Depression—causes lack of interest in self.
- Person cannot locate the bathroom.
- Water/room temperature too hot or cold.
- Fear of falling/slipping, fear of water.
- Change in bath routine.
- Unfamiliar care provider.
- Purpose of bathing forgotten.
- Task of bathing too difficult.
- Person is fatigued.
- Person is embarrassed/humiliated.

morning, whereas others bathe before bedtime. Many older persons may have bathed only once a week while growing up and this also should be considered when problems with bathing occur. Once a bath time has been established, it should be followed consistently on a daily basis. Adequate time is needed to avoid making the patient feel rushed. The bathroom needs to provide privacy and warmth.

A shower/bath chair or safety bench may prove useful for the older individual. Laying out all the needed supplies, such as soap, washcloth, and towel, will provide cues that the patient can use. In the early stages of the disease, simply reminding the patient of the bath and drawing the water may be all that are necessary to begin the routine. If the patient has mobility or balance problems, a seated shower is generally safest. If mobility and balance are not a problem and the patient can get in and out of the bathtub without great difficulty, a bath can be very therapeutic. A hand-held spray attachment can convert a bathtub into a shower and can be useful in rinsing the patient and making hair washing much easier.

Safety

Consideration also needs to be given to making the bathroom a safe environment for the patient. The patient's ability to distinguish between hot and cold water must be assessed. Temperatures on water heaters should be adjusted so that the water is not dangerously hot. Locks on doors should be removed. All containers should be plastic instead of glass. The addition of handrails in the bathtub and on the walls, the use of nonslip bath mats, and care taken to wipe up any puddles of water can help to prevent falls and broken bones. All electrical appliances such as razors and hair dryers need to be out of the patient's reach. The impaired person should not be left alone in the bath, particularly when in a tub of water.

Frequency of Bathing

The older patient usually does not need a complete bath every day; 3 times a week is normally sufficient. However, the patient does require daily cleansing of the face, hands, armpits, and perineal areas. Age changes in the skin result in reduced elasticity, moisture, and oil secretion. Daily bathing with soap can compound the problems of dry skin, itching, and fragile skin. Mild soaps and emollient lotions can be used to help decrease skin dryness. Bath oil or lotion should be applied after the patient has gotten out of the bathtub to avoid the possibility of slipping on residual oil. Special attention must be given to thoroughly drying skin creases and folds. Unscented powders and cornstarch can be used to keep these areas dry; however, care needs to be taken not to allow these powders to accumulate.

Hair Care

Washing the patient's hair may be more easily accomplished if performed separately from the bath. Many patients with Alzheimer's disease react to water running down their face and become fearful or agitated. Hair washing can be performed at the kitchen sink, or for many older women, at the beauty parlor. There are dry chemical shampoos that can be used if washing with water is not

> **—● Some Useful Strategies for Bathing**
>
> • Be consistent with the daily routine (bathe same way, same time).
> • Provide adequate lighting, privacy, warmth.
> • Lay out necessary equipment in sequence.
> • Provide verbal/visual cues.
> • Use calm, matter-of-fact approach.
> • Try shower if tub doesn't work or vice versa.
> • Engage person in conversation while assisting with bathing.
> • Have physician write a prescription for bathing: "Bathe three times a week."
> • Give the person something to handle (washcloth, etc.) during bathing.
> • Do not rush the person.
> • Tomato juice added to bath water can help with persistent body odor.
> • Phrase instructions so person cannot say "no" to bathing.

feasible. However, the dry shampoo does tend to accumulate on the scalp and should not be used for long periods without a thorough washing and rinsing.

Handling Agitation

If the patient should become extremely agitated and combative, it is generally best to stop the bath, remove the patient from the area, and try again later when the patient has calmed down. Resistive or combative behavior occurs most commonly during close contact, such as bathing and dressing. Management of this type of behavior is discussed in Chapter 12.

Regardless of the type of bath, bathing is a very personal and private activity. The loss of independence in this area can be extremely difficult for the patient. Many patients may have never undressed in front of a caregiver, and a great deal of embarrassment and humiliation may be present. Caregivers must recognize that the person with Alzheimer's disease may be experiencing strong feelings about this loss and that such feelings may be contributing to her difficulties in bathing.

DRESSING

Difficulty in dressing may be one of the problems faced by both caregivers and patients with Alzheimer's disease. The patient may no longer be able to coordinate colors, may put on a shirt backward, or may fasten buttons in the wrong order. Affected patients often put on many layers of clothes, or they may want to remove clothing at inappropriate times. The act of dressing is as complex as any of the other activities of daily living. Some possible causes for difficulty with dressing include:

• Loss of interest in self and personal appearance
• Gross and fine motor skill deterioration

- Memory loss (forgets if dressing or undressing)
- Distractions while dressing
- Too hot or too cold
- Mechanics of dressing forgotten
- Decreased attention span
- Embarrassment and humiliation over requiring assistance
- Forgotten name of body parts

Organization

In the early stages of the disease, simply organizing the patient's clothes in outfits and colors can be very useful. Labeling the closet and dresser drawers with large letters (e.g., SOCKS, UNDERWEAR) can help the patient locate certain clothing. Placing an outfit laid out in order on the bed for the patient can help avoid catastrophic reactions that may occur when the patient becomes frustrated by trying to coordinate colors or choose clothing. Eliminating clutter and distractions while the patient is dressing will help keep his attention focused on the task.

Ease of Dressing

As Alzheimer's disease progresses, the patient loses fine motor skills. A noticeable stiffening of the muscles also may occur. Both of these physical changes make the act of dressing much more difficult than it would be normally. The patient may not be able to manipulate small buttons, hooks, or zippers. Clothing that has been adapted with large zippers or Velcro closures makes dressing easier for the patient. Pull-on skirts and pants are also easier for the patient to use. Clothing that is pulled on over the head may prove problematic because of poor joint mobility but also because the patient may feel threatened if her head is temporarily covered. Clothing should also be made of easy-care fabric to lessen the burden on the caregiver since patients with Alzheimer's disease can easily go through several changes of clothing a day.

Putting away rarely worn or out-of-season clothing can help to simplify choosing what to wear. Accessories such as belts and ties should be hung with the appropriate outfit to make dressing easier. All the articles of clothing needed for an outfit can be placed in sequential order on the patient's bed to enable his or her independence. The pattern of the fabric should be relatively simple, since wild, busy prints can be distracting to the patient. Shoes should be slip-on type or have Velcro closures instead of strings or ties. If the patient wants to wear the same clothes day after day, this issue should not become a point of argument. It is generally easier to buy several sets of the same outfit to accommodate the patient.

Unusual Patterns of Dress

Some patients tend to undress frequently, which can be both embarrassing and inconvenient for caregivers. It is important to investigate the cause of this action. The patient may be too hot, the material may be scratchy, the patient may be bored,

---

─● Some Useful Strategies for Dressing

- Stick to same routine when dressing (same time, same instructions).
- Avoid interruptions and distractions once the task is started.
- Provide adequate lighting, privacy, and warmth.
- Lay out clothes in sequence.
- Hang coordinated sets of clothing together.
- Label drawers with contents.
- Place accessories such as belts and ties with outfit.
- Provide verbal cues: "Now put your leg into the pants."
- Provide visual cues—demonstrate putting arm into shirt.
- Give instructions for only one step at a time.
- Provide praise and encouragement.
- Do not rush the person.
- Replace buttons and snaps with Velcro or zippers.
- Buy wash-and-wear clothing.
- If person seems to want to wear the same thing all the time buy several sets of the same outfit.

---

or he may need to go to the bathroom. In any case, caregivers must remember that the patient with Alzheimer's disease no longer understands what is appropriate and usually is not undressing himself to be provocative. Management of this behavior is discussed in Chapter 12.

On the other hand, some patients develop a habit of putting on many layers of clothes, regardless of the weather. Again, this practice can be embarrassing to the caregiver. It also can be potentially dangerous if the environment is very warm. First, a determination needs to be made about whether the patient is cold. Is the patient shivering? Is the skin cool to touch or is "goose flesh" visible? The possibility of danger associated with the patient wearing layers of clothes should be considered. If no danger is involved, the practice can be allowed. However, if the patient needs to have several sweaters or coats removed, more appropriate clothing can be substituted. Increasing the patient's activity level can also be useful in generating body heat to help keep the patient warm. When removing the layered items, the caregiver should do so with patience and the understanding that the very same thing will need to be done again later.

TOILETING

As Alzheimer's disease progresses, the patient begins to experience problems related to emptying the bladder and/or bowel. Initially, the problem may be related to the fact that the patient no longer recognizes the body signals of a full bowel or bladder. At this point a patient with Alzheimer's disease may need to be reminded to go to the bathroom frequently to empty his bladder or sit daily on the toilet to try and have a bowel movement.

With many patients, setting up a regular schedule for toileting has proven effective in avoiding accidents. The patient may also forget where the bathroom is located, or may not recognize the toilet as the appropriate place to urinate. Such a patient will need to be taken by the hand, led to the bathroom, and seated on the toilet. Sometimes labeling the bathroom door will be helpful to the patient. Regardless of the cause, the onset of toileting problems and incontinence is distressing to caregivers and patients. The causes, treatment, and management of urinary incontinence are discussed in greater detail in Chapters 15 and 16.

Maintaining Bowel Function

Maintaining normal bowel function in the patient with Alzheimer's disease takes creativity on the part of the caregiver in addition to advice from health professionals. Generally, problems with bowel function do not arise until later in the disease; however, constipation can develop at any time. Changes in the digestive system that occur with aging tend to make the older person more prone to constipation. Constipation and fecal impaction can cause a high degree of discomfort and distress in the patient, which can lead to behavioral problems. Caregivers need to continually assess and monitor the patient's bowel function.

In initiating a bowel maintenance program, the caregiver should know the patient's usual pattern of bowel movement. This pattern includes frequency and time of day. Once this pattern has been established for the patient, all efforts should be geared toward maintaining it.

Patients should not be permitted to go longer than three days without a bowel movement because of the high risk for fecal impaction and subsequent fecal incontinence.

Taking the patient to the bathroom at the same time every day and having him sit on the toilet will help to "train" the bowel to empty at this particular time. This is often best accomplished after the morning meal.

Natural Stimulants

The next step is to use natural methods of stimulating bowel function. Diet, activity, and fluids are the mainstays of preventing constipation and preserving normal bowel function. Particular attention must be given to diet in the patient with Alzheimer's disease since chewing and swallowing problems are often encountered. Increasing the amount of whole fiber in the patient's diet is very important because fiber acts to pull water into the bowel to soften the fecal mass. Whole-grain breads, pastas, cereals, vegetables, and fruits are good sources of natural fiber. These foods should be included in the patient's diet on a daily basis.

The patient needs to be kept as active as possible because physical activity helps to facilitate bowel motion. Taking the patient for a walk twice a day, involving him

---

● Some Useful Strategies for a Bowel Management Program

- Make sure the patient is getting enough fluids throughout the day (1500–2000 ml).
- Make sure the patient is getting as much exercise as possible.
- Increase the amount of fiber in the patient's diet (fruits, vegetables, grains, etc.).
- Have patient sit on toilet every day at same time (30 minutes after a meal is often best).
- Provide comfort and privacy.
- Try a hot liquid such as coffee, herbal tea, prune juice prior to toileting.
- Use positive reinforcement (praise and encouragement).

---

or her in an exercise class (if possible), or simply moving him from one chair to another throughout the day can help add to the patient's activity level. For the bed-bound patient, turning every 2 hours and helping the patient to sit up in a chair several times during the day can aid in increasing bowel motility.

Finally, increasing the amount of fluids that the patient drinks will assist in preventing constipation. Older individuals sometimes drink less fluid to reduce urinary frequency and incontinence. Others will simply forget to drink unless the caregiver is attuned to this need. Water is definitely needed throughout the day. Some fruit juices are also good and offer nutritional value. Coffee and tea should not be used as substitutes for water because these liquids tend to act as diuretics and thus decrease body fluid. Sometimes a cup of hot liquid, such as coffee, herbal tea, or prune juice, taken approximately 30 minutes before toileting can help to stimulate bowel action.

Laxatives

If activity, fluids, and fiber are given a 2- to 4-week trial and fail to regulate bowel function, laxatives may be needed. This decision should always be discussed with the patient's physician because drug interactions may occur with some laxative preparations.

Before the use of laxatives in initiated, valid indication for the laxative should always be determined. Laxatives can lead to serious complications, such as fecal incontinence, intestinal obstruction, mental disturbances, and urinary retention. Laxatives used on a regular basis can result in a bowel that actually decreases in natural motility since it becomes accustomed to the laxative's stimulating effect. Appropriate and safe use must be followed, and continuing assessment of the patient's need for the laxative must be done.

Laxatives are generally grouped into five categories:
- Bulk-forming
- Osmotic (saline)

- Surfactant (wetting agents)
- Contact (stimulant/irritant)
- Lubricant (emollient)

The action of each varies, and the laxative chosen should be based on patient's needs.

Bulk-forming laxatives. Bulk-forming laxatives are basically fiber-containing mixtures such as bran, methylcellulose, and psyllium hydrophilic mucilloid. These agents act by retaining water in the intestine so that the fecal mass remains large and soft. This type of laxative is traditionally tried first because it tends to restore bowel function in the most natural manner. The effects of bulk-forming agents can be realized within 24 hours or may take as long as 3 days. One important factor is the need for additional fluids with these agents to prevent dehydration and obstruction. Each dose should be administered with at least 8 ounces of water. The side effects of bulk-forming laxatives include gaseousness and abdominal fullness and discomfort. Caregivers of patients with diabetes must be aware that some of these preparations contain large amounts of dextrose.

Osmotic laxatives. Osmotic laxatives act by attracting water into the intestine to soften the fecal mass. These agents work faster than bulk-forming agents, taking only 2 to 6 hours, but they have more serious side effects. Since these agents are often salts of magnesium, sulfate, or phosphorus, patients with impaired kidney functions may not be able to clear the body of the extra salt load. Also, the serum levels of magnesium and phosphate ions may rise. Lactulose is an osmotic agent that has been used a great deal. However, because it contains digestible sugars, it must be used with caution in patients with diabetes. Lactulose can also cause cramping, diarrhea, and electrolyte imbalance if taken at higher than recommended dosages. As with bulk-forming agents, additional water needs to be provided to the patient to prevent possible dehydration.

Surfactant laxatives. Surfactant or wetting agents are recommended for patients who have normal bowel tone but hard, dry stools. These agents react with the fecal mass, allowing it to be penetrated by water and fat. Dioctyl sulfosuccinates make up this category of laxatives. These agents have a relatively quick action, within 6 to 8 hours, and are recommended for temporary use. When used on a long-term basis, they do not appear to have much effect on preventing constipation. Therefore, after the immediate problem of hard, dry stool has been corrected, the patient should be given bulk-forming agents for long-term management.

Stimulant laxatives. Contact, or stimulant, laxatives are recommended only for temporary relief of constipation or for bowel cleansing before a procedure. These agents act directly on the intestinal mucosa to increase activity and mobility, stimulating the propulsion of the fecal mass. Severe cramping and diarrhea can result, and some agents remain in the system for several days, causing continued action. Chronic use of this type of laxative can lead to serious problems, such as intestinal mucosal damage, fluid and electrolyte disturbances, and malabsorption. The tablet form of these laxatives should not be crushed or chewed because this practice causes irritation of the stomach mucosa.

Lubricants. Lubricants or emollients, such as mineral oil, act by coating the fecal mass to prevent loss of water and facilitate passage of the mass through the colon. Mineral oil can interfere with the absorption of vitamins A, D, K, and E. In patients with swallowing difficulty, aspiration of mineral oil can lead to lipid pneumonia, a very serious complication. Large doses of mineral oil may leak through the anal sphincter and cause soiling of the patient's clothes and bed linens. Enemas should be used for only the most difficult cases of constipation, and they should be provided only by persons educated in proper administration. Fluid and electrolyte imbalance and perforation of the colon have been associated with the incorrect administration of enemas.

FECAL IMPACTION

If a patient begins to have small, diarrhetic stools; leakage of small amounts of feces; or abdominal cramping and pain, he or she should be checked for a fecal impaction, which often produces these symptoms. A laxative or an enema will help to remove the impaction. Once the impaction is removed, a program of preventing a recurrence should be instituted using any of the methods previously discussed. With any patient, the frequency of bowel movements should be monitored to avoid impaction, and the quantity and characteristics of the stool should be noted.

OTHER HYGIENIC TASKS

Eventually the patient will need help with other tasks related to overall hygiene. The caregiver should be alert for signs of need for assistance in these areas.

Nail Care

Fingernails and toenails should be trimmed and filed on a regular basis. They should be kept short to prevent accidental scratching. Toenails should be trimmed straight across, whereas fingernails should be rounded at the ends. An opportune time to perform nail care is after the bath since the nails are generally softer and easier to manicure at that time. The nails should be cleaned regularly to remove dirt, feces, oils, and dead skin, which accumulate under them. In the patient whose fingers are severely contracted, the nails must be kept short to prevent them from cutting into the palm of the hand. Also, the patient must have his hands thoroughly washed and dried in the palm and between the fingers to remove dirt and dead skin. If this step is not performed, the area under the contracted fingers will quickly become macerated and possibly infected.

Ears

The patient's ears should not be neglected. The outside part of the ear can be cleansed easily with a washcloth wrapped over a finger. Cotton swabs can be used, but the tip should always be visible (i.e., the ear canal should not be entered). Improper use of swabs serves only to push wax farther into the ear. The ears should be inspected periodically to detect the buildup of hard packed wax. Such buildup occurs commonly in the older person and can lead to a substantial hearing loss. This problem can be easily corrected by having the ear canal irrigated by a health professional to remove the impacted wax.

Shaving

Shaving is another task that requires safety and supervision. Once the patient's coordination and judgment have become impaired, an electric razor can be used to keep the patient independent and safe while performing this activity. If an electric razor is used, shaving should be supervised to ensure that electrical safety practices are followed (e.g., not shaving with water in the sink and correct plugging/unplugging of the cord). Rechargeable battery-operated razors can be used to avoid such hazards.

Beards and mustaches should never be shaved by a health care professional unless the family has been consulted first. Most of the time, a beard or mustache can be left, but it needs to be kept short, neat, and regularly cleaned. Because food particles often become embedded in a beard or mustache, the area should be thoroughly cleansed after each meal. Applying a small amount of after-shave lotion can help the patient feel good about himself if this has been a life-long habit.

For female patients, cream depilatories can be used on legs and underarms. However, a skin patch test should be performed before the product is used to note any sensitivity to it. Older women also may develop a growth of facial hair. This should be removed on a regular basis using either a cream depilatory or safety razor. Female patients who have previously worn makeup should be encouraged to continue the practice because doing so helps their self-esteem. The patient should be supervised when applying makeup so that it may be done appropriately. The makeup should be thoroughly removed each night to avoid skin problems. Finally, many women currently in this age group have had a lifelong habit of having their hair professionally cut and styled. All efforts should be made to continue this practice as long as possible since this routine will make the patient feel better about herself. Once the patient can no longer visit the hair salon, some stylists will come to visit the patient. Caregivers should strive to style the patient's hair each day in his or her usual fashion.

NUTRITION/EATING

Persons with Alzheimer's disease need a well-balanced diet consisting of adequate calories, protein, carbohydrates, and fat. Any dietary restrictions required for the management of other chronic problems (diabetes, hypertension, etc.) should also

---

─● Possible Causes for Difficulty in Eating

- Dry mouth
- Agitation and anxiety
- Presence of an acute illness
- Changes in taste and smell perception
- Patient forgets to eat, thinks he has just eaten
- Decreased attention span
- Constipation and depression suppress appetite
- Change in daily routine or meal routine
- No longer understands what to do
- Difficulty in using silverware
- Distractions during mealtime

---

be followed. For a more complete discussion on general nutrition, the reader is referred to the Bibliography section at the end of this chapter.

Early in the course of Alzheimer's disease, maintaining an adequate dietary intake is usually not a problem. Patients may continue to eat regular meals and caregivers should stick to the normal routine of meal preparation and serving. The patient may continue to enjoy going out to eat. Some suggestions for dining out include choosing a quiet, well-lit restaurant that has quick service, seating the patient so she faces the wall, and sticking to the foods the caregiver knows the patient likes. If the patient accompanies the caregiver to a cafeteria, it is advisable to seat the patient and have the caregiver bring the meal to her. However, as the disease progresses, patients begin to experience difficulties associated with eating. These difficulties usually stem from the continued memory loss and gradual decline in the patients' physical abilities.

Problems with Eating

When problems in eating begin to occur, caregivers should first look into possible physical problems as being the cause. Teeth, gums, and dentures should be inspected for problems that may be making chewing and swallowing uncomfortable or difficult. Caregivers should think about how long it has been since the patient had a good bowel movement, and take corrective action if needed. Certain medications can affect appetite and cause dry mouth, and should be discussed with the physician if suspected of interfering with eating.

The decreased attention span and increased susceptibility to distractions of patients with Alzheimer's disease are common causes of difficulty in eating. Noise and distractions during mealtime need to be minimized to help the patient focus on the task of eating. Patients may be more successful at mealtime if they eat alone or with only the caregiver. Table settings should be uncluttered. Brightly patterned placemats and tablecloths should be avoided. Serving one food at a time may also become necessary since the presence of more than one food on the plate may cause the patient to become frustrated with knowing what to eat.

The process of eating should be made as simple as possible. Using spoons instead of forks and bowls instead of plates may be helpful. Plates and bowls can be placed on slip-resistant materials to keep the plate or bowl from moving as the patient attempts to eat from it. Plastic utensils are generally not advisable as they are too light and could easily break in the patient's mouth. Mugs are good for serving soups and stews, and a cup with a handle should replace glasses. There is an abundance of adaptive and assistive devices, such as large-handled utensils, plate guards, and weighted cups and bowls, which can facilitate the patient continuing to feed himself. An occupational therapist can be an invaluable resource in determining which devices would assist the patient. Most medical supply stores and medical equipment catalogs have a large selection of devices. Once the patient continues to have difficulty in using utensils, caregivers can begin serving finger foods such as sandwiches and cut-up vegetables. Serving food that the patient can eat using his hands allows the patient to continue to feed himself.

For the patient who wants to eat all the time, caregivers should try serving five or six smaller meals throughout the day. Adding extra exercise and activities to this patient's daily routine will help to burn up the extra calories being consumed and can also serve as a distraction from the obsession with eating. Low-calorie snacks should be readily available for the overeater. For the patient who undereats, a glass of wine or juice prior to the meal may help to stimulate her appetite. Calorie-rich foods such as milk shakes, eggnog, or nutritional supplements can be used to get more calories into the patient in a lesser volume. This patient should be allowed to eat whenever hungry, so having nutritious snacks on hand is a must. Finally, if the patient exhibits significant weight loss (3 or more pounds per week), the physician should be consulted. There may be an underlying physical cause for the patient's weight loss.

Mealtime should be a quiet and calm time for the patient and caregiver. This will help to prevent many of the problems commonly encountered during eating. Caregivers need to be wary of food temperatures since the patient may no longer remember the meaning of hot or cold. Finally, because most patients with Alzheimer's disease eventually experience problems in swallowing, caregivers should learn the actions to take in the event of an airway obstruction or choking—the Heimlich maneuver.

SUMMARY

Hygienic practices may seem simple and well ingrained in everyone, yet each task requires decision making, judgment, memory, and coordination. Since each of these abilities is impaired in the patient with Alzheimer's disease, the caregiver must continually assess the patient's abilities and provide guidance and assistance as needed. Helping the patient to complete each task with the least amount of assistance helps to improve her self-esteem and body image and to keep her functioning longer. Eventually the patient will lose all ability to participate in her own care. At this point, patients require round-the-clock care and total assistance from caregivers. The care of the person in the end-stage, or "terminal" stage, of Alzheimer's disease is discussed in Chapter 20.

BIBLIOGRAPHY

Baum BJ: Oral health for the older patient, *J Am Geriat Soc* 44(8):997-998, 1996.

Beverly L, Travis I: Constipation: proposed natural laxative mixtures, *J Gerontol Nurs* 18(10):5-12, 1992.

Burgener S, Barton D: Nursing care of cognitively impaired, institutionalized elderly, *J Gerontol Nurs* 17(4):37-43, 1991.

Heacock P et al: Caring for the cognitively impaired: reconceptualizing disability and rehabilitation, *J Gerontol Nurs* 17(3):22-26, 1991.

Hutchinson S, Leger-Krall S, Wilson HS: Toileting: a biobehavioral challenge in Alzheimer's dementia care, *J Gerontol Nurs* 22(10):18-27, 1996.

Lee VK: Language changes and Alzheimer's disease: a literature review, *J Gerontol Nurs* 17(1):16-20, 1991.

Maxfield M, Lewis RE, Cannon S: Training staff to prevent aggressive behavior of cognitively impaired elderly patients during bathing and grooming, *J Gerontol Nurs* 22(1):37-43, 1996.

Monicken D: Immobility and functional mobility in the elderly. In Chenitz WC, Stone JT, Salisbury SA, editors: *Clinical gerontological nursing: a guide to advanced practice*, Philadelphia, 1991, WB Saunders.

Norberg A, Athlin E: Eating problems in severely demented patients, *Nurs Clin North Am* 24(3):781-787, 1989.

Robinson A, Spencer B, White L: *Understanding difficult behaviors*, Ann Arbor, Mich, 1989, Geriatric Education Center of Michigan.

Sand BJ, Yeaworth RC, McCabe BW: Alzheimer's disease: special care units in long-term care facilities, *J Gerontol Nurs* 18(3):28-34, 1992.

Souren LEM, Franssen EH, Reisberg B: Contractures and loss of function in patients with Alzheimer's disease, *J Am Geriat Soc* 48(6):650, 1995.

Stone JT: Managing bowel function. In Chenitz WC, Stone JT, Salisbury SA, editors: *Clinical gerontological nursing: a guide to advanced practice*, Philadelphia, 1991, WB Saunders.

Tanner F, Shaw S, editors: *Caring: a family guide to managing the Alzheimer's patient at home*, New York, 1985, New York City Alzheimer's Resource Center.

Van Ort S, Phillips LR: Nursing interventions to promote functional feeding, *J Gerontol Nurs* 21(10):6-14, 1995.

Yakabowich M: Prescribe with care: the role of laxatives in the treatment of constipation, *J Gerontol Nurs* 16(7):4-11, 1990.

Developing a Day's Activity

James M Turnbull
Elizabeth A Turnbull

Never tell people how to do things.
Tell them what to do,
and they will surprise you with their ingenuity.

—General George S. Patton Jr.

Since there is no cure for Alzheimer's disease, the emphasis in treatment must become care. A vital part of such care is a daily program or routine that keeps the patient's mind and body active. Although the focus of this chapter is on day treatment programs, most of the activities can be modified for the home or the nursing home.

— Day care programs for patients with Alzheimer's disease offer much more than respite for the caregivers, as valuable as that service may be.

A well-structured program provides a mechanism for the design and coordination of plans between health care providers and caregivers. Most important, it offers an opportunity for patients to maintain a sense of community and self-worth in the face of increasing isolation and an inevitable decline in abilities.

Creating day care programs for patients diagnosed with Alzheimer's disease is a simple, though multifaceted, task. Most conventional day care centers for the elderly lack important elements that are essential for patients with this disease. The characteristics of these patients impose requirements for staffing and facilities that are beyond the level that most day care centers routinely offer. The unexpected and often disruptive behavior of patients, the inability to complete tasks without step-by-step instruction, and the tendency to wander must all be accommodated.

The lack of familiarity that accompanies memory loss can lead to constant insecurity and social impotence. The strengths that patients retain are their only links with productive life. Through careful planning and guidance, these strengths may be called on, returning meaning and productivity to a life of seeming chaos.

PATIENT NEEDS

An effective program is based on a careful evaluation of each individual patient's strengths and needs. Alzheimer's disease often leaves a patient in a state of conflict, wanting to be active and involved while limited in the ability to function. The patient may react with irritability and restlessness, demonstrated in social withdrawal, a resistance to anything new, and a disinterest in ongoing activities. An effective program attempts to establish alternative modes of functioning that minimize this conflict.

Alzheimer's patients need environmental stability, and environmental influences on patient's behavior should never be underestimated. Changes in environment and overstimulation can increase feelings of anxiety and agitation. Structured and predictable environmental stimuli can be comforting and calming. This consideration needs to be part of any program at home or in a treatment center.

The hierarchy of needs developed by Abraham Maslow provides a useful framework for analyzing patient needs. The basic needs include the physiological ones, such as thirst, hunger, shelter, and warmth. When these basic needs have been met, security becomes the focus. Finally, when the need for security has been satisfied, psychosocial needs, such as self-esteem, autonomy, identity, control, and meaningful communication with others, emerge.

Meeting the security and psychosocial needs is of paramount importance in effective program planning for patients with Alzheimer's disease.

A sense of security or safety is essential. The symptoms of Alzheimer's disease make the patient's world frighteningly unpredictable. A stable, predictable, calm, and nonthreatening environment can relieve the insecurities that memory loss and perceptual impairments create, enabling the patient to make full use of the abilities that she has retained.

Nowhere is the devastation of Alzheimer's disease more profound than on a patient's identity. The deficits caused by the symptoms of Alzheimer's disease can be reversed by using the patient's remaining abilities. Tasks that the patient can still accomplish, such as drying dishes or folding clothes, can help to reinforce feelings of control and autonomy. Being included as a member of a group can deter the effects of Alzheimer's disease that often lead to social isolation and low self-esteem. These needs must be recognized in program planning. Light chores, grooming, and group activities are simple activities that can contribute to meeting both psychosocial and security needs.

ABERRANT BEHAVIOR HAS MEANING

The behaviors that Alzheimer's patients exhibit, especially the problematic ones, are attempts to communicate. Staff members can effectively work with these patients by defining and understanding these behavioral reactions. This can be accomplished by focusing on one difficult behavior at a time. It is best to focus on a problem that is potentially dangerous or is inhibiting daily functioning.

With increased cognitive impairment, agitation and combativeness increase, while verbal behaviors decrease. The most common problematic behavioral

—• **Analysis of a Problem Behavior:**

1. A note should be made specifying when the problem behavior occurs. Events preceding the behavior may be stimulating the negative response.
2. The reactions of both the patient and the caregiver should be noted in order to find patterns of stimuli that trigger the response.
3. Close attention should be paid to any reactions of caregivers that reinforce the behavior.

reactions are agitation, withdrawal, and noisiness. These problem behaviors are the result of cognitive-related dysfunctions, like confusion and disorientation, and emotional or physical distress. Anxiety is the most common emotional precipitator, and depression is second.

Physical discomfort and pain often result in restlessness and irritability. In fact, these behaviors can be attempts to convey the physical distress being experienced and they need to be addressed properly.

They may also be the first sign that activities are becoming too difficult. By altering the activities and simplifying comments, caregivers and staff can enhance the effectiveness of the activity because the anxiety or frustration resulting from the failure of the task has been alleviated or minimized. Flexibility and adaptability are crucial in any attempt to maximize patient comfort and success. Therefore, an ongoing review of environmental, physical, and psychiatric problems is crucial in order to provide a successful program.

PATIENT STRENGTHS

Although the disabilities of patients with Alzheimer's disease must be considered, programs should capitalize on their functional abilities, that is, their strengths and retained abilities, particularly emotional awareness, remote memory, primary sensory and motor functions, perseveration, and retention of well-learned or habitual tasks.

There are many ways to focus a patient's strengths. In order to help do so, the caregiver should remember that:

- Pleasant emotions can be promoted through activities such as interaction with animals or babies, group sharing sessions, and reminiscence sessions.
- Remote memory, or recollection of one's distant past, can provide pleasure by creating a link with more stable times, reaffirming the patient's self-esteem. Such life-review activities can help to create a balance between the patient's current abilities and past accomplishments.
- Music and fragrance activities are particularly effective in helping the patient recall sensory memories when abstract memory has been lost.
- Negative emotions such as frustration and anger can be diffused in vigorous physical activities.

- When a patient with Alzheimer's disease displays inappropriate emotional reactions, staff often tend to discount that person's feelings and emotions. Instead, these emotions should be acknowledged, validated, and used in the patient's behalf.

Since most primary motor and sensory functions are left intact in Alzheimer's disease, these functions can be used productively within an effective program. If perceptual problems are taken into consideration, retained strengths such as muscular control, dexterity, and strength can enable the patient to accomplish tasks and successfully engage the day care environment. Rhythm also appears to be a very effective mode of sensory stimulation. Use of these strengths is an effective antidote to inactivity and isolation.

Perseveration, the tendency to repeat a motion until interrupted, can be an asset in performing certain tasks. The ability to repeat one simple step often eliminates the frustration of forgetting the next step. Activities that require repetitive motions, such as raking leaves or vacuuming, are well-suited to this disturbance.

Habitual and well-learned activities, those that have been learned and practiced repeatedly throughout a person's life, are often retained, at least in part. Activities that incorporate these routines can be especially reinforcing because of the familiarity of the behavior and the self-confidence that performing without constant instruction imparts. Problems may occur when an inappropriate routine is evoked or when a distraction interrrupts the flow of activity during performance.

PROGRAM DESIGN

The physical environment, staffing, and selection of program activities, scheduling, and pacing of program activities should contribute to making the patient feel as productive, autonomous, and secure as possible. Several factors contribute to a successful program design.

Physical Environment

The perceptual difficulties experienced by patients with Alzheimer's disease require an effort to make the environment predictable and consistent in order to avoid confusion. Many simple techniques can promote a stable environment.

To create a helpful physical environment:
- Floors and walls should be perceptually distinct from each other (e.g., different colors) and should be clear of any markings that may be perceived as obstacles.
- Furniture should be distinct, have clear edges, and be placed outside high traffic areas, where it might become an obstacle.
- The space should be divided into specific permanent activity areas (e.g., one for meetings and another for crafts). The permanent arrangement helps the patient feel more secure and capable of getting around.
- Restrooms should be clearly marked "Men" and "Women" to avoid confusion.
- Well-marked exits are very important so that many patients do not have a sense of being trapped, but the exit should be monitored so that a patient cannot wander off unattended.

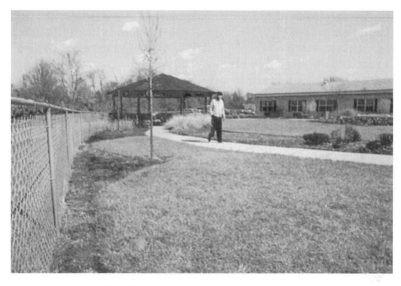

Figure 19-1   An enclosed garden allows persons with Alzheimer's disease to wander in a safe environment. (From Sorrentino SA et al: *Mosby's textbook for long-term care assistants,* ed 2, St Louis, 1994, Mosby.)

- Gardens and walking areas can be used by patients to safely work off their restlessness.
- Walking areas should be safe, fenced, and monitored in order to ensure the safety of wandering patients (Figure 19-1).

Encouragement of regular exercise with a walking companion as a regularly scheduled activity is more effective than attempting to eliminate overactive behavior. Providing safe places for masturbating and exposing parts of the body is also more effective than trying to abate the behavior. The patient can be distracted and guided to the safe area, where the behavior can be resumed in a more private and appropriate manner. Orientation to time and place can be effectively achieved by using clocks, calendars, and decorations appropriate to the current season and to holidays.

The location of the program in a nonmedical building tends to lessen feelings of anxiety on the part of patients. A large room located within a community facility, with an adjoining restroom and coat room, and having activity areas clearly segregated by furniture groupings is an ideal setting for a day care program.

When working with Alzheimer's patients, staff often face conflicts between ensuring the patient's freedom of movement and safeguarding them from social inappropriateness or harm. Historically, physical and pharmacological restraints have been used, but they often led to more staff responsibilities and patient suffering. Novel solutions have been found that utilize the faulty cognitions and misperceptions caused by the disease. For instance, when doorknobs are concealed behind a cloth panel, visual disturbances such as visual agnosia make it appear that a dead end has been reached.

Staffing

Zgola has recommended that two professional staff members (e.g., nurse, physical therapist, or occupational therapist and/or recreation therapist) and four volunteers be provided for every seven to eight patients. Although the number may vary from activity to activity, this amount suffices for most activities. The initiation period of an activity demands a one-to-one ratio that can be slowly altered to accommodate the patient's reactions and abilities. Highly structured activities such as group discussion and meal preparation may require fewer staff (two or three staff to eight patients). Having too many staff members for activities in which some staff are uninvolved tends to overwhelm patients and reduce independent activity. Uninvolved staff should withdraw, but remain available in case assistance is needed.

ACTIVITIES

Patients with Alzheimer's disease are capable of performing a variety of activities that fulfill their need to be active. These include exercise and other gross motor activities, grooming, socializing, meal preparation, housework, crafts, light work, and special events (see Box 19-1).

Physical Exercise

Exercise helps to maintain muscular strength, joint dexterity, and body awareness. It also provides a gentle cardiopulmonary workout and can be utilized to avoid the restlessness or agitation that a surplus of physical energy can cause. Simple games such as beanbag toss, shuffleboard, and bowling, which have an obvious objective and are generally considered adult games, are most acceptable. More complex games such as croquet can be used by simplifying the goal (e.g., hitting the ball the farthest.)

Grooming Activities

Grooming activities help to build self-esteem. Initiation and assistance are often required. Staff members who assist can identify helpful techniques that can be shared with caregivers for use at home.

Socialization

Socialization can be promoted in many activities (see Box 19-1). During the orientation held at the beginning of the day, patients should be encouraged to contribute to discussion and to planning the day's activities. Coffee and tea breaks offer the opportunity for self-directed interactions that help maintain good social skills. A scheduled "wind-down time" at the end of the day helps the patient to recall his accomplishments during the day's events.

Communication is difficult for many patients with Alzheimer's disease and should be facilitated by program staff. Patients need to feel safe and accepted

● **Box 19-1**

Sample Activities

Orientation
Welcome, introduce new members
Discuss/plan daily activities

Household Chores
Dust, sweep, polish, mop
Sort, fold, hand laundry
Wash and dry dishes
Water and pot plants
Rake leaves, vacuum
Organize drawers and closets

Grooming and Hygiene
Dress
Brush teeth/dentures
Comb hair, wash face, apply makeup
Polish shoes

Meal Preparation
Chop, peel, clean vegetables and fruits
Cut or shape cookies
Stir, knead, mix
Grate cheese or vegetables
Set table

Crafts
Knitting, crocheting, embroidery, making pom-pom animals
Dried flower cards, nature plaques, refrigerator magnets
Woodworking, carving, wreaths
Stenciled notes, Christmas decorations, bookmarks

Work-Oriented Activities
Staple papers, fold newsletters
Stuff/stamp envelopes
Punch holes

Special Events
Birthday and holiday parties
Outings to parks, picnics, museums
Bus trip, river cruise
Demonstrations of fashion, makeup, decorating

Gross Motor Activities
Exercise, walking, dancing
Floor games: beanbag toss, ring toss, shuffleboard, bowling

Continued

● **Box 19-1**
Sample Activities—cont'd

Social Activities
Coffee or tea break
Table games, bingo, checkers, dominoes
Sing-along, storytelling
Guided reminiscence

Sensory Activities
Perfumes, makeup
Music, art, picture books
Animals, children, touching objects (fur, fabric scraps, stones)
Rocking chair
Massage
Food tasting (hors d'oeuvres, finger foods)

---

regardless of their communication skills. Since memory loss can inhibit the recollection of material, direct questions targeted at specific information should be avoided unless it is certain that the patient can answer them. The interactions that develop among the patients within the program are probably the single most valuable benefit of participation in a day care program.

Individual Tasks

Tasks at which the patient was once proficient offer special opportunities for participation. Washing and drying dishes, dusting, sweeping, chopping vegetables, or mixing prepared ingredients can give a patient the opportunity to be useful and to accept gratitude.

Activities involving many steps need to be broken into several simple steps so that the patient can accomplish the task and proceed to the next step with confidence.

Meal preparation is most successful when recipes have assembly-line organization and do not require precise proportions of ingredients.

Crafts and Work-Oriented Activities

Crafts can be satisfying if they are modified to accommodate the limited abilities of patients with Alzheimer's disease, and have a focus that recognizes patients as adults. Work-oriented activities, such as stapling papers, stuffing envelopes, or folding newsletters, are preferred by those who are not interested in housekeeping or crafts.

Special Activities

Special activities associated with the holidays offer the opportunity to celebrate and to enjoy decorating, food preparation, and sing-alongs. These celebrations should be brief in order to avoid overstimulation and overtiring. Field trips to local points of interest are enjoyable if large crowds or bad weather are avoided. Movies are not recommended because the perceptual changes that characterize Alzheimer's disease make movies difficult to follow.

Reality Orientation Therapy

Reality Orientation Therapy (ROT) can be a very effective activity for patients with mild and moderate cognitive impairment. ROT is most effective when both forms are utilized together. The first form, informal ROT, reorients the patients with continuous reminders of who they are, where they are, and what time it is.

The second form, formal or class ROT, is a reorientation within a group. These class ROT sessions are most effective when they last around 30 minutes and are part of the patients' scheduled routines. ROT can preserve and improve orientation and memory. ROT also gives patients and staff the valuable sense that they are doing something worthwhile. The effectiveness of ROT has been linked to staff's enthusiasm and belief in the success of the therapy.

A meaningful emotional contact is made when the aim of the therapy is to understand the personal meaning of the patients' views of reality and their behavior. This goal is achieved most effectively when staff uses empathic listening and overt problematic behaviors are absent.

SELECTION OF ACTIVITIES

The plan for the individual patient should be based on a comprehensive evaluation that includes information from a variety of sources, including physical and neurological examinations, neuropsychological testing, and psychiatric consultation. A social history that includes an evaluation of the patient's home environment and support systems helps staff and caregivers to translate program gains to the home setting. The individual plan must be grounded in an accurate assessment of the individual's needs, abilities, and limitations.

Functional Evaluation

Functional evaluation assesses the patient's level of functioning in terms of basic senses and functions, cognitive and behavioral skills, interpersonal relations, self-care skills, and mobility. A useful framework for functional evaluation, developed by Zgola, includes the seven w's:
• What can the patient do?
• What does the patient do?
• In what way does the patient do it?

● Box 19-2
Sample Schedule/Communication Sheet*

Time	Type of Activity	Options
10:00 a.m.	Orientation	Make coffee and discuss plans for the day
10:30 a.m.	Housekeeping	Dust, vacuum, or fold clothes *Note:* Needs help getting started, but great at vacuuming
11:00 a.m.	Prepare lunch	Soup, sandwiches, or cake
11:45 a.m.	Lunch	*Note:* Ate well but refused soup
12:15 p.m.	Cleanup	Clear table, wash or dry dishes
12:45 p.m.	Craft	Bookmark or wreath

Modified from Zgola, JM: *Doing things: a guide to programming activities for persons with Alzheimer's disease and related disorders,* Baltimore, 1987, Johns Hopkins University Press.
*By jotting notes in the margin, staff can communicate with the patient's caregivers. Sharing this record helps keep them in touch and communicates the most effective activities, difficulties encountered, and suggestions or concerns.

- Which part of the task is the patient unable to do?
- Why is the patient unable to do it?
- Where does the patient perform best?
- When does the patient perform best?

Ongoing evaluation is essential. Staff and caregivers can assist each other by sharing perceived problems and highlighting any changes that need to be considered. A notebook containing the day's plan and notes on accomplishments (Box 19-2) is sent to and from the day care program and home, and serves as a means of communication between family members and staff on matters of importance, ensuring that the therapeutic program can be updated as the patient's needs dictate.

Appropriate activities are selected, graded according to difficulty, and analyzed in regard to each individual's capabilities and needs. An activity should be a voluntary effort. It is essential that the patient understand the activity's purpose and perceive the activity as meaningful and achievable. In addition, it is necessary for the intellectual, physical, and perceptual demands of an activity to be achievable, given the abilities of the patient.

Grading an activity permits variation of the degree of involvement of each patient, allowing a decrease or increase of the activity's demands to match each individual's abilities. If the activity is baking cookies, for example, one patient might be able to mix the ingredients (a fairly high grade), and another patient could successfully participate at a lower grade by holding the cookie sheet while the cookies are portioned for baking. The second patient is able to participate successfully even though the grade of activity is lower. Activities with several steps are preferable since individuals can work together at various levels to complete an activity.

Analyzing activities in terms of their task demands also aids in matching abilities to the individual's functional levels. Analysis can be accomplished by asking the following questions:

1. What physical abilities (dexterity, strength, flexibility, coordination) are necessary to complete this activity successfully?
2. What sensory abilities (sight, smell, hearing, feeling, balance) are required?
3. What perceptual processes (spatial relations, eye-hand coordination, visual activity) are required?
4. What cognitive functions (memory, organization, problem-solving, communication, and attention) are required?

By also analyzing an activity in terms of its potential to contribute to the patient's psychosocial needs (e.g., identity, autonomy, inclusion), the program design can ensure both productivity and social interaction even in patients with the greatest disability.

Highly repetitive activities are often very successful. They create a sense of continuity and competence through the absence of worry about the "next step." Activities that have a wide range of successful outcomes are effective in avoiding failures. The best are those that give the patient a sense of accomplishment and social interaction.

Assessment Scales

Assessment scales are effective tools for evaluating patients' functioning levels. The Bristol Activities of Daily Living Scale, BADLS, is a simple and effective assessment tool:

- It is an effective means of assessing patients' performance levels on many tasks by recording daily functions and noting unfamiliar tasks that could lead to agitation.
- It correlates well with other assessment scales, such as the Mini-Mental Status Examination, and is more effective in evaluating patients with lower education levels.
- It is an effective tool for detecting minimal to severe levels of dependence in activity, and may be usefully sensitive to changes in dependence over time.

Scheduling

Scheduling of activities should take into account the patient's fluctuating energy levels and their effects on the patient's predictability and behavior. The patient's comfort and security are often acutely affected by these changes. Since energy levels tend to be highest at the beginning of the day, it is most effective to schedule the most demanding activities in the morning.

The duration of an activity is also important. Simple nondemanding activities, such as grooming, games, singing, or simple crafts, are enjoyed for longer periods since repetitive patterns can be established after the sometimes difficult initiation phase has been overcome. Unstructured activities, such as free-flowing group discussions and free times, are usually tolerated for 30 minutes or less.

Provision of Guidance

Without the skillful guidance of the staff, patients would face numerous obstacles in attempting activities. The following aspects of supervision aid in avoiding or overcoming the problems that arrest activity in patients with Alzheimer's disease:

1. Organization and presentation of the activity
2. Assistance in initiating the activity
3. Guidance during task performance

Organization of activities helps to overcome the ambiguities that can confuse patients. Staff and volunteers need to be aware of the activity's objectives, that is, the intended benefit for the patient. The goal might involve evoking a positive emotional reaction, for example, by making a heart magnet for a grandchild or by discussing memories recalled after viewing a family photograph. The actual completion of the task is only one objective.

Next, the activity must be broken down into logical, simple steps. This approach includes checking to be sure that the proper materials are at hand, reviewing the instructions, and eliminating possible sources of interference. Staff should have already completed portions of the task that the patient is no longer able to accomplish. Last, interference can destroy a patient's focus on an activity, and therefore a distraction-free area that is already set up for the activity is needed.

An orderly, careful indexation to the activity is necessary to combat the paralyzing fears and doubts that lead to inactivity in many patients with Alzheimer's disease. A simple, concise statement ("Let's go to the restroom") with a visual or concrete tactile clue (pointing toward the restroom) is more effective than an abstract statement ("Would you like to go to the bathroom?"), which may be unclear to the patient with Alzheimer's disease.

Simple instructions that help in beginning the task, such as "Hold this" or "Sit down," can be used to overcome inertia. Fortunately, patients often experience the pattern of action taking over once the activity has been initiated.

For craft activities, a brief explanation of what will be made, its uses, and a chance to see a sample will help in overcoming patients' fear of the unknown.

> Making the purpose of the activity known (e.g., a snack for the group) helps to motivate the patient.

Each step needs to be explained, and a demonstration of how it is accomplished should be given. The patient should not be expected to remember every step, and instructions should be repeated as often as needed. This reassurance eases some of the anxiety that keeps patients from attempting new activities. Observing the staff performing an activity is often effective as a first step toward further participation, such as holding or passing something. The grading of the activity serves as a good marker for the patient's ability and his potential level of involvement. If the patient resists an activity completely, it is best to stop and move on to another activity while noting problems that the patient might be experiencing, such as fatigue, or allowing a short break.

The successful outcome of an activity largely depends on the quality of guidance after initiation has been achieved. Only as much guidance as is needed should be given. Standing back, yet being prepared to help if necessary, allows patients to fully utilize their own initiative and ability.

The prior evaluation of the patient's abilities indicates whether verbal, visual, or manual guidance is preferable for a patient. Simple cues aid in reinforcing learning and establishing a pattern. Verbal cues should be concise and simple, and repetition using the same wording should be done to avoid confusion. Cues that involve touching the patient should occur within the patient's visual range, since unexpected contact can be frightening to patients with Alzheimer's disease.

It may be helpful to prepare the patient for contact by saying, "Let me show you how to hold your fingers." Force should never be used to push or pull the patient because this approach tends to elicit either total passivity or resistance. Gentle touching or firm pressure will comfort the patient and provide guidance. All guidance should be slowly withdrawn when it is no longer needed.

Coping with problems and failures in any task is an important aspect of guidance. Staff should be able to perceive problems and effectively help the patient to overcome them. A patient with Alzheimer's disease, for example, might be asked to bring the sugar to the mixing table and find that she cannot recognize the sugar. The inactivity that results might be easily overcome if the staff member restates the direction as, "Bring the white jar with the red lid."

If a task seems to require too much guidance and too little patient participation, it is best to stop and evaluate the appropriateness of the activity or the level of participation. The activity may be attempted again with additional preparation or with the staff providing more assistance. Reducing the negative impact of failure is a critical aspect of guidance.

Effective reinforcement preserves dignity and capitalizes on the innate sense of accomplishment associated with the task. A simple nod or smile will let the patient with Alzheimer's disease know that he is doing well. The patient should not be distracted with too much praise. A simple "thank you" is preferable to overpraise, since the sense of accomplishment is the most important reward.

Assistance with Mobility

An effective program offers accommodation for a patient's impairments in mobility. Seemingly simple actions, such as walking, sitting, or rising from a sitting position, become major challenges for the patient. Selecting a route that is free of obstacles or initiating movement may not be possible without assistance. Close observation can offer clues to the cause of difficulty and reveal effective ways to assist the patient.

The following suggestions are given for those assisting patients with difficulty in walking:
1. Lead the patient with your arm rather than by pushing or pulling.
2. Break long excursions into smaller segments.

3. Clearly state the destination.
4. Warn the patient of obstacles or irregularities in the surface.
5. Create a walking rhythm with your body while holding the patient's arm to help normalize his gait.
6. Rhythmic, single-word directions such as "step, cane, step, cane" help to coordinate movement when walkers or canes are used.

The following step-by-step procedure is effective in helping patients to rise from a seated position:

1. Have the patient move forward in the seat.
2. Position the patient's feet just under the rim of the chair or toilet, with heels raised slightly.
3. Instruct the patient to lean forward, put his weight over his feet, and push off with hands on the knees.
4. Offer an arm to the patient to help him balance, but do not pull; let the patient be in control.
5. If a walker is used, place the walker in front of the patient and guide it gently while he pulls up on it.

Sitting down can also be difficult, but the following techniques are helpful:

1. Clearly direct the patient to the chair or toilet.
2. Approach the chair or toilet from the front. Help or direct the patient to bend slightly and grasp the handrail or chair arm on the opposite side. A toilet chair with rails placed over the toilet is helpful for severely impaired patients.
3. Help the patient to retain her grasp on the chair and direct her to take small, turning steps until the chair is directly behind her. Applying firm pressure to the patient's hip and nudging her in the right direction can be helpful.
4. Direct the patient to reach back for the other arm of the chair and lower herself.
5. A little downward pressure on the nape of the neck may help a patient who has trouble flexing the hips become seated.

Many maneuvers, such as getting in or out of an automobile, become even more difficult if the patient is given too much time to think about what to do. A casual distracting conversation with the patient while opening the door and gently positioning him to enter or exit can be very helpful. Established patterns tend to take over at this point. Only as much assistance as the patient needs should be given since too much assistance is as confusing as too little.

PATIENT REACTIONS

Alzheimer's disease leaves many patients with a constant feeling of insecurity and fear. These problems can persist for a long time since memory loss, perceptual difficulties, conceptual difficulties, and temporal distortions severely hamper a patient's ability to cope with change. Support for both patient and caregivers is essential during stressful periods, particularly the early stages of participation in the day care program.

Ideally, the introduction to the program is made in the patient's home by a staff member who will be a consistent contact for the patient and family. The home visit allows the staff member to effectively assess the patient's ability to benefit from the program.

▬▬● To be effective, the program must fit the needs of both the patient and the caretakers.

The patient's anxieties and fears must be acknowledged, but the staff member should point out the positive and beneficial aspects of the program and invite the patient and caretakers for an observational visit. The patient may politely agree to attend and then voice negative feelings to the family. The family should be prepared for this reaction. They should be advised to keep a positive attitude, avoid confrontations while acknowledging negative feelings, and stress the benefits that the program offers to the patient.

Leaving home to go to the program for the first time is often a highly stressful event, even if the patient is enthusiastic about participating. Patients often become ambivalent and even resistant when the actual time to leave arrives. If possible, it is helpful for the staff member who made the initial contact to accompany the patient to the program. Having family members accompany the patient during the initial visit may also help to ease the insecurity and doubt that are caused by the novelty of the situation. The staff member, sensitive to the patient's needs and anxieties, may use an approach that varies from calm reassurance to firm direction, depending on the patient's reactions.

Breaking the processes down into smaller steps is often helpful. For example, if the staff member escorts the patient on a walk during the initial home visit, leaving for the program on a later day is less unfamiliar and anxiety producing. Consistency in attendance is essential particularly if the program is held only one day per week. If the routine of preparing for and attending the program is rigidly structured, the patient adjusts to it more easily.

Some patients may continue to experience episodes of distress and anxiety. Memory loss may cause the patient to forget that he will be picked up by a loved one at the end of the day. Frequent reassurances and distracting the agitated patient by involving him in a task can decrease this distress. Caregivers of such patients are encouraged to seek psychiatric consultation; day care programs may not be well suited for these patients' needs.

Sometimes an individual will routinely become distressed at a certain time of day. These episodes of agitation can often be identified as being related to the loss of an activity always scheduled at that time in the past (e.g., early afternoon episodes may be associated with the time when the children used to get picked up from school). An engaging activity similar to the former task may be effective in combating these episodes. Sometimes a 5-minute break to allow a little respite will help the patient return to the activity more calmly.

If paranoid delusions or hallucinations frighten the patient, creating a desperate wish to leave the program, staff should be alert to recognize the episode's beginning and to distract or reassure the patient before it turns into a crisis. Staff should confirm the patient's feelings of anxiety and distress, and give support.

Physical restraint and arguments tend to increase the patient's agitation and anxiety. Unobtrusive supervision while the patient walks outside or goes to another time-out area is usually most effective. Often two staff members, one playing the role of friend and the other being directive, can stage a "rescue" without being perceived as threatening. A patient who demonstrates such persistent behaviors should be referred for psychiatric intervention and should be assured that staff will not react negatively. To prevent disruption of the program, it is essential that episodes of anxiety and distress be dealt with promptly.

Occasionally, a patient is identified who does not react positively to any activities offered and for whom the program may not be suitable. Individuals who were previously independent, demanding, and somewhat asocial may, for example, find it difficult to function in group settings that foster dependence and enjoyment of leisure activities.

CAREGIVER REACTIONS

Caregivers often need assistance in adjusting to the day care program. Rather than enjoying the respite, they may experience feelings of guilt for subjecting their loved one to the stress of a new environment and may worry that he is suffering. Patients may anxiously relate negative messages that do not pinpoint a specific cause of distress but encompass the whole experience. Caregivers must be advised that these complaints are common and should not be a reason for early withdrawal from the program. Regular meetings between staff and caregivers can provide opportunities for caregivers to feel involved. It is essential that both staff and caregivers be secure in the knowledge that the patient is receiving benefits from the program.

Caregivers are essential in providing an accurate case history since the patient's own ability to retain information and make rational judgments may be limited. Caregivers and staff must make decisions that are based on accurate evaluations of the patient's ability, emotional state, and the origins of negative emotions that are expressed. A case history should include the history of the manifestations of the symptoms, the reactions of the patient to these changes and to the diagnosis of Alzheimer's disease, an evaluation of the patient's progress in the program and at home, and a record of emotional reactions to various situations. This information aids the staff and caregivers in designing a program that benefits the patient both at home and at the program.

SUMMARY

The loss of familiar roles and tasks and the sense of self-worth that accompanied them is an inherent part of the decline facing the patient with Alzheimer's disease. Activity programs designed to accommodate both the needs and the strengths of the patient can replace the activities that have been lost, provide achievable roles, enhance self-esteem, and improve the quality of life that remains.

In addition, a well-designed program is an effective antidote to the prevalent notion that, barring the discovery of a cure, there is little of value that can be done for the patient with Alzheimer's disease. This fatalistic attitude, an important source of burnout in staff and caregivers, cannot be maintained in the face of evidence that supporting the simple activities of daily living and social interaction are powerful therapeutic tools.

The cooperative effort and mutual support between caregivers, both staff and family members, enhance the lives of patients and caregivers beyond what can be accomplished by any known drug.

BIBILIOGRAPHY

Banazak DA: Difficult dementia: six steps to control problem behaviors, *Geriatrics* 51(2):36-42, 1996.

Bucks RS et al: Assessment of activities of daily living in dementia: development of the Bristol Activities of Daily Living Scale, *Age Ageing* 25(2):113-120, 1996.

Haight BK, Burnside I: Reminiscence and life review: conducting the processes, *J Gerontol Nurs* 18(2):39-42, 1992.

Kelly BT: Alzheimer's: care does not end with drug therapy, *Geriatrics* 50(7):7, 1995.

Namazi KH et al: Visual barriers to prevent ambulatory Alzheimer's patients from exiting through an emergency door, *The Gerontologist* 29(5):699-702, 1989.

Wagner AW et al: Behavior problems of residents with dementia in special care units, *Alzheimer Dis Assoc Disord* 9(3):121-126, 1995.

Zanetti O et al: Reality Orientation therapy in Alzheimer's disease: useful or not? A controlled study, *Alzheimer Dis Assoc Disord* 9(3):132-137, 1995.

Zgola JM: *Doing things: a guide to programming activities for persons with Alzheimer's disease and related disorders,* Baltimore, 1987, Johns Hopkins University Press.

Terminal Care of the Patient

Marcia M Johnson
Mary M Lancaster

*Now it is time that we are going, I to die, and
you to live. But which of us has the happier
prospect is unknown to anyone, but God.*

—Socrates

TERMINAL AND PALLIATIVE CARE

Terminal care, palliative care, and chronic care are terms that are intermingled
and often used interchangeably. Terminal care can be defined as the care
provided to a patient with a debilitating condition that is medically incurable or
not treatable using the available technology and can be expected to cause death.
This includes conditions in which death is imminent, as well as chronic and
debilitating conditions from which there is no reasonable hope for recovery.

Palliative care is the active total care of patients whose disease is not
responsive to curative treatment. It may also be appropriate to use it to manage
suffering for patients with chronic, progressive diseases such as Alzheimer's
disease. The actual term "palliative care" has been adopted by the World Health
Organization (WHO) to describe the care of patients with advanced disease.
When cure is no longer possible, the goal is the achievement of the best possible
quality of life for patients and their families.

Chronic care is a general term that includes the care of patients with chronic
illnesses and impairments, and indicates the presence of long-term disease or
symptoms, such as Alzheimer's disease. All three of the above terms may be
referred to when discussing the end-stage care of the patient with Alzheimer's
disease.

ASSESSMENT IN ADVANCED ALZHEIMER'S DISEASE

As the patient progresses through the stages of Alzheimer's disease, he or she
becomes more and more incapacitated and eventually requires total care. Astute
observation and assessment are required because the patient can no longer
verbally communicate her needs. Difficulty with swallowing and loss of speech

and movement set the stage for serious complications such as pneumonia and pressure sores. Helpless dependence characterizes the end-stage bedridden patient with Alzheimer's disease. Caregivers become his or her lifeline. Effective terminal care involves a systematic approach to assessment and interpretation of symptoms. Because the patient has lost the ability to communicate, caregivers must anticipate needs and recognize any subtle changes in body language as evidence that something is possibly wrong. Some typical findings based on age-associated changes and the changes encountered as a result of Alzheimer's disease are listed in Box 20-1.

DAILY CARE AND MANAGEMENT OF ADVANCED ALZHEIMER'S DISEASE

The truly difficult task is to provide care to the patient who, due to a dementing illness and inability to understand, may be uncooperative, resistant, or combative during the provision of care. The caregiver must attempt to minimize the patient's fear and anxiety by using creative interventions. The caregiver should continue to talk with the patient, even if it appears that the patient does not seem to listen or understand. This dialogue should be supplemented with the comfort of touch. These interventions must be continually reevaluated in terms of the caregiver's time, psychological and economic costs involved, and therapeutic effectiveness. A challenge in meeting the basic physical needs of the patient is organizing a daily routine. Caregivers cannot rush or hurry through procedures while providing care to the cognitively impaired patient, since any sense of urgency is contagious and agitating to the patient. This can often result in an exacerbation of difficult behaviors.

MEETING PERSONAL HYGIENE NEEDS

Bathing

Complete daily bed baths are not always necessary for the bedridden, older patient. The decreased activity level of these patients, in conjunction with the decreased oil production, perspiration, and elasticity of the skin associated with aging, reduces their need for a complete bath every day. The excessive use of soap and water only adds to the extreme dryness of the elderly person's fragile skin. However, daily attention to cleansing the face, hands, armpits, and perineal areas is essential. Mild, nonirritating or super-fatted soaps and lotions or emollients should be used. It is also important to properly and thoroughly dry any skin folds. The use of unscented talcum powder or cornstarch may be helpful in keeping these areas dry, yet it is important not to allow the powder to build up in the skin folds. Fingernails and toenails should be trimmed regularly and cleansed to remove any accumulations of dirt, feces, oils, and dead skin.

The patient's ears should not be neglected. The ears can be washed with a soft cloth wrapped around a finger, or a cotton swab can be used, but care must be taken not to enter the ear canal. Cerumen (wax) may be packed or hardened and can lead to substantial hearing loss. If this is suspected as a cause of hearing loss, irrigation of the ears by a professional caregiver may be necessary to remove the impacted cerumen.

Assessment Findings

Respiratory System
Decreased cough effectiveness
Decreased chest expansion
Decreased breath sounds
Decreased depth of respiration

General Findings
Dehydration
Increased nighttime voiding
Irregular pulse
Elevated or low blood pressure
Sleep disturbances
Behavioral problems
Slower healing capacity

Musculoskeletal System
Rigidity
Diminished or absent mobility
Decreased flexibility
Decreased joint range of motion
Bone fragility
Decreased muscle mass
Decreased muscle tone and strength

Integumentary System
Thin, dry, and fragile skin
Increased wrinkles in skin
Decreased elasticity
Decreased fat content (padding)
Decreased sweat and oil
Nails thicken, more brittle

Gastrointestinal System
Atrophy of gums
Tooth loss and decay
Dry mouth
Decreased appetite
Difficulty in swallowing
Constipation and fecal impaction
Incontinence of bowel and bladder

Sensory Systems
Reduced taste and smell receptors (which can interfere with appetite)
Diminished sensitivity to pain, pressure, and heat/cold
Diminished visual acuity
Dry eyes
Decreased hearing (higher pitched sounds)

Oral Care

Oral care and hygiene must be provided for patients who are edentulous, have dentures, or have their natural teeth. Improper or inadequate care can result in serious problems within the mouth and may lead to systemic infection. The mouth should be inspected frequently for signs of tissue inflammation, swelling, or tenderness. Maintaining moisture and integrity of the gums and oral tissues will help preserve optimal dental function and patient comfort. Oral care is particularly important for patients who are "mouth breathers" or who have salivary gland dysfunction, and extensive dryness occurs.

Teeth should be brushed at least twice a day using any necessary adaptive equipment such as long toothbrushes, enlarged handle toothbrushes, or suction toothbrushes. The patient's head should be turned to the side (if lying in bed) and suction equipment should be available in the event the patient aspirates during the provision of oral care. Ingestible toothpaste should be used with the advanced Alzheimer's patient as he is likely to swallow what is in the mouth. If needed, props designed to keep the mouth open are available from medical equipment suppliers. If the patient is still wearing dentures, they should be removed twice a day and washed with a soft brush and cleanser.

All the soft tissues of the mouth should be cleansed at least once a day using a soft toothbrush, cloth, sponge, or gauze pad moistened with water. Caution should be used with antiseptic mouth rinses and lemon-glycerin products because they contain alcohol and can actually increase the drying effect. All surfaces of the mouth should be moistened regularly with water or an artificial saliva product. This helps to prevent tooth decay, gingivitis, and oral ulcerations. For the patient who breathes through her mouth or is receiving oxygen by a mask, more frequent care must be provided (usually every two hours) since the tissues dry out very rapidly. Ice chips, moistened sponge swabs, and artificial saliva can be used. The lips of these patients must not be neglected. Coating the lips frequently with a moisture barrier product such as petroleum jelly helps protect the lips from excessive dryness and cracking. Periodic examinations and routine bedside cleansing and scaling by a dental hygienist should be continued as long as possible.

Shaving

Shaving, or removal of facial hair, should be completed to help the patient feel and look better. This may also be needed in some older women since the appearance of facial hair increases as women age. Proper cleansing of beards and mustaches is necessary. Cream depilatories may be used to remove hair from the axillary areas (armpits) and legs of female patients (as desired), but should only be used after completing a patch sensitivity test. The use of cosmetics to enhance body image and self-esteem may be continued as desired.

Dressing

Dressing the patient with advanced Alzheimer's disease is more difficult due to the accompanying loss of motor skills and muscle rigidity. Clothing adapted with large zippers or Velcro straps makes dressing easier for the patient and the caregiver.

Pull-on (elastic waistbands) pants and shirts are generally easier to put on the patient. If the patient has a one-sided weakness, the affected side should be placed in the garment first, and removed from the garment last. Placing a shirt on a bedridden patient can be easily accomplished by placing the patient's arms in the sleeves, raising the arms above the head, and slipping the neck opening over the patient's head. Another way is to place one side of the shirt on, turn the patient to the side and tuck the rest of the shirt against the back, turn him or her to the other side, and then pull the shirt through. Clothing should be of easy-care fabric to lessen the burden on the caregiver since patients with Alzheimer's disease can easily go through several items of clothing a day.

Although these activities may seem simple and usual, when providing care to a person who cannot assist in the care, the time and strain involved take their toll on the caregiver. Lifting, moving, and tugging can quickly wear out caregivers. Any means of providing support to caregivers in these activities should be sought. In-home assistance may be provided by home health aides, a friend, or another family member.

Skin Care

In providing for the skin care needs of Alzheimer's disease patients, caregivers should:
- Position for prevention of skin pressure.
- Protect bony prominences.
- Keep the patient dry.
- Use support mattresses and devices.

The patient in the terminal stage of Alzheimer's disease has specific skin care needs. Because he or she is usually bedridden, or extremely limited in movement, relief of pressure over bony prominences becomes problematic. Because of aging and impaired nutrition, the patient's skin is likely to be very fragile and thin. Loss of subcutaneous fat tissue causes bony areas such as heels, hips, elbows, and sacrum to be at risk for breakdown. Therefore, special attention must be given to protecting the skin and preventing breakdown. Prevention is the key because once breakdown has occurred, it is extremely difficult and costly to heal.

Positioning

The immobile, bedridden patient must be turned to a different position regularly, at least every two hours. Turning relieves pressure on bony areas and allows the return of circulation to the tissues. A variety of positions should be used including prone (face down), back lying, and side lying. With each position, the patient should be assessed to evaluate how well he or she tolerates the different positions and the effects of the position on respirations. A written schedule is often helpful in keeping track of when to turn and what position to use. The body should always be kept in good alignment and any dependent areas, such as arms and legs, should be supported with pillows or props. The same is true for patients who can still get into a chair. In fact, patients who sit in chairs, even recliners, should have their position changed and pressure on the buttocks and coccyx relieved about every hour. This can be accomplished by helping the patient to stand for a few minutes or by encouraging the patient to use his or her arms to push up, relieving pressure on the buttocks.

In the side-lying position, the legs should be bent at the hips and knees and pulled slightly forward to prevent the patient from rolling over on to her face (Figure 20-1, *A*). A pillow or foam wedge can be placed behind the patient's back to provide additional support and to keep the patient from turning onto her back (Figure 20-1, *B*). The knees and ankles should have pillows or padding placed between them to prevent them from pressing against each other. It is not necessary to have the patient completely on her side (90 degrees), but the body should be tilted about 45 degrees. This prevents all the weight of the patient from being directly supported by the trochanter.

When the patient is placed on her back, a small pillow or towel roll should be placed under the lower leg so that the heels hang free and do not rest directly on the mattress. Heel protectors, foam, or quilted booties can also be used to protect the bony areas of the feet from undue pressure. However, doughnut-shaped props that fit around the ankle to elevate the heels should be avoided due to the increased pressure and resulting possible breakdown at the site of the prop. In the prone (face down) position, a small pillow should be placed at the lower abdomen to relieve pressure on the back and the chest wall. When the patient is turned, care must be taken to avoid dragging him or her across the bed. Friction forces that result from dragging quickly damage the skin and can lead to tissue breakdown. Lifting devices and turn sheets can be used to make this task easier and less damaging to the

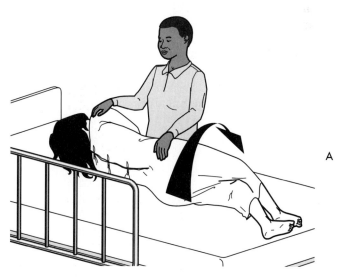

A

Figure 20-1, A   The resident is turned toward the nursing assistant. Resident's arms and legs are crossed. The nursing assistant has one hand on resident's far shoulder and the other on the far hip. (From Sorrentino SA et al: *Mosby's textbook for long-term care assistants,* ed 2, St Louis, 1994, Mosby.)   *Continued*

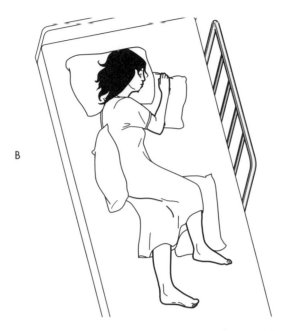

B

Figure 20-1, cont'd B   The resident is positioned on her side in middle of the bed. A pillow is placed in front of bottom leg, with top leg on pillow in flexed position; note pillow against the back. A small pillow supports arm and hand; note pillow under head and shoulder. (From Sorrentino SA et al: *Mosby's textbook for long-term care assistants*, ed 2, St Louis, 1992, Mosby.)

patient. Friction can also be reduced by the use of lubricants such as cornstarch and protective transparent barrier films that act like a second skin.

Shear is another force that is a factor in the development of pressure ulcers. Shear results when the body tissues move over the skeletal bony prominences. This is most commonly encountered when the head of the bed is raised and the patient's weight shifts downward. The skeleton remains stationary, but the soft tissues move. Therefore, keeping the head of the bed at the lowest possible position compatible with the patient's condition and medical interventions is necessary. The head of the bed can be raised for such things as meals, but should be lowered shortly thereafter.

Skin Protection

The skin, especially the skin surfaces that are against the bed, must be kept clean and dry. Any evidence of incontinence or undue perspiration should be taken care of as soon as possible, and clean, dry sheets placed on the bed. Warm (not hot) water and a mild, nonirritating cleansing agent should be used to minimize drying and irritation. Caregivers should use minimal force and friction during cleansing procedures. Incontinence pads or briefs should pull the moisture to the inner layers so that the surface next to the patient remains dry. Lotions and emollients can be applied to the skin to help prevent moisture loss. Heavier ointments, such as zinc oxide and commercially available skin barriers, can be used for the perineal area to protect the skin from the irritation of urine and feces. Linens and incontinence pads need to be kept free of wrinkles and crumbs of food or other objects. If a catheter is in place, care must be taken to avoid having the patient lie on the tubing.

All skin surfaces should be systematically assessed daily, and all bony prominences should be examined with each turning. If the redness over a bony prominence persists longer than 1 hour after relief of the pressure, the patient should not be placed back on that area until the redness has disappeared. Massaging bony prominences with each turning is a practice from the past that was widely endorsed.

> There is now evidence to support the belief that the practice of massaging bony prominences may actually cause deep tissue damage, and therefore should not be performed.

Particular attention should be given to less conspicuous areas such as ears, the back of the head, and the shoulders. Patients who are receiving oxygen should have the areas where the oxygen mask or tubing presses on skin surfaces inspected daily. Providing some padding with cotton or gauze can eliminate the development of pressure ulcers at these sites. Finally, it may be advisable to pad the bed rails to prevent blunt injury to the patient during turning or seizure activity.

Support Surfaces

Other considerations such as the support surface, environmental factors, and nutrition are also important in the prevention of pressure ulcers. All surfaces on which the patient spends any length of time (mattress, chairs, etc.) should be pressure reducing. There is a wide array of mattress overlays and mattress replacements that can be obtained through medical equipment suppliers. Some of these are foam, water, air, or gel filled and help to reduce the pressure on the patient's body. Some models are termed "dynamic surfaces," which means they change the pressure points along the patient's body. Alternating air mattresses are a type of dynamic surface that may be needed for some higher risk patients. Overlays go on top of the existing mattress to help distribute pressure more evenly, while replacement mattresses are used in place of the existing mattress. The same applies for wheelchair and recliner chair seat cushions. For patients at extremely high risk, or those who have already developed several pressure ulcers, there are commercially available pressure relief surfaces that can be purchased or rented. These products can be quite expensive and may or may not be covered by Medicare or private insurance companies.

Environmental Factors

Environmental factors that need to be considered are the humidity and temperature of the patient's environment. Low humidity and exposure to cold temperatures should be minimized. A humidifier may be necessary during the winter months. Using blankets and socks help to keep the lower extremities warm and promote circulation.

Adequate nutrition and fluid intake are also extremely important in preventing and treating pressure ulcers. Adequate amounts of protein and calories are needed to maintain the skin's integrity. Many older people do not get enough protein in their diets and commercially available protein supplements may be needed. An involuntary weight loss of more than 5% of normal body weight is associated with risk for protein malnutrition, which places the patient at an increased risk for skin breakdown. If inadequate oral intake continues, caregivers will need to determine whether an artificial means of providing adequate nutrition is in accord with their and the patient's wishes.

Elimination

As Alzheimer's disease progresses, the patient experiences problems related to emptying the bladder and/or the bowel. Options for controlling urinary incontinence are discussed in Chapter 16.

Due to decreased mobility and fluid intake that accompany advanced Alzheimer's disease, the patient is at increased risk for the development of a urinary tract infection. The caregiver can assess the presence of a urinary tract infection by noting abdominal distention or tenderness, facial grimacing by the patient when voiding, fever, increased restlessness, increased lethargy, increased confusion, and changes in the characteristics of the urine (presence of blood, change in color, cloudiness, etc.)

Patients with advanced Alzheimer's disease are prone to constipation related to immobility, variation in food and fluid intake, certain medications, and the effects of aging. In the debilitated, bedridden patient, a bowel movement can sometimes be produced by lightly massaging the lower abdomen. If this method is unsuccessful, a glycerine suppository can be used to stimulate bowel evacuation. Sometimes just digitally stimulating the anal sphincter can produce a bowel movement.

The bedridden patient does not need to have a bowel movement every day, but should go no longer than 3 days. If a patient begins to have small, diarrhetic stools; leakage of small amounts of feces; or abdominal discomfort, he should be checked for a fecal impaction. A laxative or an enema will help remove the impaction.

The frequency of bowel movements should be monitored to avoid impaction, and the quantity and characteristics of the stool noted.

Maintaining normal bowel function in the terminally ill patient requires creativity on the part of the caregiver. This involves continuous reassessment and monitoring of the patient's bowel function. A more detailed discussion on the treatment of constipation is found in Chapter 18.

Nutrition

Maintaining adequate nutritional intake in patients with end-stage Alzheimer's disease is a challenging task. Despite the best efforts of caregivers, most patients will lose weight in the terminal stage. There are several reasons for the eating difficulties these patients experience. The profound memory impairment interferes with the recognition of food, the need and desire to eat, and the mechanics of eating. Changes in the level of arousal may interfere with the patient's response to the signals of hunger. The patient may experience a return of reflex actions (sucking, biting, and tonic neck reflexes) that interfere with eating. Some patients may also resist attempts at being fed by the caregiver. As damage to the brain continues, chewing and swallowing become impaired, leading to a high risk for aspiration. In this stage of the disease, the patient becomes totally dependent on his caregivers for nutrition.

Food Choices

Choosing foods of the highest nutritional value that supply many calories becomes very important because the quantity of food and fluid the patient consumes is usually reduced. Many nutritional supplements are available to help increase the patient's intake. These supplements can be served directly from the container, or can be mixed with ice cream to make a palatable, nutritious snack. Providing foods that can be chewed and swallowed easily is also important. Caregivers need to continually assess the patient's ability to chew and swallow and then adapt foods to the patient's needs at that time. As patients experience increased difficulty with chewing, meals that include chopped or ground foods can be prepared. As even greater difficulty is encountered, table food can be blenderized and pureed. Commercially available baby food can also be used, but it tends to be less palatable and is more costly.

Often patients will experience choking on thin liquids such as water and juices. However, both are still needed to maintain the patient's hydration. Many of the patient's favorite liquids (water, coffee, juice, milk) can be thickened with corn-starch, unflavored gelatin, or commercially available thickeners. These thickeners add just enough substance to the fluid to make it easier to swallow. Gelatin desserts and flavored ice pops also can be given to provide the needed amounts of water.

As swallowing becomes affected by the disease, correct positioning for eating is extremely important. The patient needs to be placed in an upright position. The head of the bed should be elevated to the highest position tolerated by the patient. Pillows and props may be needed to help the patient maintain this position. The patient should remain sitting upright for approximately 30 minutes after the meal has been completed, and the mouth should be checked and cleansed of remaining food. Because of the danger of aspiration during eating, all caregivers, both family and health professionals, need to know how to perform the Heimlich maneuver. Equipment for suctioning the mouth and upper airway should also be available at the patient's bedside.

In this stage of the disease, a tremendous amount of time is needed to feed a patient. It may take 1 to 2 hours just to get the patient to complete one meal. This situation is problematic in nursing homes where a caregiver may have four or five patients to feed at meal time. Family members provide valuable and much needed assistance to the nursing home staff when they come in to feed their loved one. Volunteers can also be recruited and instructed on feeding patients to help alleviate this problem. Plenty of time for chewing and swallowing each mouthful is required.

Verbal cues about what to do may also be needed from the caregiver. Sometimes patients will hold the food in their mouths and not swallow. Swallowing can sometimes be stimulated by instructing the patient to swallow or by gently stroking his throat. Care must also be taken not to place too much food in the patient's mouth at one time.

Eventually the patient will not be able to take food or fluid by mouth. Family members need to recognize that this problem will eventually arise and should talk with the patient, the physician, and among themselves as to what measures will be taken when oral feeding can no longer be accomplished. If determined appropriate and in accordance with the patient's and family's wishes, a feeding tube may be used to provide nourishment and hydration. If the patient has a feeding tube, especially a nasogastric tube, it is imperative to keep the head of the bed elevated at least 30 degrees. Patients with a feeding tube receive feeding either by bolus or continuous drip. If the patient receives bolus feeding, the head of the bed should remain elevated for 30 minutes to 1 hour after the feeding and then can be lowered. However, if the patient is receiving continuous drip feeding, the head of the bed should remain elevated to 30 degrees at all times since the stomach is never empty.

Placement of the tube should be checked periodically. For bolus feedings, the tube can be checked just before each feeding. For continuous drip feedings, tube placement should be checked every 8 hours. Patients receiving either type of feeding require additional water to maintain adequate hydration. A 150-ml bolus of water can be given four to six times in a 24-hour period. The water should not be added to the feeding in a continuous drip feeding because the amount of calories the patient receives would be reduced since the caloric requirements are set by an hourly rate. Rather, the feeding should be momentarily interrupted, and the water should be given as a bolus.

Immobility

The hazards of immobility are crucial to consider when caring for the patient with advanced Alzheimer's disease. Adverse effects of being bedridden include stiffness with resulting pain in joints and muscles, muscle atrophy, and decreased strength and contractures of joints. Range-of-motion exercises are an extremely important part of daily care of the patient.

> An ideal time to perform passive range-of-motion exercises for each joint and extremity is during daily hygienic care.

These exercises should be provided two to three times a day to help combat excessive rigidity and stiffening. Additionally, with the aging process and immobility, there is an increase in loss of calcium in the bones. This predisposes the patient to bone fractures. Care must be taken during turning and other procedures, as well as in preventing the patient from falling out of bed.

Effects of immobility on the urinary system may include urinary retention, infection, and kidney stones. Immobility can also contribute to a negative nitrogen balance due to the rapid breakdown of cellular materials. It also contributes to constipation and diarrhea, a decreased metabolic rate, and possible fluid and electrolyte imbalances. Providing additional fluid intake and exercise can help prevent or reduce the seriousness of these problems.

Immobility causes pooling of blood in the lower extremities and increases the risk of blood clots. Decreased chest expansion, decreased gas exchange, and pooling of lung secretions may lead to respiratory infections and distress. If the patient has lost the ability to cough effectively, suctioning equipment to help keep the airways clear and to help prevent pneumonia should be placed at the bedside. This equipment can be purchased or rented from medical equipment suppliers.

Every effort to improve the patient's movement through position changes and range-of-motion exercises should be made. The use of mechanical hydraulic lifts is indicated for transfer from bed to a recliner chair to facilitate movement and a change of scenery. Family caregivers should be instructed in transfer techniques by health professionals prior to attempting these activities at home.

Sleep and Rest

Assessing the rest and relaxation needs of patients can alert caregivers to problems. Sleep patterns in Alzheimer's disease can be severely disturbed. Daytime sleep may be increased, while nighttime sleep is fragmented. Sleep-wake cycle disturbances are often a problem for both the patient and the caregiver. To determine if the patient has had enough rest, the caregiver can observe behaviors during the waking hours.

A patient who is excessively irritable or agitated may be sleep deprived.

The routine use of sedative or hypnotic medications is not indicated in advanced Alzheimer's disease. To help decrease transient nighttime agitation, the caregiver can reduce stimulation by providing a quiet, dark environment and by soothing the patient through therapeutic touch or massage. For further discussion on sleep disturbances the reader is directed to Chapter 12.

Comfort Needs

Meeting the patient's comfort needs can be assessed by use of an informal "checklist" to evaluate any vocalizations, motor signs, facial expressions, and behaviors indicative of discomfort. The caregiver should attempt to identify the underlying cause for the patient's discomfort and to alleviate it.

For example, yelling or loud crying may be quieted by position changes, soothing music, holding the patient's hand, and talking with the patient. Approaching the patient in a calm, confident, and unhurried manner; maintaining eye contact when possible; and using touch will help to promote a sense of security, comfort, and rest. Avoiding unnecessary chatter, speaking softly, and creating a pleasant atmosphere, perhaps with the use of personal memorabilia or a soothing mobile over the bed, may also promote serenity. If pain medication has been prescribed, the caregiver must evaluate how well the medication relieves the pain. If it does not appear to comfort the patient, the caregiver should discuss the situation with the physician.

Lethargy, anxiety, restlessness, fever, or increased pulse or respiration may be the first or only indications of an acute illness. Monitoring vital signs, regular assessment by the caregiver, and follow-up by health professionals can help identify illness at its earliest stage. A physician's attention should be sought, as necessary. As death approaches, the patient may require oxygen therapy to help maintain comfort. Attention to the patient's mouth and to areas where the mask or tubing make contact with the skin should be monitored, as was previously discussed.

Ethical Considerations

Patients and families face the tasks of accepting the reality of impending loss and death, coping with intervening challenges, and saying good-bye. The family can better prepare for the patient's death by discussing and developing a plan of action for the time of death, and by receiving education concerning the dying process, as well as the signs and symptoms of impending death. The clarification of resuscitation orders and treatment preferences, legal and financial planning, and funeral planning are all necessary components of preparing for the patient's death. Families can also benefit from bereavement counseling, which addresses feelings, emotions, and the grieving process.

As the patient enters the final stage of the disease, family members are confronted with very difficult decisions. Among these are the placement of feeding tubes to maintain nutrition, resuscitation in the event of cardiopulmonary arrest, and the aggressive treatment of infections (hospitalization, antibiotics, IV therapy, etc.). These issues need to be discussed and decided on before the onset of any crisis.

Health care professionals prefer to have decisions on these matters as soon as possible in the event that a crisis should arise when neither the physician nor the family is present. Whatever decisions the family makes, health care professionals need to remain supportive of both the patient and the family. If a health care professional feels at odds with the patient's and family's decision, another person who can work with the patient and family and is accepting of their decisions needs to be identified.

A discussion of advanced directives can be found in Chapter 22. Advanced directives help to define a common ground where the patient, family members, physician, and health professionals come to comprehend and understand the patient's and family's decisions regarding end-of-life issues. If the patient did not previously prepare an advanced directive, these decisions rest with the legally empowered family member. Paternalism, the most frequent ethical concern voiced by both elders and their caregivers, is unilateral decision making not in accord with the patient's stated wishes or value systems. Paternalistic attitudes must be avoided at the time of impending death and appropriate, informed treatment planning must be completed by the family and physician.

Family members need to be involved in the care of the patient during this final stage regardless of whether the care is at home, in a nursing home, or in the hospital. Family members need the support of others and should be allowed flexibility in visitation to help them feel part of the patient's last days. Referrals to chaplains, psychologists, or social work counselors may also aid the family in resolving any problems.

Wherever the patient receives terminal care, the last management issue to be addressed is promoting quality of life. This, too, is an ethical consideration for all people and poses a particular challenge to caregivers of the dying Alzheimer's disease patient. Promoting quality of life in the person with advanced Alzheimer's disease includes efforts that are continually directed at providing physical comfort and emotional security. The patient must be recognized as an individual. Maintaining dignity requires centering care around the unique and changing needs of the patient. Internalizing the philosophy that care is neither custodial nor performed in an assembly-line fashion assists caregivers in promoting quality of life. The appropriate approach to the management of advanced Alzheimer's disease minimizes patient suffering and provides a compassionate environment for those approaching death and for their families.

BIBLIOGRAPHY

Ackerman TF: The moral implications of medical uncertainty: tube feeding dementia patients, *J Am Geriatr Soc* 44(10):1265-67, 1996.

Agency for Health Care Policy and Research: *Pressure ulcers in adults: prediction and prevention,* Clinical Practice Guideline #3, Rockville, MD, May 1992.

Agency for Health Care Policy and Research: *Treatment of pressure ulcers,* Clinical Practice Guideline #15, Rockville, MD, December 1994.

Ahronheim JC: Nutrition and hydration in the terminal patient, *Clin Geriatr Med* 12(2):379-392, 1996.

Butler RN, Burt R, Foley KM et al: Palliative medicine: providing care when cure is not possible, *Geriatics* 51(5):33-44, 1996.

Gerber L: Ethics and caring: cornerstones of nursing geriatric case management, *J Gerontol Nurs* 21(12):15-19, 1995.

Institute for Health and Aging, University of California, San Francisco: *Chronic care in America: a 21st century challenge,* Princeton, NJ, 1996, Robert Wood Johnson Foundation.

Kovach CR, Wilson SA, Noonan PE: The effects of hospice interventions on behaviors, discomfort, and physical complications of end-stage dementia, *Am J Alzheimer's Dis* 11(4):7-15, 1996.

Morrison RS, Morris J: When there is no cure: palliative care for the dying patient, *Geriatrics* 50(7):45, 1995.

Schonwetter RS: Care of the dying geriatric patient, *Clin Geriatr Med* 12(2):253-278, 1996.

Souren LEM, Franssen EH, Reisberg B: Contractures and loss of function in patients with Alzheimer's disease, *J Am Geriatr Soc* 43(7):741-746, 1995.

Tangalos EG: Advanced directives: the role of health care professionals: sixteenth annual Ross roundtable conference on medical issues: issues in the long-term care setting, *Nurs Home Med* 3(9):203-206, 1995.

VonGunten CF, Twaddle ML: Terminal care for noncancer patients, *Clin Geriatr Med* 12(2):349-358, 1996.

Wilson SA, Kovach CR, Stearns SA: Hospice concepts in the care for end-stage dementia, *Geriatr Nurs* 17(1):6-10, 1996.

Unit 4

Those who fall in love with practice without science are like a sailor who enters a ship without a helm or a compass and who never can be certain whither he is going.

—Leonardo da Vinci

Special Issues

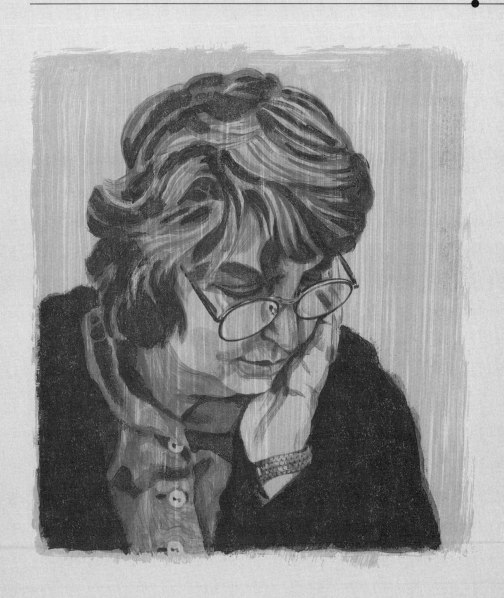

Ethical Issues

Sharon Turnbull

The three duties of a physician are: first the preservation of health, second the cure of disease, and third the prolongation of life.

—Francis Bacon

Case Study—Decisions of Life or Death

Matthew J. is 62 years old and has a wife and three grown children. Two years ago he was diagnosed as having stage 1 Alzheimer's disease and was informed of this diagnosis. He has just recovered from a mild heart attack, and his cardiologist has told him that he requires cardiac bypass surgery if he is to live. He has refused the surgery, stating, "There is no point in living." The consulting psychiatrist confirms that Mr. J. is clinically depressed in addition to having Alzheimer's disease, and believes that Mr. J. cannot make a rational decision.

Case Study—Administration of Drugs

Shirley W. is a 74-year-old patient with Alzheimer's disease who lives in a nursing home. Over the past few months she has become increasingly difficult to spoon feed because she spits, pushes the spoon away, and refuses to eat. When admitted to the home, while still coherent and clear-minded, Mrs. W. had asserted that she did not want her life prolonged by artificial means. The physician orders feeding by a nasogastric tube, which Mrs. W. frequently pulls out. In response to complaints from the nursing staff, the physician prescribes tranquilizers for Mrs. W. to make her "more manageable."

Case Study—Confidentiality

Dave S. is taken to his family doctor by his wife and grown daughter to find out why he has become so irritable. He admits to angry outbursts for no apparent reason. He also says that he has trouble remembering and is finding it increasingly difficult to add and subtract. After extensive testing, the diagnosis is confirmed: Mr. S. has probable Alzheimer's disease. The doctor tells him about the diagnosis and gives him a broad outline of what to expect. Mr. S. takes the news calmly, then states that under no circumstances does he want his wife or daughter informed.

Case Study—Patient Wishes vs. Societal Norms

Martha J.'s children have complained to the nursing home administrator that on their last three weekly visits, they have found Martha in her room dressed only in her slip.

The children have protested that "the nurses aren't even bothering to tidy her up." Actually, Martha recently had become combative each time a staff member had tried to make her dress for social activities. The nursing staff, with feelings of ambivalence, had decided to honor Martha's apparent wish not to dress as long as she was in her room.

Caregivers charged with responsibility for a patient with Alzheimer's disease continually wrestle with ethical issues. Simple day-to-day care demands a repeated confrontation with these dilemmas. Dealing with the complex problem of the elderly person with dementia arouses intense discomfort in the caretaker, especially when an ethical issue underlying the care emerges. The Fairhill Guidelines on Ethics of the Care of People with Alzheimer's Disease, a summary of a series of meetings of family caregivers, ethicists, and clinicians, provides the most comprehensive effort to date to shift the basis of ethical guidelines from the realm of theory to one of interpersonal relevance.

Yet even this valuable contribution reveals that there are no simple answers and no agreed-upon formulas that will ensure that the rights of the elderly person with dementia are maintained and that the conscience of the caretaker will remain clear. Ultimately, all caregivers have an obligation to analyze carefully the ethical principles that must guide care, to explore their own moral boundaries, and to be aware of the need for respectful consideration of the impact of ethical issues on the quality of interactions and relationships.

ETHICAL PRINCIPLES GOVERNING CARE

Moral standards and the nature of moral decision making are the concerns of ethics, and ethical reflection is an obligation of the caregiver. Moral obligations sometimes are thought of as rules and indeed may be codified into law, but ethical practice goes far beyond what can be reduced to rules.

Certain values are basic to any ethical system. These are moral obligations in the sense that, without them, no community or cooperative activity could exist. These central values include truthfulness, fairness, and respect for life.

Besides these values, there are many others, such as not inflicting harm or suffering. Caregivers often must make decisions in the face of conflicting values; for example, telling the truth about the diagnosis of Alzheimer's disease in itself may cause suffering. Rules alone are not enough. Caregivers must thoughtfully consider whether actions and policies are consistent with moral principles and rules. Care of the patient with Alzheimer's disease presents many complex challenges to these moral principles, and the "good" choice is seldom obvious. However, caregivers are obligated to consider these issues carefully and to use them to frame moral choices to guide their behavior.

Three classical ethical principles are commonly applied to the dilemmas that arise in patient care:

1. Respect for persons—that the autonomy and dignity of individuals should be preserved and promoted.
2. Beneficence—that caregivers ought to produce good, preserve life, and prevent harm and suffering.
3. Equity—that the benefits and burdens of care be fairly and equitably distributed among individuals.

There is growing concern that these principles, which have been described as the "big three" of biomedical ethics, are not sufficient to fully address the issues that the progressive nature of the dementia of Alzheimer's disease creates. Specifically, strict adherence to these principles that give centrality to the "rights of the individual," i.e., to the patient, often imperil the "rights" of others, typically the family caregivers who must bear the burden of major decisions.

A growing number of voices call for a new system of ethics that recognizes that with the progression of dementia comes the necessity for a fourth principle of biomedical ethics: negotiated autonomy, when the autonomy of the individual should be limited by consideration of the extent to which the consequences of decision making rebound to others.

PSYCHOLOGICAL REACTIONS OF CAREGIVER

The elderly patient with dementia who is seemingly bereft of relationships and cognition, is often described by family and friends as "no longer here." In this sense caregivers in the institution may have an advantage because, not having known the "former self," they may find it easier than family or friends to see the patient as a full person, albeit one who is difficult, unpredictable, and complex. The family, on the other hand, grieves for the loss of the person they once knew and loved.

Caregivers themselves often experience powerful emotional reactions that profoundly influence their ethical decisions. Besides confronting their own mortality, they may see the frailties of patients with dementia as intimations of their own future losses, mental as well as physical. If the patient does not demonstrate a strong sense of individuality, a sense that depends largely on his ability to relate, the caregiver may project certain attributes onto him—perhaps those of the caregiver's own parents—and respond to the patient accordingly.

Many of the ethical dilemmas that caregivers face place them in a double bind in which any action taken evokes guilt. For example, on the issue of forced feeding, caregivers experience conflicting demands: to preserve life (by techniques such as nasogastric tubes that may inflict additional suffering on the patient) and to respect the patient's wishes (although refusal of food will shorten life). This double bind may increase the caregivers' sense of guilt or helplessness and impede ethical choices.

Little is known about the psychological mechanisms that caregivers use to manage their own feelings in these difficult situations. Undoubtedly many flee, choosing work that is less emotionally demanding. Some caregivers distance themselves emotionally from the patient, become less sensitive to the patient's feelings and needs, and eventually reduce their perception of the person to that of "a thing . . . handled routinely and mechanically, not nursed with tenderness and understanding." Others may use denial, distancing themselves from the need for difficult actions and decisions, by steadfast refusal to acknowledge the extent of the patient's decline.

Many hospitals, recognizing the impact of the psychological reactions of their staff, have created interdisciplinary bioethics committees that facilitate discussion of dilemmas being faced and foster shared responsibility for consideration of choices and decision making. In addition, some caregivers support separate nursing ethics groups, which provide a vehicle by which all staff members have the opportunity to discuss their concerns. Similarly, self-help support groups afford family caregivers an opportunity to explore personal reactions and ethical dilemmas in an environment of mutual understanding and support.

OBLIGATION TO SUPPORT

In general, individuals are presumed to be capable of discerning their own best interest and pursuing it. Seen as autonomous and competent, a normal person has the legal and moral right to choose and to refuse. However, it is this right to make reasonable choices that is the major issue in progressive Alzheimer's disease. What degree of autonomy can be left to the patient? Who is to decide, if not the patient?

By its very nature, paternalism (limitation of a patient's freedom and authority by the "wise and loving father") exists to do good—to protect the patient from the dangers of her own freedom, such as the freedom to starve to death. Since much of the health care function is inherently paternalistic, this attitude probably cannot be totally avoided. However, an effort should be made to keep this element within proper bounds.

In a setting where most or all aspects of the patient's life are regulated by the staff, the patient's individuality is sacrificed to some extent. No longer able to select what to eat, what to wear, or when to sleep, patients often respond with either belligerence or psychological withdrawal and a steadily increasing dependence.

> Research indicates that the degree of dementia improves, or at least progresses less rapidly, when patients stay active and are allowed some role in decision making, even if only about minor aspects of their environment.

The issue of competence to decide is obviously a matter of degree. Some patients are competent to make all decisions; some, most decisions; some, only a few; and others, virtually none. Individualized assessments that are repeated periodically can limit the overzealous application of paternalism. However, such assessments require considerable effort and reduce bureaucratic efficiency. At the same time, patients have the right to refuse life-extending treatment, and incompetence does not diminish that right. When a patient, family, and clinician cannot agree on these serious matters, the decisions must be left to the courts.

The right to decide is most controversial when it involves the refusal of treatment, particularly treatment that would extend life. Recent ethical debates and court decisions have done much to clarify the patient's rights and the caregiver's obligations in decisions involving patients who are still competent. It is clear that the patient should not be forced to undergo treatment that is against her wishes, even if the treatment is for her own good.

Although caregivers have an ethical duty not to force treatment against a patient's wishes, they have the additional obligations of helping educate the patient and helping her to work through the reasons for refusal. Two criteria have been identified as morally justified for refusing treatment:
1. If the treatment is useless.
2. If it involves a grave burden for the patient or for another person.

RESTRAINT

The unpredictable behavior of patients with Alzheimer's disease is often disturbing to caregivers. Disruptive behavior, "unprovoked" assaults, and combativeness are not uncommon. If such behavior is bothersome rather than likely to injure the patient or others, restraint is viewed as unethical.

Allowing the patient to stay in his robe rather than get dressed, for example, may eliminate his resistance and prevent an assault. Unfortunately, physical or chemical restraints are often used to manage bothersome behavior, resulting in increased health risks from immobility, overmedication, and drug reactions and interactions. What are the patient's rights in such a situation? An ethical decision would demand the use of the least restraint possible to ensure safety, not consider the caregiver's convenience.

CARE AT THE END OF LIFE

Who should decide for the incompetent patient, and what criteria should be used? These questions are surrounded by great controversy. The concept of substituted judgment is increasingly being recognized by some states and validated by the courts in cases in which patients had expressed their wishes concerning care while they were still competent so that those wishes could be carried out even if they lapsed into incompetence, perhaps with the appointment of a guardian to ensure that their wishes were given weight. If the patient, while competent, does not express an intent (or if a patient has never been competent), other issues arise. In general, when the care of an incompetent patient without a guardian is debated, the courts must decide in favor of what they deem to be the best interest of the patient. However, the extent to which family members (rather than the courts) should have the right to decide among reasonable courses of action is unclear. Veatch and other authors have argued for a "limited familial autonomy" in which the family is given responsibility for carrying the patient's or the family's beliefs and values into the decision, with the physician seeking court intervention if the family is considered to be unreasonable or exploitative.

ADVANCE DIRECTIVES

Advance directives are designed to give patients an opportunity to influence their own care and to reduce the ambiguity that occurs when they cannot communicate their wishes. There are two types of advance directives in current use: a living will and a durable power of attorney for health care. Ideally, a patient should have both types. These are discussed in Chapter 22.

All caregivers should be aware of the laws governing advance directives in their own states. The specific form, process, and procedures for valid advance directives are established by state laws, which vary considerably. In many states, for example, the durable power of attorney for health care requires the notarized signatures of two witnesses who are unrelated to the patient. In some states health professionals are prohibited from serving as those witnesses. Likewise, in some states specific procedures, such as the withholding of hydration or nutrition, are not included in the definition of "life-sustaining treatments" and must be mentioned specifically. Some states do not permit the withdrawal of artificial nutrition even if the patient desires such withdrawal.

State-approved advance directive forms, including living wills, can be obtained from the Choice in Dying,* as well as from other organizations. A medical directive form that allows the patient to specify his wishes regarding medical procedures, such as invasive tests, and provides space to note additional desires can be obtained from Harvard Medical School. It is important that procedures not desired be specified because court involvement is often necessary when the patient's wishes are ambiguous. States also have varying rules regarding the longevity of an advance directive. To be kept current under the most restrictive statutes, advance directives should be revalidated every five years.

The Patient Self-Determination Act, which became effective in 1991, requires that all Medicare- and Medicaid-reimbursed agencies provide written informa- tion to patients at the time of admission concerning their rights to an advance directive for health care under their state law. In addition, the agency must document whether the patient has an advance directive and must comply with all state statues regarding these directives. The agency is not compelled to adhere to the provisions contained in a directive that is in conflict with the agency's policy. However, the agency must develop policies and provide information concerning them to the patient on admission. These policies should be detailed enough to communicate the philosophy of the institution regarding the dis- continuation of life-sustaining treatment and indicate any specific limitations the agency might place on the implementation of advance directives.

OBLIGATION TO PRESERVE LIFE AND PREVENT SUFFERING

The rigid stereotyping of professional roles, such as those of the physician and the nurse, may decrease the possibilities for successful management. Although current therapeutic measures cannot cure Alzheimer's disease, they can improve the patient's functioning and quality of life. Team efforts to resolve problems such as urinary incontinence and nocturnal agitation, for example, are often successful. Optimum care requires the involvement and collaboration of all caregivers, family members, friends, and clinicians alike. The question of what type and degree of life support should be given is a troublesome one since loss of intellect often is equated with loss of humanness. Undoubtedly, the minimum ethical requirement is that the extent and irreversibility of the loss of cognitive function be established and that the patient be kept clean, adequately hydrated and nourished, and as free of pain and discomfort possible.

---

*Choice in Dying, 200 Varick St. New York, NY 10014-4810, (212)366-5540. Harvard Medical School, Health Publications Group, Department MD, P.O. Box 380, Boston, MA 02117.

> The ethical code embodied in criminal law prohibits positive euthanasia, the performance of a lethal act, even if that act is motivated by a compassionate desire to prevent suffering. On the other hand, negative euthanasia, the decision to withhold treatment and let nature take its course, is more generally accepted.

Since criteria for decision making are not well defined, this situation creates ethical dilemmas for conscientious caregivers. The patient's wishes, if known and expressed while she was still competent, should be considered. Ethical caregivers must walk a tightrope between resisting premature requests from weary relatives or staff to stop all life-prolonging efforts up to the last and recognizing when these requests are valid. Situations in which health professionals are uncertain about what is best should be resolved in favor of extending life, where possible. This applies when friends or relatives strongly urge it. They will have to live with these decisions after the death of their loved ones, in a way that health professionals do not.

At the same time, patients have the right to refuse life-extending treatment, and incompetence does not diminish that right. When a patient, family, and clinician cannot agree on these serious matters, the decisions must be left to the courts.

PHYSICIAN-ASSISTED SUICIDE AND ACTIVE EUTHANASIA

In June 1997 the Supreme Court of the United States ruled that individuals do not have a constitutional right to have a physician assist them in ending their life. They did, however, refer the matter back to the states, which may pass their own laws concerning the matter. Given the aging of our population and the burgeoning costs of healthcare at the end of life, this issue is far from settled despite this ruling.

The debate about the morality of euthanasia has been fueled by ballot initiatives in three states (narrowly defeated in two) that would allow physician-assisted suicide. The widely publicized cases of Dr. Jack Kevorkian, a retired pathologist, including one in which he helped a woman diagnosed with Alzheimer-type dementia to self-administer a lethal injection, stimulated a growing interest in the issues surrounding the right to die. Furthermore, the book *Final Exit* by Derek Humphrey, which describes ways in which those seeking relief from terminal or debilitating illness can commit suicide, became a bestseller in 1991.

Public opinion polls consistently reveal support for the general desire for "death with dignity" and for the notion that physicians should be allowed to comply with a terminally ill patient's request for help in dying. Surveys of physicians, however, reveal support for the patient's right to die but a reluctance to involve the medical profession in the process, with most studies showing approximately 30% approval.

The issue is proving enormously divisive in the medical community. Numerous organizations, including the American Medical Association, the American Cancer Society, and the American Geriatrics Society, have presented briefs to the Supreme Court opposing physician-assisted suicide, while others such as the American Medical Women's Association and the American Medical Student Association are more supportive of assisted dying as a legal option.

Are acts of withholding treatment that allow a patient to die morally different from active euthanasia—the administration of a fatal injection, overdose, or deadly gas? This issue is the central question under debate. Those who favor voluntary active euthanasia argue that it is an individual right, the right to choose a painless and peaceful death. Opponents contend that the legalization of active euthanasia would diminish the natural value that is bound to the preservation and protection of life and raise the specter of discrimination and abuse.

If we as a society decide to honor patient requests for assistance with suicide, whose job should it be? Many in the health professions are reluctant to assume the obligation of this expanded role, which they think conflicts with their traditional roles, which are conceptualized as "life sustaining and death defying." Will a new profession be needed to carry out this role?

What safeguards are necessary to prevent abuse? Although withdrawal of treatment is a recognition of the limitations of medicine, active euthanasia raises the specter of medical omnipotence and omniscience. What controls will be needed to ensure that the physician, for example, acts (1) with the appropriate consent of the patient, and (2) only in situations in which the diagnosis is correct, life is intolerable or there is no hope of recovery, or death is ensured?

The experience in Holland, where active euthanasia and physician-assisted suicide have been allowed for 2 decades under guidelines developed by the courts, underscores the importance of adequate safeguards. The Dutch rules generally permit physicians to perform euthanasia for patients who are experiencing intolerable suffering and have no prospect for improvement, but only after consultation with an independent physician who is experienced with the disease.

Undeniably, the experience in the Netherlands where all citizens are granted equal access to health care under a national health insurance program may not be fully relevant to the United States. Given the difficulties many Americans currently experience in obtaining access to health care, as well as the apparent reluctance of many physicians, how would equitable access to assisted death be provided? Would it be a realistic option only for those with the necessary finances and persistence to find an accommodating physician?

A court-sponsored study of the Dutch experience indicated that fewer than 3% of all deaths in Holland in 1990 involved active euthanasia and assisted suicide, and that only one third of patient requests for euthanasia were honored. These figures suggested that euthanasia was not being used as an alternative to good terminal care. Most of these acts of euthanasia were conducted in the patient's home with the patient's family and physician in attendance. However, a follow-up study published in 1996 revealed an increase in both the number of physician-assisted deaths and in the number of physicians who had been participants in them. Critics point to disturbing findings amid the statistics in the study.

> Guidelines require that a patient's request be "well-considered, durable and persistent," yet in one third of the cases this standard was not met.

A separate study of deaths resulting from euthanasia indicated that the time that elapsed between the patient's request and the euthanasia was less than 24 hours in 59% of the cases.

Most worrisome was the finding that 92% of the cases in which medical decisions were made to hasten the death of the patient did not meet criteria for euthanasia. These requirements include that there be explicit and repeated requests by the patient that leave no reason for doubt concerning his desire to die; that the decision be well informed, free, and enduring; that the mental or physical suffering be severe with no prospect of relief; that all other options for care have been exhausted or refused by the patient; and that a second physician be consulted.

Only 2.9% of all deaths were recorded as euthanasia under these guidelines. However, 17.5% of all deaths resulted from the administration of opioids for the alleviation of pain and suffering at such dosages that death was either expected or intended, and an additional 17.5% of all deaths involved "passive euthanasia," or the withdrawal or withholding of treatment designed to prolong life. The finding that the physician had not discussed the medical decision with the patient in 60% of the opioid overdose cases and in 63% of the nontreatment decisions is particularly disturbing, although in many cases the patient had previously indicated a desire for euthanasia if his suffering became unbearable, even though these requests were not sufficiently documented.

Patients whose lives were terminated without documented consent tended to be those who were comatose, demented, or otherwise thought to be mentally incompetent.

In these cases physicians cited the following response for proceeding without consent: unbearable pain/suffering (30%), low quality of life (31%), no prospect of improvement (60%), and protecting the patient's family (32%).

With the Dutch studies suggesting that nearly half of the requests for euthanasia arise from issues related to suffering, it is possible that if a concerted effort were made to adequately address the issues of physical pain, psychological distress, and uncontrolled symptoms, the public demand for physician-assisted deaths might be greatly reduced. But even the best care can do little to relieve the suffering caused by the loss of meaning and personal identity and the dependence on others that may be experienced by the patient with Alzheimer's disease. Increased public pressure for a system that ensures a patient's "right to die well" will undoubtedly bring change to the American health care system.

If the legalization of euthanasia is to be adopted, it is clear that it will be preceded by vigorous, systematic deliberation and debate, and that it must be accompanied by a credible supervisory system. Alternatively, the health professions must acknowledge the widespread public dissatisfaction with many factors related to dying and increase their efforts to assist the patient in dying well—to relieve pain and anxiety; provide strength, comfort, and support; avoid burdensome treatments that are likely to prove futile; and communicate with patients and families, helping them to find meaning in their suffering.

OBLIGATION TO GIVE EQUITABLE TREATMENT

The principle of equitable treatment provides for impartiality and prevents discrimination. It ensures that the patient's rights to adequate treatment for the preservation of life or prevention of suffering are in no way diminished simply because the patient has certain characteristics, such as being elderly or having dementia. Too often the right to impartial treatment is overlooked or ignored in patients with Alzheimer's disease. When cognitive decline prevents conventional types of interaction between the caregiver and the patient, the patient often is viewed as undesirable. Yet being "undesirable" does not represent valid ethical grounds for disenfranchising a patient from the normal standard of care. Two of the numerous ways in which differential treatment can be seen involve disclosure of the diagnosis and the different management of medical problems.

DISCLOSURE OF DIAGNOSIS

In the early stages of Alzheimer's disease, the patient can understand the diagnosis and prognosis. Should he be apprised of these facts at this time? Informing a patient of a diagnosis of Alzheimer's disease presents vexing issues. Under the principle of autonomy, the patient is seen as having a moral right to know. Adherence to the principle of beneficence, on the other hand, may lead to a decision to withhold this information if it is thought that it would be detrimental to the particular patient at that time.

In a study by Erde and associates, an overwhelming majority of individuals (92%) indicated that they would want to be informed of the diagnosis. Reasons commonly given included being able to plan for financial and personal care (94%), wanting to seek a second opinion (62%), and wanting to settle family matters (36%). Those persons who wanted to know the diagnosis were even more likely to want their spouse told (89%) if for some reason the information was withheld from them. The ethical clinician balances the burden of being the bearer of bad tidings with a sensitivity to the patient's and family's needs—for timely presentation of small "parcels" of information, for support and information at times when they request it and are able to accept and process it, and for help in coping with the signs and symptoms of the disease and in preparing for its progression.

MANAGEMENT OF MEDICAL PROBLEMS

The first duty of patient care, and the least controversial, clearly is to provide care. Yet studies repeatedly have found that institutionalized persons and elderly patients with dementia seldom receive the aggressive medical care provided to patients who are more independent. Obviously, there is an ethical obligation to apply considerable effort, knowledge, and skills in reaching a diagnosis of Alzheimer's disease, particularly in searching for other possibly reversible causes of dementia.

Less clear is the extent to which medicine ought to be aggressive in the evaluation and treatment of physical illness when the patient is severely demented.

A particularly disturbing study involved a number of demented patients and revealed that although these patients were aggressively screened for signs of colon cancer, inadequate follow-up of positive findings occurred, presumably because treatment would not be offered on the grounds of medical futility. Alternately, several studies have revealed that, although intended to provide comfort rather than prolong life in the end-stage, even the use of antibiotics to combat pneumonia may inadvertently lead to medical complications that further decrease the quality of life and actually accelerate dying. Seemingly disparate, these findings suggest that simplistic guidelines for screening (such as the recommendation that all women older than 40 have an annual screening mammogram) or for treatment of illnesses do not suffice. Instead, periodic care conferences involving clinicians as well as patients and their families are required to help adapt treatment plans on a situation-by-situation basis as the patient's disease evolves and changes the goals of care.

OBLIGATION TO RESPECT THE CAREGIVING UNIT

The murder conviction in 1985 of Gilbert Roswell for the death of his wife, who suffered from osteoporosis and Alzheimer's disease (and who had frequently requested her own death), heightened debate over the need to broaden the ethical approach to address the particular concerns of community and social relationship, the very functions most poignantly threatened by the dementia of Alzheimer's disease. The view that a defined community, most often the couple or family, rather than solely the individual patient should be the decision-making agent, the unit of autonomy, is heard with increasing frequency.

Resolution of the question, Who should decide?—the former pre-demential self, the spouse, the broader family—is best conceived in terms of communicative ethics, or "negotiated consent." The caregivers should organize decision making so that family members who will be affected are invited to participate and to identify reasonable limits on their caregiving obligations.

A distinction must be made between the ability to make choices that have obvious long-term significance, such as whether or not to enter a nursing home, and those "everyday" decisions of dress and diet for which the risks and consequences may be less severe. When the dementia of Alzheimer's disease has progressed to the level where the patient becomes profoundly dependent it is obvious that the consequences arising from important decisions fall to others, most often to family members.

Ethical standards that suggest only that the patient's autonomy should be respected ignore the legitimate concerns of those who must bear the consequences of those decisions. Often it may mean either that the decisions are not carried out and the family members live with guilt, or decisions are carried out and the family members use resources for the patient that may be needed by others or by themselves.

Do group communication and decision making offer a way to prevent conflict? No, often they invite conflict rather than consensus. However, they acknowledge the ambivalence and complexity of the reality of Alzheimer's disease, the need to recognize that all parties must have their views recognized and somehow taken into account.

BROAD ETHICAL ISSUES

Numerous ethical issues surround the difficult dilemmas of Alzheimer's disease. For example:

- What special protections are needed in research on Alzheimer's disease? This disease requires experimentation on humans since no animal models have been identified.
- What is the ethical responsibility of the health care professional for ensuring that research into the cause and amelioration of this disease receives high priority?
- What are the implications for public policy?
- What choices should be made about the allocation of limited health care resources for this special group?

Underlying all these considerations, and central to the resolution of the ethical dilemmas presented by this disease, is a need for a unifying goal to serve as a guide in the care of the patient with Alzheimer's disease. Faced with a patient's inevitable disintegration into a disabling dependent state that is devoid of meaningful relationships, the caregiver must ask, What must be my goals? The answers I would suggest are:

1. To assist the family and friends in celebrating the individual personhood that once was the patient's and in grieving its passing.
2. To help make each movement for the patient as gentle, as content, and as kind as it can be.

BIBLIOGRAPHY

Badzek LA: What you need to know about advance directives, *Nursing* 42(6):58-59, 1992.

Campion EW: Ethical issues in the care of the patient involved in Alzheimer's disease research. In Melnick VL, Dubler ND, editors: *Alzheimer's dementia: dilemmas in clinical research,* Clifton, NJ, 1985, Humana Press.

Cassell EJ: Recognizing suffering, *Hastings Center Report* 21(3):24-31, 1995.

Dyck AJ: Ethical aspects of care for the dying incompetent, *J Am Geriatr Soc* 32:661-664, 1984.

Erde EL, Nadal EC, Scholl TO: On truth telling and the diagnosis of Alzheimer's disease, *J Fam Pract* 26:410-406, 1988.

Flarey DL: Advance directives: in search of self-determination, *J Nurs Admin* 21(11):16-22, 1991.

Greco PJ et al: The Patient Self-Determination Act and the future of advance directives, *Ann Intern Med* 115:639-643, 1991.

Hanks RS: The limits of care: a case study of legal and ethical issues in filial responsibility, *Marriage Fam Rev* 21(3-4):239-257, 1995.

Hersh AR, Outerbridge DE: *Easing the passage,* New York, 1991, Harper Collins.

Hertog CMPM, Ribbe MW: Ethical aspects of medical decision-making in demented patients: a report from the Netherlands, *Alzheimer Dis Assoc Disord* 10(1):11-19, 1996.

Howe EG, Gordon DS, Valentin M: Medical determination (and preservation) of decision-making capacity, *Law, Medicine & Health Care* 19(1-2):27-33, 1991.

Moody HR: A critical view of ethical dilemmas in dementia. In Binstock RH, Post SG, Whitehouse PJ, editors: *Dementia and aging: ethics, values, and policy choices,* Baltimore MD, 1993, The Johns Hopkins University Press.

Morrison RS, Meier DE: Physician-assisted dying: fashioning public policy with an absence of data, *Generations* 48-53, Winter, 1994.

Nelson JL: Pain, suffering, and other sources of support for physician-assisted suicide and euthanasia, *Pain Forum* 4(3):182-185, 1995.

Norberg A, Norberg B, Bexell G: Ethical problems in feeding patients with advanced dementia, *Brit Med J* 281:847-848, 1980.

Post SG, Whitehouse PJ: Fairhill guidelines on ethics of the care of people with Alzheimer's disease: a clinical summary, *J Am Geriatr Soc* 42(12):1423-1429, 1995.

Rhymes JA, McCullough LB: When the bill comes due for the autonomy of demented older adults, who pays? *J Am Geriatr Soc* 43(12):1437-1438, 1995.

Rouse F: Legal and ethical guidelines for physicians in geriatric terminal care, *Geriatrics* 43(8):69-74, 1988.

Sachs G: Flu shots, mammograms, and Alzheimer's disease: ethics of preventive medicine and dementia, *Alzheimer Dis Assoc Disord* 8(1):8-14, 1994.

Vand der Maas PJ et al: Euthanasia and other medical decisions concerning the end of life, *Lancet* 699-674, 1991 (see also comments in *Lancet* 338:952, 953, 1010-1, 1150).

Veatch RM: An ethical framework for terminal care decisions: a new classification of patients, *J Am Geriatr Soc* 32:665-669, 1984.

Watts DT, Howell T, Priefer BA: Geriatricians' attitudes toward assisting suicide of dementia patients, *J Am Geriatr Soc* 40:878-884, 1992.

Legal Issues for Caregivers

Lynn W Brown

Justice delayed is democracy denied.

—Robert F Kennedy

A person who learns that he or she has been diagnosed with Alzheimer's disease or any other debilitating illness is faced with important and difficult decisions regarding several very personal legal issues.

—• The progression of Alzheimer's disease will result at some point in the patient being incapable of making decisions about the type and manner of medical treatment received and of managing financial affairs.

If the patient does not make provisions for these matters while capable of doing so, these decisions will be made by a court-appointed conservator or guardian. If a person fails to make a will while still competent to do so, any property possessed at death will pass according to the law of the state in which the person is a resident at the time of death. Caregivers will benefit from a basic knowledge of the legal procedures and alternatives involved.

Legal issues for caregivers are generally focused on the needs and desires of the patient. Those issues addressed in this chapter include the following:

- What are the legal processes by which a patient with Alzheimer's disease may provide for health care and finances?
- What documents are commonly used?
- What are the provisions and limitations of such documents?
- How are documents prepared, and who has responsibility to carry out prior directives regarding health care and finances?
- When and what types of professional assistance should be sought?
- What responsibility does a caregiver have to follow advance directives of his patient?
- What is the result when the patient does not take any steps in planning for future health care and conservation of finances?

Ideally, the patient should seek legal counsel and perhaps the assistance of a financial planner as well before the effects of the illness impair competence. The technical requirements of the law of the various states and the details required in preparing the documents necessary for planned health care and finances necessitate the involvement of a lawyer.

The attorney should be involved in discussions regarding the alternatives a patient has as well as drafting documents. The better an attorney knows his or her client, the more closely the client's choices can be followed in advance directives for health care. Failure to involve a lawyer can have serious consequences for the patient and family. For example, in some states a health care power of attorney (discussed in detail later in this chapter) must contain very specific language to be valid, which is required by state law.

POWERS OF ATTORNEY

A power of attorney is a legal document that allows one person to act for another. For example, depending on the terms of a power of attorney, an agent may be given authority to sign bank checks, invest money, transfer funds, convey land by executing a deed, or make decisions regarding health care. This document generally does not remain effective if the principal, the person giving power to another person to act for him or her, becomes incompetent.

A DURABLE power of attorney, however, provides that the agent given the authority to act for the principal continues to have authority to act after the principal becomes incompetent. A durable health care power of attorney gives the agent the authority to make decisions regarding health care, such as choosing among alternative treatments or medical procedures or determining in which nursing care facility the principal is placed when he or she is not capable of making such decisions.

The agent under a power of attorney is also referred to as the "attorney in fact" for the person who has executed such a document. An agent (attorney in fact) under a health care power of attorney is usually not a lawyer, but a close friend or relative of the principal. The legal term "execute" means to put into effect by an act, such as the signing of a document, with the understanding of the contents of the document and its effect.

The laws of the various states impose different requirements of witnesses or a notary public for the execution of a deed, will, living will, or power of attorney. An agent under a power of attorney has only the power to act as specifically delegated by the principal and is limited accordingly. A health care power of attorney should provide for a successor agent in the event the first named agent is unable to act.

A person who desires that no extraordinary medical procedures be used to sustain his or her life should make specific provisions in a living will, which is discussed later in this chapter. However, since there remains the problem of who will put a living will into operation, it is prudent to provide in a durable health care power of attorney that the agent has the authority to see that the provisions of the living will are carried out as directed by the patient. Usually, a person should execute both a durable health care power of attorney and a separate living will. The durable health care power of attorney should then make specific reference to the living will.

One problem is that a patient is very often given both of these documents to sign by an admissions counselor at the hospital when he or she is admitted. Under the stress of hospital admission for a serious medical procedure, the patient may focus on the living will and the fear of "pulling the plug," resulting in fear about signing any document.

> The best time for a patient to make difficult health care decisions is before a crisis or hospitalization occurs.

Some nursing homes will not admit any person who has not executed a durable health care power of attorney. Accordingly, a patient may be pressured into making decisions regarding future health care without taking the time and reflection appropriate for such decisions. No thoughtful person will find it easy to contemplate and make detailed provisions for his or her eventual loss of mental acuity, gradual physical decline, and death. When possible, physicians, nurses, and other caregivers should direct their patients to an attorney with experience in these matters before a hospital or nursing home admission.

An attorney in such matters should be familiar with not only the legal issues and documents involved, but also with problems involving health care for the elderly, long-term care planning, and public benefits including Medicaid, Medicare, and Social Security. Although still allowed in some states, the patient should usually avoid hiring an attorney who charges a fee based on a percentage of the patient's assets for advice and preparation of the documents necessary for the patient's anticipated health care and distribution of assets. In addition the lawyer should be able to quote a reasonable hourly fee with an anticipated total cost for legal services. A lawyer's hourly rate pays for the lawyer's support staff, library, computer services, and other office expenses as well as for the lawyer's time.

The field of elder law is becoming a recognized specialty for attorneys; some states now certify lawyers in elder law. A local or state bar association may be able to refer a patient to attorneys in this specialty. Information may also be obtained from the National Elder Law Foundation, 1604 North Country Club Road, Tucson, Arizona 85716.

The decisions a patient makes in the provisions of a power of attorney will differ markedly depending on the family, close friends, and financial circumstances of the patient. Usually a spouse, child, or close friend of the patient will be designated as agent under a durable health care power of attorney. The agent cannot be a provider of health care to the patient. The patient will often designate an agent under a durable health care power of attorney, saying the agent "knows what I want regarding health care." But often the agent, when faced with a patient who is incompetent and unable to communicate, is uncertain or unknowledgeable about what the principal would want.

Ideally while still competent, the patient and his designated agent should both be made as fully aware as possible of the disease with which the patient is afflicted, including its course and progression. The patient should communicate to the agent his or her desires regarding preferred treatment and care. Any caregiver who provides medical advice to such a patient should take the time to involve the designated agent under the health care power of attorney. The attorney in fact should be prepared to consider the principal's personal and religious beliefs regarding likely decisions for medical treatment, since the agent is informed by caregivers. The agent has the right to examine the principal's medical records in making such decisions.

It is of great importance for a patient to understand that so long as he remains mentally competent and can state an opinion regarding a health care decision, his decision must be honored by the health care provider. A patient's informed decision overrides any request by his or her agent.

> Only when the patient's mental functioning becomes such that he cannot understand alternatives, make decisions, and communicate them does an agent under a durable health care power of attorney have authority to make decisions for the patient.

The problem for the health care provider is in determining whether the patient is competent to make a health care decision, and thereby determining whether to ask the patient or the agent to make a decision regarding health care. During the course of an illness, a patient may for given time periods be incompetent, interspersed with periods during which she is competent. Some patients do not go into incompetency without a struggle. Our society teaches us to value our freedom of choice, and the freedom to choose treatment and decide health care alternatives is usually the last right taken away from a person.

Caregivers should be aware that an agent under a durable health care power of attorney has only such power as is provided in the written terms of that power of attorney. What an agent requests must not conflict with those provisions. A patient may give advance directives for treatment in his durable health care power of attorney, which the agent must then follow. Generally, a patient can orally revoke the appointment of an agent under a health care power of attorney.

The question of whether the patient is competent may be a major problem when there is disagreement between the patient and the agent. The patient may not have the mental ability to revoke the designation of an agent. If a principal designates a spouse as agent under a health care power of attorney and the parties divorce, this act generally removes the agent from all authority. As circumstances change, a competent patient may decide to execute a new health care power of attorney, changing the designated agent, successor agent, or advance directives regarding health care.

A hospital or nursing home can refuse to recognize any advance directive contained in a power of attorney, but must transfer the patient to a facility that will comply with the terms contained in the power of attorney or the directive of the designated agent if this is possible. Generally, the agent must present the <u>original</u> of a durable health care power of attorney with the raised seal of a notary to the appropriate caregiver; a copy is not sufficient. Therefore, an agent should take care to preserve the original health care power of attorney. Also, the agent should not give an original health care power of attorney to a hospital clerk and risk it being lost or misfiled, but a copy may be provided to a hospital or nursing home for the health care provider's information.

■ Caregivers should be careful to determine the proper identity of any agent under a durable health care power of attorney.

A nurse should not hesitate to ask for a photo identification. If a person comes in and says to a caregiver on night shift that he is the patient's son with power to act for the patient under a power of attorney, a prudent caregiver will note the means of identifying the agent in the patient's chart. A well-drafted health care power of attorney will include the name and address of each agent and successor agent for the health care provider to contact when a decision needs to be made.

A person does not have to sign a durable power of attorney for it to be effective. Generally, the person's initials or any mark made by him is sufficient, so long as the witnesses have observed the person and are satisfied as to his mental capacity and intent. These requirements will vary from state to state, but the law usually prohibits any health care provider from serving as either a witness to or agent under a durable health care power of attorney. This is a result of the potential conflict of interest for a provider of health care. A nursing home might find its best interest in keeping a patient alive (because he is a paying client) beyond the patient's wishes. On the other hand, a hospital may have a contrary interest based upon lack of insurance or funds to cover care and the allocation of funds for the curable. While it would be uncommon for such interests to affect a patient's health care, it is worth noting that the best interest of the institution and the patient may differ.

Notations in the chart regarding the patient's mental state, such as that a patient is lucid and conversational, are very appropriate and helpful any time the patient is requested to execute a document, whether it is a power of attorney, living will, or otherwise. Generally, a high degree of mental functioning is not required, but the patient must understand the consequences of executing a durable health care power of attorney and be able to designate an agent.

A person executing a durable health care power of attorney will usually give her attorney in fact broad powers to make health care decisions with limitations or advance directives such as the following options regarding life-sustaining treatment:

1. I specifically direct my agent to follow any health care declaration or "living will" executed by me.
2. I do not want life to be prolonged nor do I want life-sustaining treatment to be provided or continued if my agent believes the burdens of the treatment outweigh the expected benefits. I want my agent to consider the relief of suffering, the expense involved, and the quality as well as the possible extension of my life in making decisions concerning life-sustaining treatment.
3. I do not want my life to be prolonged and I do not want life-sustaining treatment:
   (a) if I have a condition that is incurable or irreversible and without the administration of life-sustaining treatment, expected to result in death within a relatively short time.
   (b) if I am in a coma or persistent vegetative state that is reasonably concluded to be irreversible.

4. I want my life to be prolonged to the greatest extent possible without regard to my condition, the chances I have for recovery, or the cost of the procedures.

Additional directives may be made regarding specific treatment such as discontinuing dialysis for kidney failure when the person goes into a coma, determined by caregivers to be irreversible. The use of experimental treatments may be allowed or disallowed by such prior directives. The patient may also wish to choose health care facilities as a prior directive. Some principals exclude certain facilities in their health care power of attorney, for example by prohibiting placement in a certain nursing home.

A patient may also provide advance directives in his health care power of attorney for religious services, burial arrangements, or cremation. The problem with providing for funeral arrangements in a will is that it is usually not read until after the person who made it has been buried.

The principal in her durable health care power of attorney may choose options regarding nutrition and hydration provided by means of a nasogastric tube or tube into the stomach, intestines, or veins, such as the following:

1. I intend to include these procedures among the "life-sustaining procedures" that may be withheld or withdrawn under the conditions previously stated.
2. I do not intend to include these procedures among the "life-sustaining procedures" that may be withheld or withdrawn.

A competent patient and her family should be informed in advance by the caregivers of the course of withholding feeding tubes. After removal of these tubes, several days to a week may pass before the patient dies. Caregivers should prepare a patient's family and designated agent for what will likely be a very unpleasant and emotionally stressful situation if the patient has chosen to refuse nutrition and hydration as an advance directive.

Although we have focused on health care powers of attorney, a person's financial situation may require management by an attorney in fact (agent) under a general durable power of attorney. While a person usually chooses a close friend or relative as agent under a health care power of attorney, a financial adviser, bank, or trust company may be the appropriate agent for financial management. For a person with either substantial assets or sizeable income beyond social security, the execution of both a general durable power of attorney for management of the person's finances and a durable health care power of attorney is recommended.

A person's situation may result in the designation of a different agent in each power of attorney. A bank's trust department with expertise in managing money will not want to serve as agent under a health care power of attorney. Seeking counsel and advice from a lawyer with experience in elder law is highly recommended.

Living Wills

The legislatures of the various states have acknowledged the right of every person to die naturally and with as much dignity as circumstances permit by the creation of a legal document that is usually referred to as a living will. Generally, a living will takes effect only when the patient is in a terminal condition and the attending physician has determined there is no reasonable medical expectation of recovery, regardless of any treatment that may be administered.

> A living will provides that the life of a patient who is dying shall not be artificially prolonged under circumstances decided upon by the patient.

The living will differs from a durable health care power of attorney in that the health care power of attorney allows the attorney in fact to act on behalf of the incompetent or unconscious patient who is not in a terminal condition. Like the durable health care power of attorney, a living will may authorize the withholding or withdrawal of artificially provided food, water, or other nourishment or fluids, resulting in what statutes refer to as a "natural death." Only medicine or medical procedures necessary to provide the patient with comfortable care or to alleviate pain would then be administered. However, other than providing for such artificial support, a living will cannot usually direct medical care, procedures, or facilities as in a durable health care power of attorney. A living will is a much more limited document; the patient has much broader choices in prior directives in a health care power of attorney. A living will takes effect only at the end of life as a specific directive to the health care provider; a health care power of attorney, on the other hand, provides for ongoing care such as a nursing home and gives an agent discretion to make health care decisions. Usually, state law also allows a living will to contain provisions for the donation of organs to be transplanted after death.

A patient must be competent, which means able to understand the nature and consequences of deciding whether to accept or refuse treatment, in order to execute a living will. Usually, a living will does not require the exacting language and warnings of a durable health care power of attorney to take effect. Since the law of each state is different, and because a living will should not conflict with a durable health care power of attorney, the advice of a lawyer is suggested in preparing both documents.

State law often requires that a copy of any living will be delivered to the patient's attending physician or health care provider. Some states require the physician to place a copy of any living will in the patient's medical record. Any person who executes a living will should give a copy of it to several people so that it will be available if and when needed. A person's wishes in this regard should be communicated to close relatives or important friends before the person is incompetent. Anyone may generally revoke a living will by either written or oral statement. A health care provider who refuses to comply with the provisions of a living will must notify the patient, or the patient's next of kin or legal guardian if the patient is not competent, and then make every reasonable effort to transfer the patient to a facility or provider who will comply with the terms of the living will.

WILLS AND ESTATES

Wills and estates are not of as great a concern to professional caregivers as the previously covered topics that relate directly to health care. However, any caregiver should have a basic understanding of these matters in order to assist patients and their families.

> A will is a legal document that provides for the disposition of a person's property after death.

A will takes effect only upon the death of the person who has made it, and cannot provide in any way for the health care of the person while living. As with the other documents that have been discussed, to be valid the execution of a will requires certain legal formalities, particularly regarding witnesses to the will. These requirements vary from state to state. A will should be prepared by a lawyer to ensure its validity. If a will is not properly executed, a court may declare it to be invalid, in which case any property of the deceased person would be inherited as provided by the law of the state in which the person resided at death. Inheritance of property without a will is called interstate succession.

The aggregate of all property owned by a person at death as well as the person's debt is called the person's estate. The terms of a will provide for a person to serve as executor of the estate of the deceased. The executor has a legal obligation to determine the assets of the deceased, account for them, pay the just debts of the deceased, and then distribute the remaining assets as provided by the terms of the will. Usually, a final accounting of all the property of the deceased is required by the probate court.

A will may require the named executor to post a bond with the probate court to ensure that these obligations are correctly completed. If a person dies without a will, a relative or a creditor of the deceased may petition the probate court to appoint an administrator who will complete the same tasks as would an executor. The court will require the administrator to post a security bond, usually in the amount of the total value of the estate. An executor or administrator may be required to file both state and federal tax documents. If the estate has income, he or she may also be required to file both state and federal income tax documents.

A person must be mentally competent to execute a will. The ancient phrase, "of sound mind and disposing memory," requires that to be competent, a person must be aware of both the property he or she owns and the natural recipients of such property. A caregiver should not be involved in suggesting who should inherit a patient's property.

TRUSTS

A trust is a legal entity in which one person (or a corporation) holds property for the benefit of another person under written provisions and directives. The person holding such property for another's benefit is called the trustee. A trust can be created by the gift of property while the donor is alive, or be a provision of a person's will. For example, a person may give a child a sum of money in trust, to be used for the child's education and support until the child reaches a certain age. Banks are often named as a trustee and usually have a trust department to administer assets held by the bank in trust. A bank will charge a fee to administer a trust, usually based upon a percentage of the value of the assets in trust.

The law usually requires an annual accounting of the assets and income of a trust as well as annual income tax reporting. Because of their complexity, trusts usually involve sizeable amounts of money or other assets. Placing assets into a trust may result in loss of Medicaid eligibility for several years. Advice of a lawyer in such matters is indispensable.

COURT-APPOINTED GUARDIANS

If a person's mental faculties deteriorate to a point that he is no longer competent to make decisions regarding his health care or finances, the laws of the various states provide for court proceedings to determine whether a guardian should be appointed to manage the person's finances and make health care decisions. These court proceedings would be instituted only when a person has failed to execute a durable power of attorney for financial matters and/or a durable health care power of attorney before becoming incompetent. The law of some states uses the word "guardian" only to refer to a person with supervisory duties over the affairs of a minor, and the term "conservator" for a court-appointed manager of an adult's affairs. Although the distinction is important, depending upon the particular state, this chapter will use only the term "guardian" in this regard.

State law generally provides that any person, which in practice is usually a relative or friend of the disabled person, may file a petition in the appropriate court requesting that it appoint a guardian. The filing of a petition usually requires the assistance of a lawyer. Sometimes a hospital or other health care facility will petition the court to have a guardian appointed for a patient. Usually, the court will appoint a guardian ad litem, meaning a guardian for the purpose of the litigation, to protect the rights of the disabled person.

The guardian ad litem is commonly an attorney, and must not be the lawyer who prepared and filed the petition. She has the duty to consult with the allegedly disabled client as soon as possible after appointment by the court. The guardian ad litem must generally explain to her client the substance of the petition, the nature of the guardianship proceedings, the client's right to protest the appointment of a guardian by the court, and the identity of any proposed guardian. She also has the duty to independently investigate the physical and mental condition of the client. The court order of appointment will usually allow the guardian ad litem access to all of the financial and medical records of the client. A court may authorize the guardian ad litem to have her client undergo an independent mental or physical evaluation. Although the terms sound similar, it is important to understand that the guardian ad litem and the proposed guardian are two different people with two different roles.

The duties of the guardian ad litem end when the legal proceedings are concluded, the point at which the duties of the guardian, if one is appointed by the court, begin.

Usually, the fee for the guardian ad litem as well as for court costs and the cost of any evaluation will be paid out of the assets of the client.

State law usually requires that the guardian ad litem present the court with a written report of his investigation including whether the client wishes to contest the appointment of a guardian or the person proposed as guardian. Also, a proposed property management plan and proposed plan for health care are often presented to the court at this time. The judge in the proceedings then has the duty to determine (following the trial) whether or not a guardian should be appointed, who the guardian should be, and whether there should be limitations on the guardian's authority. The judge sometimes also must approve a plan for health and financial care of the incompetent person. The court may require the guardian to post a bond to guarantee preservation of the assets of the disabled person.

If a guardian is appointed, he must usually file an inventory of the property of the disabled person, as well as a plan for the management of those assets. As the guardian makes regular reports to the court, he or she will be paid a reasonable fee for the management of such assets in an amount approved by the court. The guardian must also file appropriate state and federal income tax returns for the disabled person.

Many states or local jurisdictions have provided for a public guardian for the elderly in situations in which there are no willing and responsible family members or friends to serve as such or when the disabled person does not have sufficient resources to compensate a guardian and pay court costs.

SUMMARY

Advance planning by a patient who is diagnosed with Alzheimer's disease is preferred. A court-appointed guardian in some situations may be a person completely unknown to the patient. Although difficult to consider under such circumstances, a durable health care power of attorney and living will allow a patient to choose a plan for health care and provide advance directives for medical care that will remain effective as the disease progresses. However, the decisions of an agent pursuant to a durable power of attorney for financial matters are not supervised by a court as would be a guardian. An agent must be selected most carefully because of the potential for ineptitude or less than adequate attention to financial details. The trust placed in an agent pursuant to a durable health care power of attorney allows the agent to decide the most personal matters of health care for the principal who has become incompetent. Difficult decisions under the best of circumstances become more difficult and less informed as Alzheimer's disease progresses.

Appropriate counsel, information, and advice will result in protection of the assets of the patient, and most importantly, the assurance that the wishes of the individual are carried out as health fails.

Stress in Caregivers

Chapter 23

Linda J Kerley
James M Turnbull

You don't get ulcers from what you eat, you get them from what is eating you.

—Vicky Baum

Stress has been defined in a number of ways. Hans Selye, probably the most famous writer on the subject, referred to stress as a physiological state that results when an organism is influenced by a stressor. Stressors include both physical stimuli (e.g., noise, heat, cold, pain) and psychosocial stimuli (e.g., death of a relative, moving into a nursing home, changing jobs).

Human response to stressors is mediated, or influenced for good or ill, by personality, coping skills, and awareness of what is happening (insight). Thus the stress of the job of caring for a patient with Alzheimer's disease is influenced by a variety of factors.

THE FAMILY CAREGIVER

Of the over 4 million Americans who suffer from Alzheimer's disease, 70% live at home. They are cared for by loved ones and friends of the family. Additionally, families pay an average of $12,500 to hire outside help, usually from home health agencies, on an annual basis. The burden of this caregiving disproportionately falls on women—wives, daughters, daughters-in-law, and granddaughters. Caregivers, most of whom are middle-aged women, are at high risk for becoming secondary victims of the illness. They may concurrently have responsibility for their own children, work outside the home, be pursuing a career, or be in college. Caring for a relative with dementia leaves little time or energy for self-care. Thus the demands of the job may cause caregivers to neglect exercise, nutrition, socialization, and even sleep.

316

The spectrum of potential negative effects experienced by family caregivers is called "caregiver burden." This burden may be either physical or emotional, or both.

Physical Burden

The physical burden includes all the tasks that are needed to meet the personal needs of the family member with Alzheimer's disease. In the early stages the caregiver needs to assist in such tasks as balancing the checkbook, paying bills, answering correspondence, doing special shopping (Christmas, birthdays, etc.), and ensuring that medical, dental, hairdressing, and other appointments are kept. Later in the course of the disease the relative will require assistance with feeding, bathing, dressing, walking, and toileting. Problematic behavior such as wandering, sleep/wake reversal, crying, and being combative become more apparent. Compulsive and repetitive questions, such as Where are my glasses?, and unrealistic demands, such as I need to go to the store right now!, are extremely wearing.

> The physical demands of caregiving and burden generally increase as the body and mind of the Alzheimer's disease patient progressively decline.

The response of caregivers differs with respect to the tasks demanded of them. Some fare better with relatives who are in the early stage of the disease, while others are more tolerant when dealing with the physical needs of a later stage. Some even gain a degree of personal satisfaction in caring for a relative with severe dementia.

One of the major difficulties experienced by most caregivers, especially those who work full-time or who manage a busy household, is the disruption of sleep. The relative who awakens at night, stumbles to the bathroom, switches on the lights, or attempts to make a cup of coffee disturbs the whole household, but it is the caregiver who takes responsibility for settling the person down and putting her back to bed. This is at the expense of the caregivers own need for sleep.

Emotional Burden

The emotional burden of caregiving is a direct response to the change in personality, demeanor, and behavior of the loved one. A kind, generous, loving father becomes a petty, moody, irascible tyrant. A competent, caring, and sympathetic mother turns into a scatterbrained, helpless, and seemingly self-centered harridan. The response of caregivers to these changes in someone they love is directly related to three major factors:
1. Their own emotional and physical well-being.
2. The degree of support they receive from siblings and other relatives.
3. How well they take care of themselves.

Isolated, depressed caregivers who receive little or no support from the rest of the family develop feelings of frustration, despondency, and even impotent rage, which can result in a giving-up syndrome or even physical/psychological abuse of the Alzheimer's disease patient.

Male Family Caregivers

Men are living longer but women are more likely to suffer from Alzheimer's disease. Thus there are times when a man may become the caregiver for his mother, wife, or aunt. Many men have little or no experience with household chores. Thus cooking, cleaning, and changing diapers are skills that have to be learned from scratch. Taking a female relative to the bathroom or bathing her may provide extreme discomfort for the male caregiver.

While some men embrace the new experiences of caregiving cheerfully, others are resentful of the burden placed upon them and the unfamiliarity of the role. Particularly painful is the social isolation from their male peers that many of these men experience. Male bonding is generally accomplished through activities—golf, playing cards, and watching football. Unlike women, men rarely meet other men to chat, exchange world views, or engage in neighborly gossip. The man who is now confined to the home and is unable to participate in activities outside may find himself totally cut off socially. This sense of isolation leads to a feeling of being abandoned and lowers self-esteem and self-worth.

Sickness in Caregivers

Caregivers who are themselves sick with chronic illness often experience more stress than do healthy caregivers. Less free time available for leisure and social activities lowers the amount of social interaction and may also lower resistance to infections. Caregivers may have to reduce their work hours or quit their jobs.

Studies that have compared caregivers for stroke with those looking after relatives with Alzheimer's disease find more depression and anxiety in the latter group. Much of this is related to the cognitive and behavioral changes taking place and the steady, downhill decline so characteristic of the disease.

Caregiver Reactions

The caregiver undergoes a variety of psychological reactions in response to the combination of accepting their new role and their changing attitude toward their ill relative. These include guilt, powerlessness, anger, and hopelessness.

The guilt arises from feelings of anger and frustration resulting from lack of patience, the failure of the ill person to meet expectations, and the role reversal in which the parent or spouse becomes a child. Anger and exhaustion then result from the amount of time rendered in care, the lack of appreciation for such care, and the feeling of being tied down. Powerlessness results in pessimism and lack of ability to make personal choices.

The feeling of hopelessness is one of the symptoms of depression and results from an overwhelming sense of loss. The caregiver realizes that the person he or she once loved is present in body but not in spirit. Communication is poor, the future looks bleak, and fond memories of good times are all in the past. The caregiver is confronted by the stark reality that his or her relative is no longer the same person he or she once knew.

Coping Skills

Coping skills are enhanced by the following:
- Strong family support
- Taking time for self every day
- Utilizing community resources
- Respite care
- Strengthening spiritual life
- Support groups

A number of formal services are available to help reduce the stress of caregiving. These are described in Chapter 26. Various services provide respite for the caregiver, help the caregiver cope with the emotional demands of caregiving, and provide assistance when the demands of caregiving become overwhelming. It should be noted, however, that none of the formal services has been demonstrated to alleviate the emotional burden of caregiving, which continues regardless of the supports utilized.

Respite Care

Respite care is professional short-term care in a hospital, a nursing home, at home, or in an adult day care center. During respite care, the caregiver is given an opportunity to rest and attend to selected personal tasks. Respite programs vary in length and the benefits are different among programs. The use of in-home and adult day care respite care has been associated with less emotional burden, reduced personal distress, a more positive outlook, and enhanced feelings of being able to cope with the situation.

The reduction in personal stress provided by respite care may be short term and, in some situations, may affect patient outcomes. In one study, a 2-week in-hospital respite was associated with reduced emotional stress of the caregiver only during the time of respite care. The relief experienced during respite was short term and did not last after the respite was over. In addition, some care recipients declined in their ability to perform activities of daily living and their health worsened.

Support Groups

Several types of support groups are available to help the family caregiver manage the emotional stress involved with care. The Alzheimer's Association support groups provide information about dementia and care receiver management, share coping strategies, and provide support in discussion groups with other caregivers. This type of support group may be more important to caregivers who are concerned about the future of relatives who are in the later stages of dementia.

Educational support groups are self-limited and provide information to assist caregivers. These groups provide information about dementia; patient care; legal and financial resources; and available community services. Caregivers who have relatives in the early stages of Alzheimer's disease may be more inclined to favor educational groups rather than Alzheimer's Association support groups.

Stress management support groups help caregivers identify stressors and develop strategies to cope with the stresses of caregiving. Time management, communication, and relaxation are discussed. Caregivers in a stress management support group have used more effective coping skills at home but have not reported reduced stress. Support groups are further discussed in Chapter 25.

Caregiver Training

The difficult family responsibility of caregiving may be lessened through training for the task. One model assists the caregiver in managing the environment to reduce the anxiety and agitation of the care receiver. Routines and strategies are simplified to reduce fatigue, change, demands, multiple and competing stimuli, physical stressors, and affective responses to perception of losses. The goal of this model is to improve the family's ability to manage the care receiver and thus to reduce caregiver stress.

Nursing Home Placement

Nursing home placement is a consideration when the demands of caregiving exceed the personal resources of the caregiver. In the later stages of Alzheimer's disease, cognitive confusion and physical problems may create a demand for 24-hour care. The strenuous physical activity needed for helping the individual and caregiver burden may create the need to seek institutionalization. Particularly among children and among some spouses, the necessity or desire to maintain outside employment may prevent in-home caregiving. Families with adequate financial resources are more likely to seek nursing home placement.

Caregivers may choose to institutionalize their relative with Alzheimer's disease for personal reasons. A sense of role captivity (being an unwilling, involuntary incumbent of the caregiver role) has been demonstrated to increase the chances of nursing home placement. Role captivity was more apparent in white caregivers who were adult children rather than spouses. Role captivity was made worse by loss of relationships with the care receiver, role overload, problematic behavior, and problems with relationships.

Care recipient characteristics affect the likelihood of nursing home placement. Nursing home placement is desired more frequently when the caregiver is older, more services are used, the spouse exhibits a high level of forgetfulness, and the spouse/caregiver has a poor relationship with the relative. The longer the spouse is involved in the caregiver role, the more likely he or she is to keep the individual at home rather than place him/her in a nursing home.

The primary advantage of nursing home placement is allowing the caregiver time for family and social activities. Caregivers of institutionalized family members have reported a more stable family network and more frequent participation in social activities than do in-home caregivers.

While nursing home placement may provide the caregiver with more time for participation in social activities, the emotional stresses of caregiving may not be relieved, especially if the caregiver maintains frequent contact and visits with the care recipient. Nursing home caregivers reported more stress associated with assisting their relatives with activities of daily living, with the relative's behavior problems and memory loss, and with lack of caregiving support from family and friends than did in-home caregivers.

A disadvantage of institutionalization is the increased risk of decline in the care recipient. In one study, care recipients had an increased risk of death following institutionalization. This risk was unchanged even when health status was controlled.

Pastoral Counseling

Pastoral counselors may assess and provide coping skills for caregivers. They can assist the caregiver to examine and reframe relationships, appraise and look for ways to improve self-efficacy, and help him or her find and use social support.

STRESS IN PROFESSIONAL CAREGIVERS

Long-term care is long, arduous work. Both in nursing homes and in home health agencies the professional staff (i.e., paid workers) are certified nurses aides (CNAs). They give 80%-90% of the care, and are almost always women, minimally trained, and poorly paid. Their patients are also mainly women who are ill, sometimes in pain, and frequently both disoriented and abusive. Apart from the person she is caring for, the aide most frequently comes in contact with the patient's family, who often treat her as a domestic servant.

Staff turnover is a real problem in nursing homes. Between 1992 and 1994, turnover rates in nursing homes averaged 46% annually, while in home health agencies the rate was 10%.

Low wages, poor benefits, the emotional and physical demands of the job, lack of organizational training, and the absence of opportunities for advancement—all lead to "burnout." Worker "burnout," which is the direct result of stress, is fairly common among people who care for patients with dementia. Burnout is a process that consists of three stages. The first stage of burnout involves an imbalance between the internal resources of the caregiver and the demands placed on them. In other words, whether the individual is a health care worker or a family member, the demands placed on her exceed her ability to deliver.

For example, a CNA who is also the single mother of two teenage children undergoing their own life crises is suddenly faced with the illness of a co-worker who is unable to stay on the job. Doing the work of two while a replacement is being sought, she spends extra hours at work and is unable to attend to the needs of her children, and their surliness and uncooperativeness increase. The CNA finds herself experiencing demands beyond her ability to meet them.

The second stage is the immediate (short-term) emotional response. It is characterized by tenseness, anxiety, and feelings of exhaustion.

The third stage consists of several changes that the CNA undergoes. These include a tendency to treat the patient in a detached and mechanical fashion or a cynical preoccupation with having her own needs met.

Burnout is a transactional process. In other words, it is an interaction among many different factors—in this example, between job stress, the strain on the aide, and the way the individual accommodates psychologically to the whole process. What happens is that a previously committed person disengages from her work and develops a series of signs and symptoms of burnout.

CNAs are often unaware of their own health risks, despite being able to identify the major stressors in the workplace and at home, ethical conflicts about appropriate patient care, team conflicts, role ambiguity, workload, organizational deficits, marital and family disputes, and financial concerns.

INSTITUTIONAL SETTINGS

In an institutionalized setting, the signs and symptoms of burnout can be summarized in the following way:
- A highly resistant attitude toward going to work every day, characterized by frequent tardiness or even absenteeism
- A feeling of being overwhelmed by the thought of going to work when getting up in the morning
- A sense of failure
- Anger and resentment, directed particularly at supervisors, the institution itself, and sometimes residents

These feelings are followed by guilt and blame, discouragement and indifference, social isolation and withdrawal, and negativism toward life in general. Individuals who are burned out spend time watching the clock during the day and feel tremendously fatigued after work.

They come home and are unable to engage with their own families in any meaningful way. Another sign of burnout is a loss of positive feelings toward patients and a tendency to group them all together. The CNA is unable to concentrate on or listen to what the patient is trying to say. Instead, she has a feeling of immobilization, of being unable to do anything about the situation. She then becomes cynical and blames the patients, as if it were their fault that they are in the institution.

> The burned out professional demonstrates a tendency to go by the book, to follow instructions in a mechanical way, and to do only the very minimum amount of work to get by.

A series of psychosomatic complaints then follows, including insomnia, avoidance of discussing work with colleagues, and self-preoccupation. The CNA develops frequent colds, viral infections, headaches, and upset stomach. She becomes rigid in her thinking and resistant to change.

Some individuals even become paranoid about their co-worker and the administration. At this stage the health care professional may use drugs and alcohol, begin to have marital and family conflicts, and show a heightened rate of absenteeism.

STRESS AND PERSONALITY

Individuals respond to the stresses of their job according to their own personality traits, what they want to do with their lives, what sort of experiences they have had, and the quality of their life outside work.

> Individuals who have an external locus of control are more vulnerable to burnout than those who have an internal locus of control.

Individuals with an external locus of control project all problems onto the environment and see themselves as victims. This attitude applies to their whole life. These people are not self-motivated but require tremendous amounts of support to continue doing their job. Individuals who start out being extremely humanitarian tend to burn out in institutions such as nursing homes because they do not see their work resulting in changes for good.

On the other hand, individuals with an internal locus of control consider themselves the masters of their own destiny and require much less positive feedback to feel good about themselves. The person with an internal locus of control feels much less stressed about caring for a patient with Alzheimer's disease than does his counterpart with an external locus of control.

Patients with Alzheimer's disease are rarely, if ever, openly appreciative of the tremendous amount of work done for them by family members and aides. If being thanked, praised, complemented, and rewarded in some way is of paramount importance to an aide's well-being, the professional will be sorely disappointed in caring for these patients.

Worker burnout always affects patient care. It is well known in psychiatric hospitals on inpatient units that high rates of suicide attempts, high rates of elopements from the unit, high rates of depression, and general misery among patients occur when the staff members are demoralized. This patient reaction, in turn, increases the degree of stress that the staff feels, and a vicious cycle has begun. Attempts to improve staff morale can turn this situation around. As staff members begin to feel better, patients begin to do better.

JOB SATISFACTION

CNAs who care for patients with dementia expect a certain degree of job satisfaction. Traditionally, nursing homes have not been high-prestige work locations; little glamour is attached to working in such institutions. In fact, sometimes the relatives of residents are abusive toward and demanding of staff members who are working as hard as they can. Although this type of abuse reflects guilt and shame, it is difficult for staff members not to take it personally. Therefore it is important for nursing homes to be able to attract professionals who are content to work with chronically ill individuals and who are not burned out and cynical about their job.

Much of the job satisfaction experienced by CNAs comes from the professional endorsement they receive from their colleagues and the fact that they like their co-workers. The friendships that they make at work can create an important and highly sustaining support system.

PREVENTIVE MEASURES

How can burnout be prevented in people who care for patients with dementia? There are two aspects of prevention: individual and organizational. Interventions designed to alleviate burnout include the following measures:
1. Reduction or elimination of excessive job demands (people must not be expected to do more than they can reasonably accomplish).
2. Change in personal goals and preferences to meet the reality of the situation.
3. Increase in the resources for meeting the demands of the task.
4. Provision of coping substitutes for the withdrawal characteristics of burnout.

> Burnout in an institution is a highly contagious disorder and requires tremendous efforts to achieve reversal.

Such efforts are often met with resistance by a pessimistic and thoroughly demoralized staff. In almost no other situation is the adage "an ounce of prevention is worth a pound of cure" so appropriate.

Since work overload is a common cause of burnout in many human services agencies, one of the simplest solutions is to hire more staff. However, the tendency to define the solution solely in terms of more resources has some very serious flaws. Researchers have suggested that tremendous changes in staff-patient ratios are necessary before any substantial change can occur if this is the only step taken. Burnout has many other causes, such as role conflict, ambiguity in the definition of work, lack of variety, lack of autonomy and control over one's work, and destructive norms. These factors have nothing to do with the number of people hired.

STAFF DEVELOPMENT

One of the first ways in which intervention is possible and necessary is staff development, which has three main objectives:
1. Reduce the demands that workers impose on themselves by encouraging them to adopt more realistic goals.
2. Encourage the people who work in an institution to adopt new goals that might provide alternative sources of gratification.
3. Help the workers develop new monitoring and feedback mechanisms that reflect short-term gains—for example, reporting regularly to someone who listens to what a person has been able to accomplish and getting positive feedback.

Staff development should also seek to provide frequent opportunity for in-service training designed to increase role effectiveness. It should attempt to teach staff members coping strategies such as time-study and time-management techniques.

In our early work with patients, one thing that we learned was to be pleased with relatively small gains. New staff members frequently expect to be "world shakers" and to make tremendous gains with patients very early in their careers. However, CNAs who work with the elderly, particularly those with Alzheimer's disease, do not make many such gains during their careers.

CNAs must learn to work with patients' relatives, who may give some positive feedback. In-service training provides opportunities to learn new techniques for working out problems with patients or to redefine old techniques.

WORKLOAD

Another way in which burnout can be prevented is to change job and role structures. This type of change can be made by limiting the number of people for whom staff members are responsible at any one time. This approach is particularly important for settings in which CNAs work with groups of ill patients. For example, suppose a program has 12 patients and 3 staff members. Either the staff members can share the responsibility for all 12 patients, or they can each take responsibility for 4 patients.

> Researchers have found that overload is lessened when responsibility is divided.

Even though the patient-staff ratio is no different, there is less stress when the group is divided into three smaller groups, with certain staff members assigned to each one. The staff members also feel a greater sense of personal responsibility and control when they are solely responsible for a smaller number of patients.

It is important to carefully select the mix of patients assigned to staff members. In general, the most difficult patients should not be assigned to any one staff member. Newly hired staff members are often given the most difficult patients, but patients who are repugnant, resistant, abusive, very withdrawn, or severely disabled should not be assigned to new staff members who have had limited training.

TIME-OUT

Most jobs in the human service industry allow little opportunity for reflection and thought. Yet both are vital to effective coping. Time-outs, which allow staff members to escape temporarily from the demands of their role and to think about what they are doing without interruption, reduce workload and strain.

One way of ensuring that time-outs will be available is to use auxiliary workers such as volunteers or part-time employees. Vacation time policies also can be used to provide relief. Sometimes employees need to be encouraged to take frequent vacations. The tendency to allow vacation time to accumulate and to regard this time as a kind of status symbol should be discouraged. Flexibility must be maximized so that people can take vacations on short notice whenever they need to.

Another difficulty arises over the matter of part-time workers. We think that part-time workers are extremely beneficial to an institution. Unfortunately, most institutions do not provide fringe benefits, such as medical leave, medical coverage, and insurance, for part-time workers.

ADMINISTRATIVE SUPPORT

Administrators of institutions need to think about ways to make life more pleasant and work more enjoyable for their staff members. One such approach is career ladders. Lack of career ladders has been identified as a major source of dissatisfaction among people who are not professionally trained. Career stages do alleviate burnout by enhancing the individuals' vicarious sense of competence.

Competence is one of the most important factors leading to self-esteem on the job. However, human service work is expected to be more than just a job. It is considered a calling in the truest sense of the word. A CNA who wants to work on an Alzheimer's unit or in a nursing home must prepare more than someone who wants to become a factory worker, bartender, or postal employee. The greater preparation is emotional as well as financial and intellectual. Yearly merit raises that are given automatically are not enough to reinforce an aide's confidence. A true career ladder requires advancement in the form of meaningful increases in responsibility, privileges, and status.

Administrators and managers must know how to do their jobs properly. They must make their goals clear, develop a strong and distinctive guiding philosophy, and make education and research a major focus of the program in which they are involved. Most of all, administrators and managers must make the staff who are working for them and with them understand that they are doing a good job.

Although supervisors may feel uncomfortable saying thank you or acknowledging that their staff members are working hard in unusually trying circumstances, offering such support is one of their most basic and vital responsibilities.

SUPPORT GROUPS

The Nurse Aid Project at New England Research Institute attempted to reduce stress and turnover by conducting support groups for nursing assistants. The model was the groups conducted for nurses in intensive care units. It was felt that nurses aides often missed out on opportunities for collegiality, education, affirmation of a job well done, and information sharing. The meetings lasted an hour, were conducted biweekly by trained leaders, and went on for eight weeks.

In the support group the most frequently discussed topics were:
• Problems communicating with peers
• Difficulty obtaining help from supervisors
• Working with a "short" staff
• Managing difficult residents
• Salaries and benefits

One of the side benefits was the bringing together of people of different races and cultures. Many CNAs in urban areas are recent immigrants to the US and have a poor command of English. These groups provided a means for improving language skills and other forms of communication.

Although modest improvements were made in reducing staff turnover, many of the participants improved their problem-solving and communication skills and also felt better about their jobs and themselves. Many also went on to leadership roles in the institution.

BIBLIOGRAPHY

Adler G, Ott L, Jelinski M et al: Institutional respite care: benefits and risks for dementia patients and caregivers, *Int Psychogeriat* 5(1):67-77, 1993.

Aneshensel CS, Perlin LT, Schuler RH: Stress, role captivity, and the cessation of caregiving, *J Health Soc Behav* 34:54-70, 1993.

Barrett JJ: Counseling those who care for a relative with Alzheimer's disease, *Past Psychol* 42(1):3-9, 1993.

Boykin A, Winland-Brown J: The dark side of caring: challenges of caregiving, *J Gerontological Nursing* 21(5):13-18, 1995.

Chappel NL, Novak M: The role of support in alleviating stress among nursing assistants, *Gerontologist* 32(3):351-359, 1992.

Conlin MM, Caranosos GJ, Davidson RA: Reduction of caregiver stress by respite care: a pilot study, *South Med J* 85(11):1096-1100, 1992.

Farran CJ, Keane-Hagerty E: Interventions for caregivers of persons with dementia: educational support groups and Alzheimer's Association support groups, *Appl Nurs Res* 7(3):112-117, 1994.

Feldman PH: 'Dead end' work or motivating job? Prospects for frontline paraprofessional workers in LTC, *Generations* 5-10, Fall 1994.

Fisher L, Lieberman MS: Alzheimer's disease: the impact of the family on spouses, offspring, and inlaws, *Fam Process* 33:305-325, 1994.

Gerdner LA, Hall GR, Buckwalter KC: Caregiver training for people with Alzheimer's based on a stress threshold model, *IMAGE: J Nurs Sch* 28(3):241-246, 1996.

Gruetzner H: *Alzheimer's: a caregiver's guide and sourcebook,* New York, 1992, John Wiley & Sons, Inc.

Kaye J, Robinson KM: Spirituality among caregivers, *IMAGE: J Nurs Sch* 26(3):218-221, 1994.

McDonald C: Recruitment, retention and recognition of frontline workers in long-term care, *Generations.* 41-42, Fall 1994.

Reese DR, Gross AM, Smalley DL. et al: Caregivers of Alzheimer's disease and stroke patients: immunological and psychological considerations, *Gerontologist* 34(4):534-540, 1994.

Selye H: *Stress in health and disease,* Sydney, 1976, Butterworths.

Williamson GM, Schulz R: Coping with specific stressors in Alzheimer's disease caregiving, *Gerontologist* 33(6):747-755, 1993.

Wilner MA: Working it out: support groups for nursing assistants, *Generations* 39-40, Fall 1994.

Elder Abuse

Chapter 24

Curtis B Clark
Lynda Weatherly

My son, take care of your father when he is old;
grieve him not as long as he lives. Even if his
mind fails, be considerate with him; revile him
not in the fullness of your strength.

—Sirach

THE "UNENDING FUNERAL"

Caregivers have referred to Alzheimer's disease as an "unending funeral." Cognitive function does not improve, and a general decline that may take 7 to 10 years can be expected, although some individuals have been known to survive as long as 20 years.

Relationship to Caregiver Stress

This disease does not discriminate according to race, religion, or socioeconomic status. Caregivers or the middle-aged children of the "sandwich generation" are caught between the competing demands of their own lives, such as responsibilities to their spouse, children, and work demands, and the burdens of caring for a frail, elderly parent with dementia. Although a caregiver's intentions may be good, the strains of a relationship may develop over a long period and result in abuse. The theory of the stressed caregiver emphasizes the importance of stress in triggering abusive behavior and reinforces the idea that the care of a family member with Alzheimer's disease is, indeed, a "36-hour-a-day" burden.

In addition to the theory of the stressed caregiver, the increase in dependency by patients who suffer from Alzheimer's disease seems to be a crucial factor in elderly abuse. Both abused and nonabused patients tend to have a similar degree of physical impairment; however, abused victims seem to have significantly greater cognitive impairment. Thus recent onset of an increased dependency state places a patient with Alzheimer's disease at much higher risk.

AGEISM

In our youth-oriented society, the elderly experience a great deal of "ageism." Ageism can be defined as systematic stereotyping of and discrimination against people because they are old. It is comparable to racism and sexism, which are forms of stereotyping and discrimination based on skin color and gender. Older people are commonly categorized as senile, rigid in thought and manner, garrulous, and old-fashioned in morality and skills.

Many advertisements and cartoons depict the elderly as being "roleless" and useless to society. Such stereotyping may cause some persons to be inconsiderate of the elderly. Physicians and nurses can aid the elderly by understanding both their capabilities and their limitations as individuals and by acting as enlightened advocates for them.

Ageism encourages professionals to adopt a paternalistic attitude toward older people. Such an attitude prevents professionals from allowing elders the privilege of making their own decisions. Ageist attitudes are often shared by elderly people themselves and may help to explain their greater acceptance of abuse than would be expected.

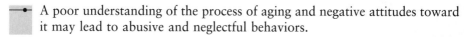

A poor understanding of the process of aging and negative attitudes toward it may lead to abusive and neglectful behaviors.

Education is the key to dispelling the ignorance and negative attitudes associated with the process of aging and elder abuse. Many potentially explosive situations can be defused if knowledge of the existence of elder abuse and of its causes are provided to society.

INCIDENCE OF ABUSE

Fulmer and Wetle suggest that 500,000 to 1.5 million cases of abuse and neglect occur annually in the United States. The incidence of elder abuse is difficult to determine, but it seems to lie somewhere between 4% and 10% of persons older than 65 years. The persons abused and the criteria used are not universally accepted, and this disparity may account for the variation in the prevalence of elder abuse from investigator to investigator. Unfortunately the problem of elder abuse is likely to grow as the percentage of those afflicted with Alzheimer's disease increases along with population growth.

Only recently has attention been focused on abuse of the elderly. In a 1981 report the U.S. House of Representatives Select Committee on Aging said that elder abuse was "alien to the American ideal." The report further stated that "the abuse of our elderly is at the hands of their children and, until recent times, has remained a shameful and hidden problem."

Elder abuse was not given attention until the 1960s, and significant work in this area was not begun until about 1978, when several investigators began studying the problem. Pillemer focused on 42 physical abuse cases, and researchers found that 64% of the abusers were financially dependent on their victims and 55% were dependent on the victim for shelter. Abusers are most likely to be close family members, usually an adult child of the patient. Sons more often than daughters are prone to feel that their parents should continue to support them in their old age, even though these parents may have developed mental impairment or physical disabilities. Since such sons continue to expect parents to provide the nurturing and parental role, they may be having difficulty accepting the fact that their parents are aging and failing in health.

DEFINITION OF ELDER ABUSE

Although definitions of the problem vary widely, the American Medical Association has proposed the following definition of elder abuse:

> *"Abuse shall mean an act or omission which*
> *results in harm or threatened harm to the*
> *health or welfare of an elderly person. Abuse*
> *includes intentional infliction of physical or*
> *mental injury, sexual abuse, or withhold-*
> *ing necessary food, clothing, and medical*
> *care to meet the physical and mental health*
> *needs of an elderly person by one having the*
> *care, custody, or responsibility of an el-*
> *derly person."*

A number of terms have been used in an attempt to define and describe the phenomenon of elderly abuse. Elder mistreatment, elder miscare, old age abuse, nonaccidental injury, granny bashing, and granny battering have all been used by various researchers and writers. Regardless of the term that one chooses to describe this phenomenon, elder abuse is a form of family violence that has some similarities with child and spouse abuse. Elder abuse and neglect are forms of family violence that have been addressed by elder abuse reporting laws in at least 30 states.

Although child and spouse abuse have been recognized and addressed by the courts for many years, the same type of abuse of an elder citizen has only recently been recognized as significant, worthy of reporting, and requiring appropriate treatment, care, and prevention. One significant difference in the handling of child abuse and elder abuse cases is that the elder patient, if competent, can refuse protective services. At times the moral and legal aspects of abuse may be in conflict. If the elder person is incapable of giving consent, the health care provider should contact the adult protective services or local law enforcement for assistance. Individual rights must be honored at all times, and such a conflict is well suited to an interdisciplinary approach for resolution.

Examples of abuse are active physical assault, verbal and psychological assault, denial of rights, inadequate nutrition, misuse of drugs, financial exploitation, sexual abuse, and withholding of basic life resources. There may be a pattern of intrafamilial violence with reports to the authorities of children and wives also being abused.

Although uncommon, sexual abuse of the elderly does occur. Cases have been described in which a son who had previously been the caregiver of his mother was discovered sexually abusing his mother in a nursing home. In another case a male orderly in a nursing home, who was responsible for feeding a cognitively impaired female, was observed fondling the patient at feeding time.

RECOGNITION OF ABUSE

Abuse of the elderly can be a most difficult diagnosis to make. Such behavior is not only problematic to determine but it is also even more difficult to prove. There is a fine line between the normal deterioration of a patient and what can be a "bona fide" abuse situation. Physical signs of abuse, such as bruises, welts, and cigarette or rope burns caused by involuntary confinement, may be difficult to evaluate adequately because patients with Alzheimer's disease who have cognitive dysfunction are poor historians. Lacerations are more straightforward indications of abuse. Neglect can be subtle and more difficult to determine than gross physical abuse.

Many abused elders are at home, and the caregiver who has charge and custody can keep the elderly person's injuries from becoming apparent to outside individuals. In addition, the person may be denied medication or even basic medical care. Since the abused elderly may have physical disabilities, he or she may be kept as a prisoner and not allowed to have any contact with the outside world.

Gradually, but certainly, patients with Alzheimer's disease lose the capacity to perform any activity of daily living. The period of total disability and the need for total care may continue for years and, contrary to popular belief, most of these patients are not placed in nursing homes. As patients become more dependent, they are more likely to be abused in some manner.

ABUSER PROFILE

Estimates suggest that 40% of abusers of persons with Alzheimer's disease are spouses and 50% are children or grandchildren. Since this disease is such a devastating and prolonged illness, caregivers play an extensive role in the day-to-day care of these patients. In abusive situations the average length of time that the relationship has existed is approximately 9.5 years. Studies have shown that the least socially active individual in the family is usually given the responsibility of caregiving.

The family members who are responsible for the care of the patient may not realize the tremendous time, effort, financial burden, and exhausting activity involved in the responsibility that they have accepted. Early in the illness caregiving that seems to be simple may develop into a complex, time-consuming, and stressful situation. There is evidence that abusers of women and children frequently perceive themselves as being powerless. Being perpetrators of abuse gives them a feeling of power and assists them in compensating for their feelings of inadequacy. This situation also may be true for elder abuse and neglect because the adult child is aware that he or she is not fulfilling the expectations of society. Striking out or inflicting abuse may make the person feel powerful again. In their book, *The 36-Hour Day*, Mace and Rabins provide an excellent guide for families who struggle with the frustrations involved in caring for a family member with Alzheimer's disease and related dementia illnesses.

Many times abusers are family members who have a fixed income and may transfer the funds of the patient to their own personal account for expenditures. Diversion of funds to the caregiver may sometimes result in denial of life-saving medications for the patient. In some instances such diversion results in a situation in which there are no funds to purchase the basic necessities. Such circumstances have been known to result in the death of the patient.

Caregivers may find themselves not only caring for an elderly parent but also having the continuing responsibility of rearing and nurturing their own children. The many demands made on their time and finances can bring great stress and exhaustion. Often there is only one parent in the family, due to divorce or death of the spouse, who becomes not only the breadwinner but also the caregiver of several individuals in the family. The average woman can expect to spend at least 17 years of her life in nurturing and caring for her children and an equal number of years caring for her parents and/or the parents of her spouse. Today men comprise about 30% of the caregivers. This figure is gradually increasing. Women remain the caregivers of approximately 70% of elder parents.

As the need for assistance with activities in daily living increases, so does the danger for abuse and neglect. Caregivers may be experiencing other problems in the family, such as an unwanted pregnancy, drug abuse, or another stressful situation that adds to the likelihood that they will become over stressed and strike out at the dependent parent. Role reversal can cause considerable difficulty in a relationship since the parent may not wish to give up the authoritarian role. The dependent child may find this conflict stressful and experience difficulty in accepting his or her role as the decision maker in the family. In such situations the relationships between parent and caregiver/child may have never been satisfactorily defined. The children may take on the responsibility of caregiving because of guilt, or they may be fearful that they will be harshly judged by family or acquaintances if they do not assume this role.

It is important to emphasize that some of the abuse may be involuntary and result from the caregiver not using existing services in the community and not caring for themselves in a way that is needed to effectively care for others. This can be especially true of family members, especially if personal support systems are lacking. These issues are discussed further in Chapter 23.

VICTIM PROFILE

The overwhelming majority of victims of elder abuse are women. The typical abused patient is a white widowed female over age 75, who is financially, physically, or mentally unable to live alone. She is more dependent on the caregiver for assistance with activities of daily living than her nonabused counterpart.

DIAGNOSIS OF ABUSE

Abused patients are likely to have special problems, such as incontinence, nocturnal shouting, wandering, or symptoms of paranoid delusions. Some of the traits generally thought to be prevalent among elders, such as stubbornness, hypercritical attitudes, and somatization, which may represent attempts by the patient to deal with his or her new dependency role, are also irritating to caregivers.

Abused patients have considerable difficulty accepting the fact that someone they have reared and nurtured is now abusing them. In addition, many barriers exist that prevent elderly citizens from asking for help. These victims may fear retaliation from the abuser. They also may feel shame, guilt, and failure and may blame themselves for the abuse. Since they feel guilt and embarrassment in admitting to society that this abuse is occurring, they may choose to suffer in silence. Many times patients stay in an abusive situation because they are fearful of the unknown. If institutionalized, they fear that they will be alone and are uncertain about the care they might receive. In other situations persons have grown up in an abusive environment and consider abuse to be a normal behavior.

With elder abuse being subtle and difficult to diagnose, it is made more problematic because many physicians do not take the time necessary to collect a detailed medical history. Although data obtained from the nurse's history may indicate possible abuse, the attending physician may choose to ignore or explain away the nurse's assessment by indicating that such injuries were most likely caused by an accident. Evaluating and diagnosing abuse can be a time-consuming and delicate process that requires a great deal of detective work. Nurses as well as physicians are professionals bound to report suspected abuse for investigation by the proper authorities. If a health care team member feels that abuse is likely, it is recommended that the individual be firm and kind but professionally persistent in communication.

Rarely will the elderly patient be able to assist in the diagnosis of abuse. Patients with cognitive dysfunction or short-term memory loss cannot give an adequate history and may suffer from fear or emotional blocking. If abuse is suspected, the health care professional may find it necessary to initiate legal actions that are contrary to the wishes of the patient and family. The professional must be prepared to deal with abuser hostility, threats, or harassment. At times, even the patient may manifest such behavior.

In evaluation of suspected abuse, it is important to assess the patient for social and/or environmental isolation. For example, is the patient not allowed to have outside contact through visits to family and friends or even telephone calls? Such control by an abuser can be successful in keeping family, friends, and other contacts out of the home, ensuring continued isolation of the patient and very little likelihood that the abuse will be detected.

It is also important to assess the interaction between the patient and the caregiver. The caregiver's behavior can be evaluated by obtaining answers to two main questions: Is the caregiver overprotective or unwilling to leave the patient unattended with medical, paramedical, or nursing staff? Does the caregiver try to "shadow" the patient closely at all times to prevent appropriate questioning?

In addition to assessing the caregiver's behavior, it is important to note the patient's behavior, especially in front of the caregiver. The patient may appear to be nervous, fearful, apprehensive, or depressed. He may cringe, back off, or dodge as if expecting to be hit. The nonverbal communication between patient and caregiver also should be observed closely. If the caregiver manifests a disinterested attitude toward the patient by not obtaining medications or not securing adequate care at appropriate time intervals, this attitude may also be an indication that the patient is being abused.

PHYSICAL INDICATORS OF ABUSE

Injuries that have not been treated appropriately and fractures that have not been set as necessary should arouse suspicion. Pallor, sunken eyes and cheeks, dry lips, excessive weight loss, and extreme dehydration may be indicators of abuse or neglect. All these factors must be closely monitored to achieve the appropriate index of suspicion that the patient is failing to receive the care that is necessary. Many times it is necessary for the health care provider to see the patient on repeated occasions in order to establish a rapport. This approach reassures the patient that the provider is compassionate and caring and is willing to serve as an advocate without betraying confidentiality.

> Physical indicators that are particularly important to evaluate include bruises on the face, shoulders, or arms; burns from cigarettes or rope; lacerations; human bites; and fractures that have been left untreated.

Bruises may be noted in different stages of the healing process. Welts may be observed, often inflicted by the use of belts or other objects used for corporal punishment. Rope burns, which are commonly found around the wrist or ankles, can arise from the use of crude restraints.

The provider should employ a calm, unhurried, persistent, empathic approach that is balanced with skepticism of stories told by the family when investigating suspected abuse. Interviewers who have problems with confrontation and tend to believe everything that they are told should not be the investigators of cases of suspected elder abuse.

Severe head injuries have occasionally been inflicted by the caregiver, but unless an appropriate history is obtained, this type of injury can be easily explained as an accident. Emergency technicians and ambulance drivers are an asset in providing valuable information for evaluating the circumstances of injuries, as noted when they arrive at the scene. Repeated trips to the physician's office or emergency room should create suspicion of abuse, particularly if there is a pattern of going to a different physician on each occasion.

Food and fluid deprivation that result in malnutrition and dehydration are more subtle forms of elder abuse. There is a fine line between expected deterioration of the patient and failure to feed the person appropriately, either at home or in a nursing home. Therefore, before either condition is attributed to abuse, the patient must be adequately evaluated since many disease states can be responsible for malnutrition and dehydration.

GERIATRIC ABUSE INTERVENTION TEAM: A METHOD FOR INTERVENTION

The geriatric abuse intervention team (G.A.I.T.) team was organized in 1980 in a family practice setting. It consisted of members from the community with interest, skills, and dedication to the service of the abused elderly. The original team consisted of a medical educator, a family practice resident, a medical student, a social services student, two nurse clinicians, a pharmacist, a social service director of the local department of human services, a psychologist, and a family practice physician who served as both member and coordinator.

The assessment process of G.A.I.T. was very effective, providing evaluations that proved to be accurate in diagnosis. The primary focus of the team was the needs of the patients. No problems arose to elicit intraprofessional conflict that could have defeated the purpose of G.A.I.T. Professional services of the team members included accompanying the client to court, when necessary, in order to serve as a witness.

The composition of G.A.I.T. has changed over time since various team members have completed their training, changed employment status, or relocated to other communities. Three members of the original team are still active in the G.A.I.T. organization. However, the team is now under the control of the local and state adult protective services. It currently serves in a consultation role for an 11-county area and becomes involved only in those cases in which there is no apparent solution for the resolution of adult protective cases.

Although all cases of abuse and neglect may not be resolved, the overwhelming majority of them can be stopped or reduced to livable circumstances. Every geographical area has enough caring, motivated, and knowledgeable persons to form an effective team that will care for the abused and neglected individuals. A community team such as G.A.I.T. can be effective in investigating and solving cases of abuse and neglect.

The case examples presented in this chapter are illustrations of abuse or potential abuse. These case histories, which are composites of patients and families, are intended to reinforce the significance of elder abuse as a social problem and to dispel the myths associated with it.

● Case Study—Physical Neglect

A 93-year-old woman was brought to the emergency room in the early evening hours. She was suffering from severe dehydration; had multiple decubitus ulcers on her hips, shoulders, and heels; and was in a comatose state. Bruises were also noted on both breasts. Her son, who had her brought to the hospital, identified himself as the primary caregiver but admitted that he was gone a lot of the time since he worked. When asked why he had neglected to obtain medical care for his mother for so long, he stated "She never complained. I never noticed anything wrong until my own son said, 'Dad, Grandma smells bad and looks really sick.'"

G.A.I.T. was never able to determine whether any of the injuries had been inflicted by this patient's caregivers. However, this case was one of the most severe examples of neglect that the abuse team had ever seen. After consultation between the police officers and the team, it was concluded that G.A.I.T. could not prove beyond reasonable doubt that intentional abuse had occurred. No criminal charges were filed.

● Case Study—Unintentional Medical Neglect

Mr. J. was a 67-year-old man who was admitted to the nursing home because he could no longer care for himself and had no available person who could assume responsibility for his care. The patient came to the attention of the nurse practitioner and physician team while they were making routine visits in the nursing home. Mr. J. was noticed because of the loud noises that he was making. On investigation, it was discovered that he was restrained but persisted in asking to go to the bathroom. The nursing home staff reported that the patient was suffering from agitation and had been given antipsychotic medication for sedation. It was soon discovered that his bladder was distended to a severe degree because of a nonfunctional indwelling catheter. When the bladder was drained, the patient became calm.

● Case Study—Financial Abuse

A 65-year-old widower who lived alone was seen in the dementia assessment unit after referral by an interested neighbor. The patient was determined to be suffering from early dementia, but much of his conversation made perfect sense. He repeatedly said, "My kids are ripping me off. I don't know how, but I can sense it." When the unit social worker visited his house, she discovered that the man had written several checks for groceries in the past month, some amounting to $200, but there was no food in the house. It was learned that since the man could no longer drive a car, his son and daughter-in-law did all the shopping for him. However, they gave him only a fraction of the groceries that he was paying for and used the rest themselves.

SUMMARY

Elder abuse is not uncommon and may be perpetrated, sometimes unintentionally, by people who would not be suspected of such behavior toward their own loved ones. Often the circumstances that lead to abuse evolve insidiously and imperceptibly. As the relationship between the patient and the caregiver gradually deteriorates, a breaking point may be reached and abuse occurs. Health care professionals must know the signs of abuse and intervene to protect the patient.

If the potential for abuse is to be minimized, the caregiver must be supported in his or her role. The burden of caring for patients with Alzheimer's disease should not be confined to a single caregiver. It should be shared with other family members and with society as a whole.

BIBLIOGRAPHY

American Medical Association: *Elder abuse and neglect: diagnostic and treatment guidelines,* Chicago, 1992, The Association.

Benbow SM, Haddad PM: Sexual abuse of the elderly mentally ill, *Postgrad Med J* 69 (816):803-807, 1993.

Bosker G: Elder abuse: patterns, detection, and management, *Res Staff Phys* 36(3):39-44, 1990.

Bourland M: Elder abuse from definition to prevention, *Postgrad Med* 87(2):139-144, 1990.

Clark-Daniels C, Daniels RS, Baumhover L: The dilemma of elder abuse, *Home Healthc Nurse* 8(6):7-12, 1990.

Conlin MM: Silent suffering: a case of elder abuse and neglect, *J Am Geriatr Soc* 43(11):1303-1308, 1995.

Cooney C, Mortimer A: Elder abuse and dementia, a pilot study, *Int J Soc Psychiatry* 41(4):276-283, 1995.

Council on Scientific Affairs. American Medical Association white paper on elderly health, *Arch Intern Med* 150:2459-2469, 1990.

Coyne AC, Reichman WE, Berbig LJ: The relationship between dementia and elder abuse, *Am J Psychiatry* 150(4):643-646, 1993.

Forte D: Elder abuse: myth or reality? *Nurs Eld* 12(2):14-15, 1990.

Fulmer T, Wetle T: Elder abuse screening and intervention, *Nurse Pract* 11(5):33-38, 1986.

Grafstrom M, Nordberg A, Hagberg B: Relationships between demented elderly people and their families: a follow-up study of caregivers who had previously reported abuse when caring for their spouses and parents, *J Adv Nurse* 18(11):1747-1757, 1993.

Grafstrom M, Nordberg A, Winblad: Abuse is in the eye of the beholder. Report by family members about abuse of demented persons in home care. A total population-based study, *Scand J Soc Med* 21(4):247-255, 1993.

Jogerst G: Diagnosing and managing elder abuse, *Iowa Med* 86(1):29-31, 1996.

Kurrle SE, Sadler PM, Cameron ID: Patterns of elder abuse, *Med J Aust* 157(10):673-676, 1992.

Lachs MS, Pillemer K: Abuse and neglect of elderly persons, *N Engl J Med* 332(7):437-443, 1995.

Mace N, Rabins PV: *The 36-hour day. A family guide to caring for persons with Alzheimer's disease, related dementing illnesses, and memory loss in later life,* Mass Market Paperback, 1994, Warner Books.

Mendonca JD, Velamoor VR, Sauve D: Key features of maltreatment of the infirm elderly in home settings, *Can J Psychiatry* 41(2):107-113, 1996.

Paris BE, Meier DE, Goldstein T et al: Elder abuse and neglect: how to recognize warning signs and intervene, *Geriatrics* 50(4):47-53, 1995.

Pillemer K, Suitor JJ: Violence and violent feelings: what causes them among family caregivers? *J Gerontol* 47(4):S165-172 1992.

Quinn MJ, Tomita SK: *Elder abuse and neglect,* New York, 1986, Springer Publishing.

Ross M, Ross PA, Ross-Carson M: Abuse of the elderly, *Can Nurse* 81(2):36-39, 1985.

Rounds L: Elder abuse and neglect: a relationship to health characteristics, *J Am Acad Nurse Pract* 4(2):47-52, 1992.

US House of Representatives Select Committee on Aging: Elder abuse: an examination of a hidden problem, 97th Congress, Committee Pub No 97-277, Washington, DC, 1981, US Government Printing Office.

Unit Five

Example is not the main thing in influencing others, it is the only thing.

—Albert Schweitzer

Community Support

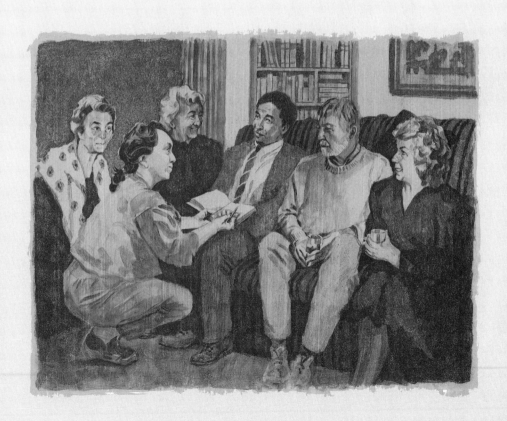

Caregiver Education and Support

Mary M Lancaster

We are all strong enough to bear the misfortunes of others.

—Duc de la Rochefoucauld

Although a cure for Alzheimer's disease is not yet known, there is an abundance of management information for the disease that caregivers need to carry out their role. Each member of the health care team must take it upon himself or herself to become involved in the educational process and to lend knowledge, expertise, and support to caregivers.

Education of caregivers is the foundation for successful day-to-day management of Alzheimer's disease. Armed with the necessary information, caregivers will possess the sense of support and competence needed to continue in their caregiving role. This information and support is vital regardless of whether the caregivers are family members or health care personnel. In fact, the basic educational needs of both family and professional caregivers are very similar. The overall objectives of caregiver education can be generalized into three main categories, as shown on p. 342.

INFORMAL VERSUS FORMAL TEACHING

Informal Teaching

Education can be carried out both formally and informally. Meetings with health care professionals are good mechanisms for informal teaching. These meetings offer a good way to identify the specific behavior that is most troublesome, how the caregivers explain the behavior, what solutions have been tried, and the effectiveness of their solutions. Family meetings are also an opportune time to discuss more sensitive issues such as legal and financial matters, wills, burial

---

—● Educational Objectives for Caregivers

1. To provide information on the disease itself
2. To teach the fundamentals of day-to-day care and management
3. To offer information on relevant community resources

---

arrangements, and advanced directives. These matters must be discussed, and the assistance of the health care team makes the discussion easier.

Informal education also can be carried out at the bedside, in the home, over the telephone, or walking down the street. Role modeling is an excellent way to provide informal education for both family and professional caregivers. Having a professional caregiver and a family caregiver work side by side, a visiting nurse in the home or a family member in a hospital or nursing home, affords each the opportunity to learn from the other.

Education is a two-way process. For instance, the family caregivers may be able to provide information about the best way to gain the patient's cooperation, and the professional caregiver can teach the family how to incorporate range-of-motion exercises into daily activities. Usually, the family caregiver has taken care of the patient at home for quite some time and is very knowledgeable about the idiosyncrasies of the patient.

—● Professional caregivers must be accepting of the family's knowledge and experience and apply this information to care planning.

Frequently family caregivers have already discovered a solution to a problem that may be perplexing to the staff, and vice versa. Both family and professional caregivers should be encouraged to contribute to the patient's plan of care.

Formal Teaching

Formal teaching can take place in support group meetings, seminars, training classes, and in-service programs. Many of the same topics are covered in formal classes; however, these classes do not generally allow as much hands-on demonstration, feedback, and interaction as does informal teaching. Formal teaching is helpful for health care professionals and family caregivers alike. A critical area is continuous education about aging in general and other problems or diseases that the patient might have. Caregivers will need instruction about how to assess the patient for acute problems such as infections, pain, constipation, or fractures. They must be taught that the cognitively impaired person may not be able to relate signs and symptoms of acute conditions and that continuing physical assessment of the patient is vital.

Caregivers in long-term care facilities have special needs for education. Federal and state regulations require approximately 75 hours of training for Certified Nursing Assistants, which must include information on aging and working with the cognitively impaired patient. In addition, staff assigned to Special Dementia Units must also meet requirements for annual continuing education and training on dementia and working with the patient with dementia.

Written Materials

Education can be accomplished through verbal interaction, that is, by sitting and talking. However, verbal information must be supplemented and reinforced with written information. Numerous pamphlets, videos, and books are available through the local Alzheimer's Association, support groups, the Alzheimer's Disease Education and Referral (ADEAR) Centers, doctor's offices, and university-based Gerontology Centers. These resources are another vehicle for presenting necessary material, and they provide hands-on information that caregivers can refer to at later times.

Written or videotaped materials serve as a reminder of the information that was presented verbally and can be used as a step-by-step guide. Written information can be individualized to meet the patient's and caregivers' needs by adding specific instructions and information in the margins of the pamphlets and books. Research has shown that much of the initial information caregivers receive from the physician or nurse is lost because the individual is overwhelmed and confused by the diagnosis and because attention is not focused on learning. Pamphlets, videos, and books allow the caregivers and other family members to review the information at home when they are more attentive and can absorb the information at their own rate.

Education of caregivers goes beyond learning about the day-to-day management of the patient and the disease. It must also involve education about what can happen to the caregivers and other family members and the impact of caregiving on family roles.

> Caregivers are often very interested in possible cures and treatments, and therefore are susceptible to media coverage of "breakthroughs" and "cures."

Caregivers need to recognize that the media frequently sensationalize this type of information. Caregivers must be informed that some people will take advantage of their desperate situation.

It is vital to encourage caregivers to investigate any advertisements carefully and to discuss them with the patient's physician. They should be made aware of the side effects that can result from experimental treatments and the quality-of-life issues involved in the treatments. Caregivers need to know that it takes many years for research to be completed on a new drug and for that drug to be approved by the Food and Drug Administration and then made available to the public. However, there are legitimate research programs in progress throughout the country, and frequently subjects are needed for these studies. Caregivers and patients should have the option of becoming involved in such studies if they meet the criteria. Involvement in these programs offers the caregivers a sense of doing something to help patients and others who may be afflicted with Alzheimer's disease in the future.

> ─● **Caregiver Baseline Assessment:**
> * Current emotional state
> * Current physical state
> * Sources of stress
> * Educational level
> * Current knowledge of disease
> * Misconceptions
> * Readiness to learn

BASELINE INFORMATION

To address the educational needs of the caregivers appropriately, baseline information about the caregivers and the caregiving environment must be obtained. This process begins with an assessment of the caregivers' current emotional state. If the caregiver is in emotional crisis, the situation must be resolved or diffused before learning can take place. Caregivers who are still in denial must first be assisted in accepting the diagnosis. Other sources of stress impinging on the caregiver (e.g., unresolved financial or legal matters) also must be handled. In addition, caregivers should be assessed for their ability to adapt to ever-changing needs and demands. If the caregivers are unable to adapt their daily lives to meet changing roles and demands, they may be unable to use the information provided or to apply it to their own situation.

Caregivers must be able to understand the information they are given. Asking the caregivers what they know about the disease is a useful tool for determining the educational level of the caregivers. It is also an excellent opportunity to find out what misinformation and misconceptions they may have about the disease and its management. Many of the problems and crises that caregivers experience evolve from misinformation or lack of information. Finally, it is important to find out if the caregivers are ready and willing to learn.

Once the baseline assessment has been completed, caregivers must be involved in developing a support and education plan. Although many are overwhelmed and confused when first involved in the learning process, their investment in developing the learning plan helps to set realistic goals for themselves and the patient. The gathering of the baseline assessment and the development of the plan will be educational in themselves for the caregivers. In general, caregivers need to understand the disease, and know how to cope with daily management and where to find support in the community in which they live.

INFORMATION ON ALZHEIMER'S DISEASE

Initially, caregivers should be taught about the disease, its course and symptoms, and the available treatment options. Since Alzheimer's disease has several stages, educational efforts should concentrate on the symptoms, problems, and behaviors associated with the various stages. Other topics that will need to be addressed include information about the aging process, common problems resulting from the emotional stress of caregiving, and general information about the progression of the disease. All this information should be provided slowly, over an extended time period, since research has shown that most people can absorb only small amounts of information at any one time.

Much of what is known about the treatment and management of Alzheimer's disease is the result of trial and error. No one has all the answers to Alzheimer's disease. Educators must admit to themselves and to the caregivers that because of the nature of the disease, the solutions and management strategies offered are not going to work in every situation. There will be times when the phrase "I do not know but will try to find out" may be the best response. Getting back to the caregiver with an answer is particularly important for maintaining a good, ongoing relationship with him or her, one that is centered on trust and honesty.

A continuing relationship with a health care professional offers caregivers a real sense of support and security. They need to feel that there is someone they can turn to with their questions and problems. In general, caregivers need a piece of information or an answer to their question quickly; waiting until the next appointment with the physician may be too late. Caregivers should be encouraged to keep a notebook on hand for jotting down questions, incidents, and problems. This notebook can then be reviewed with a health care professional or at a support group.

Anticipatory Guidance

Anticipatory education, or information before the events occur, is vital. It may help to alleviate unnecessary emotional conflict and strain if caregivers have an idea of what the future may hold. Caregivers generally function on a fairly even plateau, and since patients with Alzheimer's disease tend to deteriorate slowly, the caregivers usually have time to adapt to the changes. However, as the disease progresses, each additional impairment that the patient develops adds to the overall strain on the caregivers. This situation can continue until at some point even a very minor additional stress (e.g., the patient loses the car keys) makes the situation intolerable and leads to a crisis. Through anticipatory guidance and education, the caregivers can be assisted to delay or possibly avoid this type of spiraling crisis.

When the patient has new problems or difficulties or when his condition is changing, providing the caregivers with information on what behaviors may lie ahead and providing them with management strategies can help allay their fears, frustrations, and anxieties. Caregivers must learn to react to the catastrophic and emotional overreactions of the patient and themselves by remaining calm and separating the patient from the upsetting situation. Having strategies for dealing with problems in advance will help to achieve the desired response from the patient and the caregivers when a difficulty arises.

Education on behavior management of the patient is probably one of the most important and most difficult tasks because behaviors vary so greatly among patients. Well-meaning caregivers sometimes evoke a severe reaction from the patient through lack of information on how to deal with certain behaviors (see case study that follows). The reader is referred to Chapter 12 for an in-depth discussion on managing problem behaviors.

● Case Study—Reaction Cause by Caregiver

The crisis

Mrs. M. was diagnosed as suffering from Alzheimer's disease 4 years ago. She is currently living with her daughter and son-in-law. One Sunday morning Mrs. M.'s daughter instructed her mother to get dressed for church. Mrs. M. had always been able to manage dressing herself. Yet 15 minutes before they were to leave, the daughter found Mrs. M. crying in her room. She said that she did not want to go to church. The daughter, feeling rushed, insisted that her mother get dressed and go with the family. The daughter hurriedly tossed three of Mrs. M.'s favorite dresses on the bed and told her mother to hurry. Moments later Mrs. M. began screaming and tearing at her clothes. The daughter, angry at her mother for being so slow and childish, took one of the dresses and began to help her mother get dressed. Mrs. M. immediately began to fight with her daughter.

The explanation

Mrs. M. was suddenly faced with her inability to dress herself. If her daughter had been prepared for this event, both mother and daughter might have reacted differently. Instead of rushing her mother, who was already distressed, the daughter could have simply asked her mother what was wrong and if she needed help. In addition, by forcing a choice on her mother (which dress to wear), the daughter added to the stress. The whole situation may have stemmed from Mrs. M.'s inability to decide what to wear. To avoid the confrontation that eventually occurred, it probably would have been most effective to redirect Mrs. M.'s attention to some other task, such as applying makeup or fixing her hair. Once her mother had calmed down, the daughter would have been able to help her get dressed.

Preparing Caregivers for Emotional Reactions

Caregivers also need to know that they are human, with feelings and emotions like everyone else. They need to know that, despite their best efforts, they may occasionally react to situations based on their emotions rather than brains. They need to know that this is a natural reaction to stress, so that their guilt feelings about how they reacted can be minimized. Through anticipatory education and helping caregivers to analyze their interactions with the patient, they can be assisted to see that their behaviors may be contributing to the patient's troublesome behaviors. Discussion of some of the reactions of caregivers that may be detrimental to patients and to themselves follow, along with strategies that can be used to educate caregivers.

PREVENTION OF EXCESS DISABILITY

Well-intentioned caregivers can effectively block the patient's competence and capabilities by expecting too little (or too much) from him. Caregivers inadvertently cast the patient in a role of being unable or disabled to perform. The expectation of the patient to participate in activities of daily living are replaced with an expectation "to do for" the patient. The end result is that patients do not do as much for themselves as they are really capable of doing. This negative effect can be seen not only in patients with dementia, but also in patients who have had a stroke or who suffer from other chronic disabling conditions. This is commonly referred to as "creating excess disability."

> Being overly helpful can promote apathy, dependence, and deterioration in the patient.

If this practice of doing everything for the patient continues over an extended time period, the patient's abilities quickly diminish. Caregivers may need guidance about ways to allow the patient maximum self-sufficiency while offering just enough assistance to compensate for her real limitations. A delicate balance between doing too much for the patient and doing too little must be achieved. The overall goal is to consistently allow the patient to do as much for herself for as long as possible, even if the way things are done needs to be adapted.

Caregivers should allow the patient to be involved in decision making and performing to her maximum capacity. Supporting lost abilities while challenging and using remaining abilities allows the patient to continue to be involved in her own self-care. This in turn helps to maintain the patient's sense of self-esteem and pride.

Case Study—Supporting Remaining Capabilities

Mr. K. is a certified nursing assistant on an Alzheimer's unit. Today he is caring for Mrs. S., a 78-year-old patient with Alzheimer's disease. After reminding Mrs. S. several times to brush her teeth, Mr. K. finds Mrs. S. wandering in the hallway. Mr. K. takes Mrs. S. to her bathroom and again instructs her to brush her teeth. Thirty minutes later, he finds her still in the bathroom, teeth unbrushed. Since it is nearing visiting hours, Mr. K. goes ahead and brushes Mrs. S.' teeth for her. The same scenario occurs the next week.

At a team meeting the following week, it is reported that Mrs. S. can no longer perform her own oral care. The nurse specialist inquires about what measures were used to assist Mrs. S. in performing her own oral care. Finding that no plan of action had been implemented to enhance Mrs. S.' ability to provide oral care for herself, the nurse specialist suggested the following plan of action:

1. Take Mrs. S. to the bathroom each morning.
2. Obtain a wide grip toothbrush.
3. Lay out the needed equipment on the sink.
4. Stand by and provide verbal instruction in a step-by-step manner (open toothpaste, put paste on brush, etc.).
5. Remain with the patient and provide verbal/visual guidance as needed.

When the plan was implemented the following day, it was found that Mrs. S. only needed help in gathering the equipment together and a few verbal cues to get started.

OVER INVOLVEMENT

Over involvement in the care of the patient commonly occurs with caregivers who are trying to compensate for the patient's disabilities and losses. When involvement with the patient is carried to an exaggerated extent, the caregivers may sacrifice many aspects of their own personal health and welfare. In such situations, the caregivers become the "second victims" of Alzheimer's disease.

Over involvement can lead to the emotional and physical breakdown of the caregiver. Educating caregivers about this tragedy and explaining that they must take care of themselves is of utmost importance. Becoming emotionally and physically drained can actually hinder caregiving and interaction with the patient and others. Offering the caregivers stress management strategies provides them with tools they can use to keep themselves well balanced (see Chapter 23).

ROLE REVERSAL

Role reversal and changes in role functions are likely to occur with Alzheimer's disease. Caregivers should understand that they may need to assume some of the roles of the person who has the disease. Assuming the patient's roles and place within a family can be very difficult and emotionally charged. Some caregivers may need to learn how to manage the day-to-day business of cooking, cleaning, doing laundry, and running a household. Others may need to be educated on legal and financial business, taking care of the car, or finding a job. Through education, caregivers can be helped through these changes and instructed in ways to lessen the impact of these changes on themselves, the patient, and others.

DAY-TO-DAY MANAGEMENT

Caregivers need to know how to maneuver through the increasing personal care demands posed by a loved one or professional charge as Alzheimer's disease progresses. Knowledge of hygienic care, dressing, nutrition, maintenance of bowel function, and many other details can "make or break" the caregiver's self-esteem and ability to deal with the stressors of caregiving. Tips and techniques for preventing catastrophic reactions to simple daily care are invaluable to the caregiver and the patient. Much knowledge has been gathered through experience in the area of daily care. Detailed descriptions of strategies to aid the caregiver and the patient are found in Chapter 23.

INFORMATION ON RELEVANT COMMUNITY RESOURCES

Support Groups

Education and support should not be separated. They are currently the backbone of patient and caregiver management. Caregivers need the support of others to be able to assimilate the information they have received and put it into practice. Research has demonstrated that providing information alone, without meeting the support needs of caregivers, is not nearly as successful as a combined approach. A study conducted at Duke University in the early 1980s demonstrated that the mere *feeling* of being supported had a greater impact on reducing caregiver strain than the amount of actual outside help the caregiver received.

Support groups have a long history of providing mutual aid to their members through the sharing of common experiences and problems.

Members of support groups develop ties with one another based on the commonality of their emotions and experiences.

If caregivers can openly discuss their problems and share their emotions in support groups, the physical and mental stress of providing care can be eased. Knowing that there are others in the world in similar situations provides a sense of being "able to make it."

Most support groups develop from the caregivers' needs to receive information and emotional assistance. Because no one person possesses all the knowledge or answers to Alzheimer's disease, the support group serves as an open educational forum for both professional and family caregivers. The informal format of most support groups allows everyone to learn from one another. For example, I have gained a great deal of knowledge about caring for victims of Alzheimer's disease and the associated stresses on caregivers from leading a support group for 10 years. Support groups provide the time needed for relaxed discussion and problem solving.

The members of a support group have varying roles within their community and families. They may be spouses, adult children, grandchildren, health care personnel, and friends of persons with Alzheimer's disease. However, the common interest and caregiving experience place the group members on a similar level. A technical aspect to be considered in developing or participating in a support group is the caregiver-patient relationship. The varying relationships give rise to different needs, viewpoints, and emotions on the part of the caregivers and the patient. Separate groups may be necessary to adequately meet the needs of the various members. Having separate support groups can help avoid a potentially disturbing situation, such as having the spouse and the adult child of a patient attend the same meeting.

In this situation the freedom to express true feelings and emotions may be hindered by the presence of the other family member. In one of the support groups I was involved in, the daughter of a patient was attending the same group as her father (the mother was the person with Alzheimer's disease.) One day the daughter came to me to express her concern about attending the group. She felt unable to discuss her real feelings and emotions openly and honestly within the group because they differed from those of her father. Since her father was the primary caregiver, she felt that she had to let him do what he considered best. After a lengthy discussion, she decided that she would attend another support group for herself and also attend the one with her father in order to keep the lines of communication open with him.

Health care personnel who work with Alzheimer's patients often become involved in support groups. These persons can provide informational and administrative support to the group. They can lend their expertise and knowledge of various fields at the meetings. Some health care personnel attend groups to share their own frustrations and problems in providing care to Alzheimer's patients in the institutional setting. These health care workers face many of the same problems that family caregivers do. Other health care personnel may attend in order to better understand the problems full-time caregivers face and how they can assist those caregivers. It must be remembered that regardless of education and experience in caring for patients with Alzheimer's disease no one "knows it all" or is immune to the stresses and strains of caregiving.

Benefits of Group Involvement

Participants of support groups work through various stages of involvement in the group. Initially, the interactions may be superficial and may center around telling one's own story. Most often, new members attend a group session because they are in need of an immediate solution to a problem or some information.

> **—• Positive outcomes of support groups:**
> - Enhanced education of group members
> - Respite—time away
> - Stress management
> - Enhanced socialization and decreased isolation
> - Ability to work through emotions
> - Problem solving

However, after attending the meetings several times, they begin to develop a basic trust and understanding with the group. As this process takes place, the members grow and mature, and begin to recognize and discuss their personal feelings, emotions, and needs.

> **—•** Eventually, this type of discussion enables the members to assist one another in identifying and resolving problems and conflicts.

This is the ultimate goal of a support group. While receiving support and guidance from one another, the members are also lending support and guidance to others.

Support groups provide caregivers a time to bring before the group a new problem that they have encountered. Frequently someone in the group has experienced the same situation and suggests a solution. Support groups also offer a time for socialization for the caregivers. Isolated by the necessity to be with the patient 24 hours a day, caregivers rarely have an opportunity to visit with other people. In addition, if the patient is in an advanced stage of the disease, his ability to carry on a real conversation has been lost. Therefore the caregivers may have little opportunity to make conversation. I frequently hear caregivers say, "I went so stir crazy that I was talking to pictures, the walls, anything that would stay still and listen. If it had not been for this group, I don't know if I could have held out much longer." The support group offers a time to meet new people, to develop friendships, and to get away. In addition, having the meeting revolve around the care of the patient can help ease the guilt caregivers may feel about having taken time for themselves.

Negative Aspects of Support Groups

Although support groups have been shown to increase the caregiver's sense of support and knowledge about Alzheimer's disease and community resources, there are potential dangers associated with support groups. Of primary concern is that some support groups may begin to view themselves as a replacement or substitution for professional psychotherapy.

> **—•** Lay support groups cannot provide professional counseling or psycho-therapy.

However, through a caregiver's interactions and participation in a group, individuals who are experiencing a great amount of stress or difficulty in coping can be identified and referred for professional help.

A second potential danger is one of dependency, either on the group itself or on the leader of the group. In the event that the group disbands, caregivers who have become totally dependent on the group for information, social interaction, and support may find themselves at a great loss. This sort of dependency also can focus on the group's leader. Because of their high visibility in the group, their interest in combating Alzheimer's disease, and their knowledge of the disease, leaders are primary targets to take on the responsibility of the other group members.

Many group leaders have said that a great deal of their time and energy are expended on the problems and needs of the group members. This situation can be especially dangerous if the leader is also a caregiver, one whose time and energy are already stressed to the maximum. This additional responsibility can lead to burnout for the leader, which leaves the group members stranded. Through careful guidance, group members can be helped to find additional sources of support outside the group.

Sometimes group members become so familiar with the behavior, problems, and symptoms of the disease that they tend to forget the individual nature of the disease and start "packaging" information and solutions. Yet this type of packaged information may not apply to another person's situation. Along with this familiarity comes the potential for diagnosing friends and relatives, and recommending treatment plans without the proper medical evaluation, diagnostic workup, and advice.

When a group has been meeting for a long time, a great deal of freedom, trust, and understanding develop among the group members. They can talk openly about their problems and what may be ahead for them. They are able to discuss life-and-death issues, funeral plans, and autopsy. This openness is one of the goals of the group, but it must be kept in mind that newcomers may be present at any meeting.

New members of the group, especially if the patient has been recently diagnosed, become easily frightened and upset when they hear about the problems that caregivers and patients face in the last stages of the disease.

They may become so overwhelmed with fear and distaste for the group that they never return. One solution is the development of a group for newcomers. If this approach is not reasonable, new group members can meet with an especially sensitive caregiver while the regular group members continue with their discussions. There is a delicate balance in trying to meet all the needs of caregivers who are experiencing various stages of the disease at the same time.

Group leaders need to have training in group dynamics and group processes. Situations arise that can be highly disruptive to the group. Some individuals talk so much that they monopolize the entire meeting, whereas others never get the opportunity to speak. The group leader will need to know how to draw a very shy, quiet individual into the conversation. Arguments can develop, and some members may appear particularly hostile or abusive. Involving group leaders in workshops on group process can help them feel more comfortable with their role and more assured in handling difficult situations. In addition, professional caregivers who are experienced in group process can be called on to assist in the meetings.

Developing, implementing, and leading support groups can be stressful and time consuming. Yet there is great satisfaction to be found in taking this responsibility. Support groups are for all the members. Involving caregivers in a useful and meaningful interaction with one another yields personal rewards for everyone.

● Case Study—The Importance of Group Leader Training

During one group meeting the topic of terminal care came up in the discussion. The caregivers present began to discuss such concerns as tube feeding, CPR, and artificial ventilation. As the discussion progressed, caregivers started expressing their own beliefs and feelings regarding what should occur at the end of life. One particular caregiver, Mr. A., gradually became louder and more defensive of his beliefs and his plans for his wife's care. Several professional caregivers attempted to confront Mr. A. with the futility of his desires for his wife's care. Forty-five minutes into the group meeting, Mr. A. got up and left. The new group leader followed Mr. A. into the hallway to find out why he had left.

If this new group leader had been through some training prior to assuming the role of group leader, the above scenario may have been avoided. The group leader most likely would have recognized the escalating emotional climate and been able to intervene. Understanding that the topics being discussed are ethical issues and without a "right" or "wrong," the group leader could have introduced this into the conversation, stating that the topics are emotionally laden and prefacing the growing tension with a statement that each person holds his/her own beliefs and whatever he/she believes is "right" for him/her. Finally, sensing Mr. A.'s frustration and growing uneasiness, the group leader could have stepped into the conversation and possibly prevented the confrontation that occurred.

SUMMARY

Persons adapt to and cope with situations based on their knowledge and experience. If the amount of stress and demands outweigh their competence (knowledge and experience), the person is likely to be unable to handle the situation. This inability to cope for a long time can result in the physical or psychosocial breakdown, or burnout, of the individual. However, if the person possesses the competence to handle the situation, his stability can be maintained and tragic results can be prevented.

Through education, experience, and support, caregivers can be provided with the competence needed to handle the various problems and situations that arise in their lives as caregivers. All members of the health care team (M.D., R.N., Social Worker, L.P.N., C.N.A., etc.) must work together to facilitate the exchange of information and support that professional and family caregivers require to continue their job as essential providers of care to Alzheimer's disease patients.

BIBLIOGRAPHY

Anderson KH et al: Patients with dementia: involving families to maximize nursing care, *J Gerontol Nurs* 18(7):19-25, 1992.

Buckwalter KC, Abraham IL, Neundorfer MM: Alzheimer's disease: involving nursing in the development and implementation of health care for patients and families, *Nurs Clin North Am* 23:1-9, 1988.

Davies HD: Dementia and delirium. In Chenitz WC, Stone JT, Salisbury SA, editors: *Clinical gerontological nursing: a guide to advanced practice*, Philadelphia, 1991, WB Saunders.

George LK: The burden of caregiving: how much? what kinds? for whom? *Adv Res* 8(2):2, 1984.

Given CW, Collins CE, Given BA: Sources of stress among families caring for relatives with Alzheimer's disease, *Nurs Clin North Am* 23:69-82, 1988.

Gwyther L: Caregiver self-help groups: roles for professionals, *Generations* 53:37-38, 1982.

Hayter J: Helping families of patients with Alzheimer's disease, *J Gerontol Nurs* 8(2):81-86, 1982.

Katzman R, Jackson JE: Alzheimer's disease: basics and clinical practice, *J Am Geriatr Soc* 39:516-525, 1991.

Kuhlman GJ et al: Alzheimer's disease and family caregiving: critical synthesis of the literature and research agenda, *Nurs Res* 40:331-335, 1991.

Lawton MP: Competence, environmental press, and the adaptation of old people. In Lawton MP, Windley PG, Byerts TO, editors: *Aging and the environment: theoretical approaches*, New York, 1980, Garland STPM Press.

Ory MG: Families, informal supports, and Alzheimer's disease: current research and future agendas, *Res Aging* 7:623-544, 1985.

Powell L, Courtice K: *Alzheimer's disease: a guide for families*, Reading, Mass, 1986, Addison-Wesley.

Ruppert RA: Caring for the lay caregiver, *Am J Nurs* 96(3):40-46, 1996.

Salisbury SA: Preventing excess disability. In Chenitz WC, Stone JT, Salisbury SA, editors: *Clinical gerontological nursing: a guide to advanced practice*, Philadelphia, 1991, WB Saunders

Sharpe PA, Koerber ME, Macera CA et al: Training former dementia caregivers to provide peer education and social support, *Am J Alzheimer's Disease* 11(4):16-24, 1996.

Shibal-Champagne S, Lipinska-Stachow DM: Alzheimer's educational/supportive group: considerations for success—awareness of family tasks, preplanning, and active professional facilitation, *J Gerontol Soc Work* 9(2):41-48, 1986.

Simank M, Strickland K: Assisting families in coping with Alzheimer's disease and other related dementias with the establishment of a mutual support group, *J Gerontol Soc Work* 9(2):49-58, 1985-1986.

Sommers T, Zarit S: Seriously near the breaking point, *Generations* 10:30-33, 1985.

Stolley JM, Buckwalter KC, Shannon MD: Caring for patients with Alzheimer's disease: recommendations for nursing education, *J Gerontol Nurs* 17(6):34-38, 1991.

Zarit S, Todd P, Zarit J: Subjective burden of husbands and wives as caregivers: a longitudinal study, *Gerontologist* 26:260-266, 1986.

Social Services

JoAnn Cox

We criticize and separate ourselves from the process. We've got to jump right in there with both feet.

—Dolores Huerta

Because Alzheimer's disease is a slow, insidious disease, caregivers often become so involved in caring for their patient that they forget to look to the social support systems provided by their community. As the patient with Alzheimer's disease gradually deteriorates, the demands on the caregivers gradually increase until the situation becomes unbearable. Often, caregivers are embarrassed to seek the help that may be available. They may have had no experience with social services and may equate them with "being on welfare." Also, they may resent having strangers enter their homes or may feel that by involving a public agency they are being disloyal to their loved one.

It is imperative for health care professionals to know about the social services and benefits available to the elderly. Much has been said about the "fragmented" systems that abound, and often when people do seek help, they are confused and overwhelmed about where to go. This situation is especially true for caregivers of the patient with Alzheimer's disease. This chapter will hopefully provide information about what services are available and how to access them.

AREA AGENCY ON AGING

One major resource that is readily available is the Area Agency on Aging (AAA). Money that is distributed by the federal agency, the Administration on Aging (AOA), and provided through Title III of the Older Americans Act is allocated to each state based on its number of residents 60 years of age or older. The state units on aging then distribute the funds to each AAA with the proviso that the money be used solely for the benefit of people 60 years of age or older, with emphasis on serving those in greatest social and economic need. There is no charge for programs offered under The Older Americans Act, although participants are encouraged to contribute to the program so that more people can be served.

▸ Each AAA is autonomous, but the same services for the homebound elderly are available in most communities.

These include home-delivered meals, a homemaker program, personal care and chore services, minor home repair, transportation, legal assistance, a long-term care ombudsman, respite care, adult day care, hospice, senior center services, such as telephone reassurance and friendly visiting.

The Title III program utilizes case managers to provide a thorough assessment in the individual's own home. This determines what services are necessary to enable that individual to remain in his or her own environment. A care plan is then developed and arrangements are made to have the services begin. Follow-up is done on a regular basis to assure the services are working and are still appropriate. The Title III case management program also provides information and referral services to assist older people in finding solutions to other problems.

The Area Agency on Aging is listed in the local telephone directory, and through the local senior citizen center. The toll-free number for senior services is 1-800-677-1116.

NUTRITION PROGRAMS

A few years after the Older Americans Act was passed in 1965, a nutrition program was started and has become the largest funded service delivered through the AAA network. Both congregate and home-delivered meals, which operate out of senior citizen centers and other community buildings, must provide one-third of the required daily dietary allowance for older people. The congregate meals enable the individuals to get out of the house and socialize with their peers. The home-delivered meals enable the frail, elderly individuals to live at home for as long as possible.

Programs vary from state to state, but most Title III nutrition programs provide meals five days per week, usually at noon. In metropolitan areas, breakfast, evening, and weekend meals may be available. Low-sodium menus are usually provided and in areas with large specific ethnic populations, menus reflect those tastes. Special diets are often available. Eligibility is the same for all Title III programs.

▸ No person is refused on the basis of ability to pay and most programs accept food stamps.

Many programs and nutrition sites also offer other services such as nutrition education, special diets, shopping assistance, food co-ops, and mobile food supplements.

The home-delivered service is called Meals on Wheels. It is another program authorized by the Older Americans Act that provides meals to persons 60 years of age and older who are homebound. Meals are delivered directly to the homebound frail elderly usually by volunteer workers. Having the meals delivered to the individual on a daily basis can also provide a way for someone to check on the elderly person and notify the necessary family or emergency personnel if something is amiss.

Information on all meal programs can be obtained by contacting the Area Agency on Aging or local senior citizen center.

RESPITE CARE, ADULT DAY CARE

A respite program provides family caregivers with intervals of relief from the demands of their caregiving. Respite care has been provided for many years through informal support systems—relatives, friends, and neighbors who are willing to come in and "sit" with the patient while the caregiver runs errands, goes to the doctor, or takes time for himself or herself. More formal types of respite care include services that can be provided in the patient's own home or in churches, community centers, private homes other than the patient's home, and even nursing homes.

Most respite centers provide personal care, some centers provide social and recreational activities, and a few programs are tailored to each patient's individual needs. Others have a 24-hour, on-call physician and 24-hour nursing care. Some respite care is covered by insurance plans and many have a sliding scale fee for private pay individuals.

Respite care at home involves a home care worker or volunteer who stays with the impaired individual in his or her own home while the caregiver takes an extended break. A major advantage of in-home respite care is that the patient can remain in familiar surroundings. At home, respite care can usually be provided on short notice during an emergency, such as the hospitalization of a caregiver.

Some social service/health agencies will arrange for a trained home care worker to come to the home a few hours each day or week. Fees are usually manageable and based on ability to pay.

In addition, the Alzheimer's Association has been instrumental in establishing volunteer in-home respite programs. Volunteers are recruited, screened, and trained on how to care for individuals with dementia. These individuals provide companionship and simple social and recreational activities.

Some hospitals and nursing homes provide overnight, weekend, or longer respite care in their facilities. This service allows the caregiver to go out of town or have some free time. This has several advantages in that the patient will have 24-hour medical and nursing services as well as a more structured, contained environment. This alternative can also be helpful in preparing the patient and her family for permanent institutional care.

Information regarding overnight, weekend, or more long-term nursing care can usually be found through contacting local nursing homes directly, the local Alzheimer's support group, the national Alzheimer's organization, or the local Area Agency on Aging.

ADULT DAY CARE

Adult day care, geriatric day care, dependent care, and therapeutic adult care are some of the names for community-based programs.

> Adult day care offers family caregivers an opportunity for a much-needed rest for several hours a day, several days per week.

In the adult day care environment, patients receive supervision and are involved in social and recreational activities that are developed especially to meet their needs. Most programs are open 2 to 7 days a week and last from 3 to 12 hours each day. They usually provide lunch and nutritious snacks. Activities may include arts and crafts, music, exercises that are suited for older individuals, gardening, picnics, outings, and discussion groups. This is discussed further in Chapter 19. One of the most important aspects of adult day care programs is that they provide the impaired individual an opportunity to get out and socialize on a regular basis. Many programs accept clients on a drop-in basis but some require that the person be enrolled for a minimum number of days each week. Some programs provide transportation.

> There are two distinct models of adult care—social and therapeutic.

Social day care may supervise medication and focus more on recreational and socialization activities. The social model may not accept patients who are incoherent. In contrast, the therapeutic model administers medication, will generally provide some medical and psychiatric consultation, and is usually supervised by a registered nurse or other professionally educated and trained staff. Although there are an increasing number of adult day care centers opening in communities across the nation, only a few will accept individuals who are in the latter stages of the disease.

In 1990, the National Council on Aging's National Institute of Adult Day Care (NCOA's NIAD) drafted standards and guidelines for adult day care. Some states have not adopted these standards and have no licensure requirements, except for compliance with local and state fire, health, and safety building codes, making the selection process difficult for the caregiver. In a community or state that has no adult day care standards, it is advisable for the caregivers to make unannounced visits to the center at various times of the day (e.g., during meal time, at mid-morning, and mid-afternoon) to observe the quality of meals being provided or activities offered. Attention should also be given to the ratio of staff to participants. The NCOA recommends a minimum of 1 staff person per 6 clients but a study of adult day care done by NCOA'S NIAD shows that national averages range from 1 staff person per 12 to 25 participants.

HOSPICE CARE

Hospice care is primarily a comprehensive program of care delivered to someone who has been diagnosed as having a terminal illness whose life expectancy is six months or less. Statistics indicate that approximately one percent of patients seen in hospices are patients with Alzheimer's disease. It is the purpose of hospice to offer effective management of pain and other symptoms of terminally ill patients and their families. Physical, emotional, social, and spiritual needs of the patient and family are addressed, as a way to offer hope and prepare the patient and family for the dying process, death, and the period of bereavement. The primary location for hospice is the home setting. It is in the patient's own familiar environment that the greatest level of security and comfort can be felt. Hospice teams usually consist of highly qualified nurses, social workers, chaplains, and community volunteers to provide the support needed in the home. Assistance in the form of nursing care, personal hygiene, homemaking, and equipment are available to the patient and their caregiver as needed. Every effort is made to keep the patient at home, but short-term hospitalization or placement in a skilled nursing facility can be arranged. The hospice team remains involved with the family and physician to make changes in the patient's care plan on an ongoing basis.

The primary care physician can identify if and when hospice care may be appropriate. Medicare, private major medical, and supplemental insurance plans will usually cover most hospice costs. More information can be obtained by calling the National Hospice Organization's toll-free number: 1-800-658-8898.

HOME HEALTH CARE AND IN-HOME SERVICES

Home health care and in-home services are two of the fastest growing industries in this country. These services can provide a vast array of in-home nursing care; physical, occupational, or speech therapy; medical social services; home health aides; homemaker services; and medical supply services. They are vitally important in enabling frail, disabled elderly people to remain at home. These services can be provided by a wide variety of individuals, and often are reimbursable by Medicare, Medicaid, Medigap insurance, private health insurances, or long-term care insurance.

Examples of some of the various types of home health and in-home care available in today's health care environment are:

Volunteers

In addition to family, neighbors, and friends, there are many sources of volunteer help in every community (e.g., senior citizen centers, religious organizations, churches, synagogues, fraternal organizations, and civic organizations). Volunteers can help in ways such as shopping for groceries, running errands, driving the person to appointments, consulting with medical and legal experts, handling forms and financial matters, making telephone calls, assisting with both inside and outside home maintenance, or even spending a few hours each day with the patient

Senior Companions

This is a nationwide program in which volunteers (usually senior citizens) take the sick person out for a walk and encourage him or her to do simple exercises, games, or other activities. The local chapter of the American Association of Retired Persons (AARP) or the Alzheimer's Association can refer caregivers to a Senior Companion Program.

Home Aides or Homemaker Chore Services

These individuals are paid, part-time workers who do light household chores, shopping, meal preparation, transportation to appointments, and various other supportive services. In 1996, the average cost was $50 to $70 for a 3-to 4-hour visit, depending on the locale. A freelance home aide usually charges $10 per hour.

Home Health Aides

Similar to the home aides described above, these individuals usually have more technical duties. For example, their duties may include changing dressings, supervising baths, physical therapy, and monitoring vital signs and medication. These individuals usually have training and certification in basic areas of health care, safety, and first aid.

In 1996, the annual average cost was $20 per hour, depending on the locale. In some states, Medicaid programs help defray the costs.

Visiting Registered Nurses and Licensed Practical Nurses

These professionals oversee the patient's vital signs, administer medication, and supervise the care provided by the home health aide. Nurses can also detect new medical problems that may occur and help the primary caregiver decide whether more intensive treatment is needed. They can also monitor any ongoing physical problems, carry out physician orders, and prepare medications.

In 1996, the annual average cost was $80 for a 3-to 4-hour visit, depending on the locale. These services are almost always covered by Medicare, Medicaid, and even some private insurances.

Title III of the Older Americans Act also has several in-home services available. These services include homemaker services that may do housecleaning, laundry, grocery shopping, meal preparation, and running errands. Most Title III homemakers can provide assistance in bathing, dressing, and hair care.

Also available through Title III is a chore service program. This service may include heavy cleaning, outdoor work such as bringing in wood or coal, and yard work. Repairs to steps, construction of wheelchair ramps, and replacement of windows and door screens are examples of eligible minor repairs. Any major repair work (i.e., roof replacement) is usually referred to a reputable company in the hope that the work will be performed at a reduced fee.

Closely related to home repair is the Weatherization program, which is federally funded under another entitlement. This program provides eligible people with storm windows and insulation for their home to cut down on energy costs.

Eligibility for the Title III program is based on age and need. In communities that use volunteers to provide similar services, there are organizations such as Shepherd

Centers, Good Samaritan, and Carpenters Helpers. Many of these organizations are part of local churches and/or civic organizations. Generally, information regarding these services is located in the local telephone book or can be found by calling churches within a community.

Housing Alternatives and Nursing Home Care

Sooner or later most caregivers are faced with the situation of no longer being able to care for or cope with the demands of the patient at home. At this juncture a decision must be made about alternative housing arrangements. There are a number of options available, which include sheltered settings where, if possible, the individual can manage alone for a time; environments where a couple may be able to manage more easily together; and other environments in which the seriously ill or the individual in the latter stages of Alzheimer's disease receives complete skilled care.

EXAMPLES OF HOUSING ALTERNATIVES/LIVING ARRANGEMENTS

Retirement Villages and Senior Citizen Apartments and Condominiums

These environments are usually planned for retired individuals who can function more independently. Residents usually pay a monthly mortgage plus a monthly fee for maintenance of the building and grounds and sometimes for transportation to doctor appointments and shopping. These forms of housing often have emergency call services and easy access to medical facilities. Generally, these housing alternatives are not appropriate for the more confused or ill person unless a caregiver will be sharing the residence with them.

Assisted Living or Sheltered Housing

These settings are appropriate for individuals who are unable to live independently but do not need constant supervision. These settings may provide security systems and transportation; may offer meals and social service assistance, and employ staff who will regularly check on residents. In order to live in these settings, it is usually necessary for the individuals to be capable of providing their own personal care, and not be disruptive to the other residents or wander. An individual in the early stages of Alzheimer's disease would be able to live without much difficulty in one of these settings. This type of housing is somewhat scarce, resulting in long waiting lists.

Life Care Facilities

These offer a living environment somewhat like the retirement village. In return for an initial entry fee or down payment, individuals can move into the facility and expect to be cared for, regardless of their decline in health, for the rest of their lives, even if their financial resources run out. It is important that family members investigate these homes thoroughly because once they invest their financial resources into the facility, there may be no flexibility.

Adult Foster Homes

In this setting, the patient lives with an individual who offers a room, and provides meals, transportation, access to social work, assistance, and supervision. In these homes, residents are cared for like members of the family. There are several types of adult foster care. Some will not care for patients with Alzheimer's disease, but others specialize in the care of these patients. There are no federal or state quality assurance requirements.

If this type of living arrangement is chosen, the quality of care must be carefully monitored.

Boundary Homes, Domiciliary Homes, Personal Care Homes, Homes for the Aged

These homes usually provide a room, meals, some supervision, and other types of basic assistance. Again, there are no federal or state quality assurance standards.

When evaluating any type of alternative housing, it is important to consider these areas:
- Cleanliness of the physical environment, particularly the kitchen, eating areas, and bathroom
- The fees and what is covered, especially the "extra" charges
- Staff training and understanding of Alzheimer's disease and dementing illness
- The type of care provided
- The kind of supervision provided
- The types of recreational, social support, and medical support provided
- How meals are prepared and secured to include how any special dietary needs are met
- How holidays (Christmas, Thanksgiving, Hanukkah, birthdays) are celebrated
- The person responsible for administration of medications
- The type of medical care provided in an emergency
- The safety plans (fire alarms, evacuation plans)
- Unpleasant odors (such as urine)
- Under what conditions a resident would be asked to move

Finally, the contract needs to be carefully reviewed, and at times legal advice may be required.

Quality care is very difficult to find. Many alternative living facilities, especially the most reputable ones, have waiting lists. It is wise to begin looking for options long before they are needed. This will give an opportunity to make a well thought-out decision rather than hastily taking what is available at the last minute.

Quality care costs a lot of money! The cost may be the responsibility of the individuals and/or their family, charitable gifts, or governmental programs. In many cases, individuals will use a large portion of their monthly Social Security checks.

FINANCING NURSING HOME CARE

Making the decision to place a family member in a nursing home is a very difficult decision and needs to be carefully made. (It is discussed in Chapter 23.) Once the decision has been made to utilize nursing home placement, the following steps are recommended:
• Investigate all funding resources
• Locate a suitable home
• Obtain a thorough physical/medical exam for the patient

Although nursing homes are alike in many ways (e.g., have similar purposes and regulations), there are differences that make one nursing home better suited to a particular patient. It is important to know that some nursing homes are not equipped to care for the patient with Alzheimer's disease, and Medicaid will not pay for the level of care sometimes required with Alzheimer's disease. When a private pay patient on an Alzheimer's disease unit reaches the stage where custodial care is needed, the nursing home will transfer the person to a regular nursing home bed. When the person runs out of financial resources and becomes income eligible, Medicaid will start paying the costs.

Some private insurances will pay for nursing home care or at least a portion of the care; however, some policies contain clauses that exclude people who have Alzheimer's disease or dementing illnesses from average, long-term care. Insurance is available but is often expensive and offers limited benefits. In some situations, part of the nursing home care is covered by Medicare, but only for a limited time.

Information regarding nursing home care can be found through the local Alzheimer's Association or the Area Agency on Aging. Another useful resource is the local Department of Human Services, Division of Adult Services. Comprehensive guides to nursing home care are also available in most states.

TRANSPORTATION SERVICES

One of the most important, yet often unavailable, services for any impaired individual is transportation. The kinds of transportation available are as diverse as the communities in which we live. Some agencies and organizations provide transportation to and from appointments. For example, the Department of Human Services will arrange and pay for transportation to and from health care appointments. Some areas have rural mass transit programs that are based in each county. Vans are operated in an efficient manner by two-way radios. Reasonable fares are charged to riders, regardless of age. Most of the vans are equipped with wheelchair exits and the drivers are trained in transporting people with disabilities to medical and other appointments. Additional information regarding the availability of transportation can usually be obtained from pertinent treatment centers, the local Department of Human Services, local senior citizen centers, or the local Area on Aging Office. In some communities, churches and religious groups also offer this service.

CASE MANAGEMENT SERVICES

Case management is a set of services provided by many different community organizations. These include the Area Agency on Aging and other social and health agencies in the community. The case manager identifies the needs of the individual, develops a service plan with her and her family, and assists in accessing services specific to their needs.

Case management includes assessment (evaluation of the individual's current behavioral, social, and vocational status), service planning, assistance in daily living (providing, advocating, and assessing supports to enhance the individual's ability to live independently in the community for as long as possible), linkage/referral, and support and crisis intervention.

INSURANCE AND MEDICAL BENEFITS

One of the most confusing issues an elderly person or his caregiver must contend with is health insurance. Health insurance and major medical insurance plans may help to defray some of the costs for home care or needed appliances. Health insurance policies sometimes contain clauses or exclusions that affect payment for dementing or chronic illnesses. It is important to know what insurance covers. The major types of insurance and health care coverage available for older people today are briefly described in the following sections. It should be noted that these may change.

Medicare Hospital Insurance (Part A)

This insurance program helps pay for medically necessary inpatient care in a hospital, skilled nursing facility, or psychiatric hospital and for hospice and home health care once the deductible has been met. Any person who has paid into this system is automatically eligible upon reaching age 65.

Medicare Supplementary Medical Insurance (Part B)

This insurance picks up where Part A leaves off. It pays for a wide range of medical services and supplies, but most importantly, it helps pay doctor bills. In addition, Part B will help pay for outpatient hospital services; ambulance transportation; physical and occupational therapy; flu, pneumonia, and hepatitis B immunizations; and durable medical equipment (wheelchairs, walkers, hospital beds, and oxygen equipment ordered by a physician). When using Medicare Part B, the patient is responsible for paying the first $100 each year of the charge approved by Medicare. This is called the Part B annual deductible. The current monthly premium as of January 1997 is approximately $43.

Qualified Medicare Beneficiary (QMB)

The QMB program is for persons with limited resources whose incomes are at or below the national poverty level. It covers the cost of the Medicare premiums, coinsurance, and deductible that Medicare beneficiaries normally pay out of pocket. To be eligible in 1996, single seniors need to have incomes below $665 and assets of less than $4,000; married seniors need to have incomes below $884 and assets of less than $6,000.

Generally, those individuals who receive both Medicare Part A and B and QMB insurance need no other health insurance.

Additional information can be found by contacting the local Social Security office for a free copy of The Medicare Handbook. The toll-free number is: 1-800-772-1213.

Social Security

Most people think of Social Security as a retirement program, but only about 60% of recipients are retired. Other individuals receive Social Security benefits because they are disabled, are a dependent of someone who receives Social Security, or are a widow, widower, or child of someone who has died. In 1996, employee and employer each paid 7.65% of the gross salary up to $62,700.

Social Security is based on a simple concept. Taxes are paid into the system while the individual is working, and after retirement, or becoming disabled, the individual, spouse, and dependent children receive monthly benefits. These are based on lifetime earnings, and survivors collect benefits when the individual dies. Social Security benefits are not intended to meet all financial needs. Other sources of income, such as savings or a pension, are needed. Social Security is basically a foundation on which to build the future. More information can be obtained by requesting SSA Publication No. 05-10024, January 1996, from the nearest Social Security office.

Veterans Affairs Benefits (VA Benefits)

VA benefits are available to any veteran who did not receive a dishonorable discharge. Dependents and survivors of veterans may also be eligible. In applying for benefits, it is important to have birth certificates, death certificates, marriage licenses, insurance polices, and record of military service. The VA provides, on a limited basis, skilled or intermediate-type nursing care in the VA facility or private nursing homes for convalescents or persons who are not acutely ill and not in need of hospital care. Additional benefits may be available for veterans who are permanently housebound in nursing homes or in need of regular aid and attendance. More information can be found by contacting the local Veterans Affairs office.

Long-Term Care (LTC) Insurance

Long-term care can be very expensive. This is true for both nursing home care and in-home care. LTC insurance is best suited for those aged 65 to 75 years who have significant disposable income and who believe that peace of mind is more important than a good investment decision.

When shopping for a LTC policy, it is important to consider the following issues:

- Choose a policy only after comparing information from several companies.
- Does the policy provide coverage in home settings as well as in a nursing home or extended care facility?
- Does the policy limit the number of years of coverage? If so, how many?
- Does the policy have a built-in factor to offset the inflationary increases in the costs of care?
- Are there any restrictions on preexisting conditions?
- Are there any restrictions on the types of conditions that are not covered?
- Does the policy begin paying on the first day of a nursing home stay?
- Consider the age and present health status of the individual.

All these factors will affect the amount of the premium. The Health Insurance Association of America offers a very informative pamphlet entitled "The Consumer's Guide to Long-Term Care Insurance." (See Appendix A for some useful addresses.)

OTHER SUPPORT SERVICES

Alzheimer's Association

This national voluntary organization with local support groups was founded in 1990 and designed to help families affected by Alzheimer's disease. The Alzheimer's Association is described in Chapter 27. For more information regarding the organization, call their toll-free number: 1-800-621-0379 or 1-800-272-3900.

Senior Citizen Centers

There are more than 12,000 senior centers across the United States. All of them offer social and recreational programs. Some centers serve as community centers for many services, including Meals on Wheels, adult education classes, day care, health screening, transportation, and social services. Some centers are directed toward serving independent older persons in the community. Others have a comprehensive program that provides services for both well and frail older people. Its members not only receive services but they also provide services by visiting the homebound or making daily phone calls to be sure the homebound persons are all right. Caregivers can also gain access to low-cost legal care and free help with medical and tax forms. Most services provided at senior citizen centers are usually free or low cost.

Self Help Alzheimer's Caregivers Training and Information (SHACTI)

SHACTI is a nonprofit group that concentrates on classes, workshops, and training seminars for anyone who lives with or cares for an individual with Alzheimer's disease. Founded in 1989, the organization has trained caregivers, respite workers, facility staff, and family members. SHACTI's director is Frena Bloomfield, who is available as an educator for groups, facilities, or family members and can be reached at 541-547-3140.

Department of Human Services

The local Department of Human/Social Services can provide information about adult protective services, social work services, food stamp programs, Meals on Wheels, and state-funded health care services for the low-income individual. The telephone number is located in the telephone directory.

BIBLIOGRAPHY

Cohen D, Eisdorfer C: *Caring for your aging parents, a planning and action guide,* New York, 1995, G.P Putnam's Sons.
Commonwealth Fund Commission on elderly people living alone, Baltimore, 1987, Commonwealth Fund Commission.
The consumer's guide to long-term care insurance, Washington, DC, 1992, Health Insurance Association of America. Health Insurance Association of America, 1025 Connecticut Avenue NW, Washington, DC, 20036-3998.
The consumer's guide to Medicare Supplement Insurance, Washington, DC, 1992, Health Insurance Association of America. Health Insurance Association of America, 1025 Connecticut Avenue NW, Washington, DC, 20036-3998.
Goldsmith SB: *Choosing a nursing home,* New York, 1990, Prentice-Hall.
Gruetzner H: *Alzheimer: a caregiver's guide and source book,* New York, 1992, John Wiley and Sons.
Lindeman DA et al: *Alzheimer's day care: a basic guide,* New York, 1991, Hemisphere Publishing Corporation.
Mace N, Rakins P: *The 36-hour day,* Baltimore, 1992, The Johns Hopkins University Press.
The Medicare Handbook 1996, Health Care Financing Administration, Pub No HCFA 10050, revised April 1996.
Medicare, Medicaid, and Medicare supplement insurance: what you need to know to protect yourself, Nashville, TN, 1992, Legal Services of Middle Tennessee, Nashville Legal Aid Society.
Medicare Savings for Qualified Beneficiaries. Pub No HCFA 02184, revised April 1996.
Portnow MD et al: *Home care for the elderly: a complete guide,* New York, 1987, McGraw-Hill.
Social Security: Understanding the Benefits, SSA Pub No 05-10024, January 1996.
Standards and guidelines for adult day care, Washington, DC, 1990, The National Institute on Adult Day Care (The National Council on Aging).

The Alzheimer's Association

Nancy Erickson
Sheryl Williams

Leave the dreams of yesterday,
take the torch of knowledge,
and build the dreams of the future.

—Marie Curie

In the late 1970s, Alzheimer's disease was a term few people knew. The general public and most health care professionals equated the symptoms of this disease with the outdated term "senility," believing that its occurrence and course were common elements in the aging process.

THE ORIGINS OF THE ALZHEIMER'S ASSOCIATION

In an attempt to find definitive information about the disorder affecting their loved ones, to learn how to cope with its progression, and to gain hope for the discovery of its cause and cure, seven independent caregiver groups joined together in 1980 to form the Alzheimer's Disease and Related Disorders Association, now called the Alzheimer's Association. From a handful of dedicated family members and researchers with an initial budget of $85,000, this association has become the nation's leading nonprofit health organization (with a combined national and chapter budget of more than $60 million) serving individuals with Alzheimer's disease and their families.

ORGANIZATION OF THE ALZHEIMER'S ASSOCIATION

This charity is anchored by a 60-member volunteer board of directors representing family members of individuals with Alzheimer's disease, health care professionals and practitioners, and business leaders. In addition, there is a Medical and Scientific Advisory Board of physicians, scholars, and researchers in clinical, social, and biological sciences who oversee the research programs and scientific information projects.

The foundation of this association is its chapter network of more than 200 chapters in all 50 states. Each chapter is guided by a volunteer board of directors and operates with a budget that may range from less that $25,000 to over $1 million. More than 35,000 volunteers nationwide participate in providing services, such as leading one of the 1,800 support groups, raising scarce dollars for the association's research programs, providing support groups, and educating the public about the effects of Alzheimer's disease. As the network has evolved and chapter operations have become more sophisticated, state councils have been formed for the primary purpose of addressing the legislative and regulatory concerns of individuals with Alzheimer's disease.

> Many chapters began in the living room of a caregiver who was answering phone calls from other caregivers who desperately needed help in caring for a memory-impaired spouse or parent. Although many chapters have moved their operation from a home to an office, their focus on the needs of the individual and the family has not wavered.

MISSION OF THE ALZHEIMER'S ASSOCIATION

The Alzheimer's Association's mission declares its dedication to research for the prevention, cure, and treatment of Alzheimer's disease and related disorders and to providing support and assistance to people with the disease and to their families. The association's mission is carried out by:
- Investigating the causes, prevention, and treatment of Alzheimer's disease and related disorders
- Offering programs and services to individuals and families affected by the disease
- Maintaining a nationwide network of chapters to provide family support in local communities
- Educating and informing the public and health care professionals
- Advocating for research funding and legislative support for families

A synopsis of key areas suggests the breadth of the programs, services, and resources offered by the association and its chapter network: Research, patient and family services, education and public awareness, and public policy form the nucleus of the defense and support of the individual and family members fighting this devastating disease.

RESEARCH ACTIVITIES

In July of 1989, President George Bush officially declared the 1990s the "Decade of the Brain." This designation signified a pledge by the federal government to focus vital resources on brain research. This pledge stems from the needs of more than 50 million Americans with disorders and disabilities of the brain, 4 million of whom suffer from Alzheimer's disease. For the latter group, the estimated cost to society equals $100 billion each year.

The remarkable advances that occurred in brain research in the past decade, coupled with this timely support from the federal government, promise exciting opportunities throughout the rest of the decade. The federal government, still the major funding source for Alzheimer's disease research, provided over $310 million for research in 1995. In 1996, the Alzheimer's Association, the largest private funding source, funded approximately $7.8 million in research grants.

Highlighted research projects include those breaking new ground in understanding how the brain controls certain cognitive abilities (e.g., comprehension, speech and language, reasoning) and what happens to these abilities when the brain undergoes degeneration. Other research examples note that preliminary studies, combined with epidemiological research, suggest that estrogen replacement therapy could have a significant effect on delaying the onset of symptoms and altering the course of the disease. The association joined with the Women's Health Initiative, a program of the National Institutes of Health, to launch an ancillary Memory Study, to verify the effectiveness of estrogen as a preventive treatment for Alzheimer's disease.

The association supports numerous studies focusing on developing methods for the early diagnosis of Alzheimer's disease. One study used positron emission tomography (PET) to examine individuals who had not shown symptoms of Alzheimer's disease, but whose apolipoprotein E (APOE) genetic makeup suggested they were at high risk. The PET scans revealed they had the same brain abnormalities as those showing disease symptoms. Another study of elderly nuns found that those who demonstrated poor linguistic skills at an early age experienced greater cognitive decline in later years, opening up another avenue for investigation of early indicators.

Despite this strong program, a much more aggressive research effort is urgently needed. By the middle of the next century, 14 million Americans will have Alzheimer's disease unless a cure or prevention is discovered. If research can find a way to delay the onset of symptoms by five years, the number of people afflicted by the disease can be reduced by half, adding years of greater independence and saving billions of dollars.

The association's research grants program relies on the strength of the Medical and Scientific Advisory Board, a group of 40 internationally recognized scientists representing many fields of study, including neurology, psychiatry, molecular neurobiology, and research on nursing and caregiver issues. The expert advice of this community enables the Alzheimer's Association to fund a well-balanced group of research projects that are likely to enhance our understanding of Alzheimer's disease.

Through its research grants program, the association has built a sound research investment portfolio:

- As a short-term investment—studies in patient care, caregiver respite services, and behavioral interventions will make the lives of persons with Alzheimer's disease more comfortable and the burden of the disease on families more bearable.
- As a long-term investment—research into basic functions of the brain, chemical reactions, and genetics will improve our understanding of the processes that occur in both the normal brain and the brain of a person with Alzheimer's disease.

This knowledge creates a firm foundation for future research to find the cause(s), effective treatments, and, eventually, methods of preventing Alzheimer's disease. Along the way, we can expect large dividends from our midrange investments in the form of better diagnostic techniques and drugs to help relieve symptoms of this disorder.

Research Programs

The association's research programs began in 1982 with the goal of encouraging more and better research into the cause, treatment and management, prevention, and cure of Alzheimer's disease and related disorders. By the end of 1996, grants and awards totaling more than $50 million were funded by the association through these programs.

Structured to complement the United States Public Health Service funding programs, the research program is designed to encourage investigators to engage in research on Alzheimer's disease and related disorders. Proposals are solicited for biological, clinical, and social research relevant to degenerative brain diseases such as Alzheimer's disease. The proposed research need not directly involve Alzheimer's disease, but must have the potential to add to knowledge about issues relevant to the disease.

Targeted Research Grants

These grants are designed to support research into specific areas that the Medical and Scientific Advisory Board considers vital. They can be either 1-year pilot grants ($25,000) or 2-year grants for a maximum of $45,000 each year. In 1995, the Alzheimer's Association granted funds for two special targeted studies:
• "Mechanisms to Stop or Slow the Progression of Alzheimer's Disease"
• "The Effectiveness of Services and Interventions in Caregiving"

Zenith Awards

The Zenith Awards represent a milestone in the association's efforts to keep talented scientists in the field of Alzheimer's disease research. The researchers receiving these awards have already demonstrated impressive track records in asking the right questions about Alzheimer's disease, and in developing methods to find the answers. The association has granted 19 Zenith Awards since the program was created in 1991. So far, $3 million has been given through this program to scientists who are pioneering new territory in Alzheimer's disease research.

All awardees are working at the leading edge of molecular and cell biology in their attempts to unlock the mysteries of Alzheimer's disease. Their projects address reasons for and mechanisms of the fundamental problem in the brains of patients with Alzheimer's disease: massive nerve cell degeneration and death, and possible ways to correct them.

In addition to providing research support to the scientific community, the association has a commitment to communicating the results of this research and working with scientists and government agencies to accelerate research.

The Reagan Institute Initiative

The association has formed the Ronald and Nancy Reagan Research Institute to accelerate research. The mission of the Reagan Institute is to delay the progression of the disease and reduce the number of people afflicted by Alzheimer's disease by focusing on three major objectives:

- To find the cause of Alzheimer's disease
- To develop safe and effective treatments so afflicted individuals can continue to function independently for 5 to 10 years longer
- To prevent Alzheimer's disease

PATIENT AND FAMILY SERVICES

Alzheimer's disease is often called the "family disease" because the caregiving provided by families can be overwhelming. Family members give most of the care at home. One of every three families is affected by this progressive disease, and the financial and emotional burdens often make caregivers "second victims" of the disease.

Because the progression of Alzheimer's disease can range from 3 to 20 years, the needs of people with the disease and their family members vary with their individual circumstances.

Programs, services, and resources—support groups, helplines, the Safe Return Program, and educational programming—are a sampling of the key activities that draw families to the Alzheimer's Association. Physicians, nurses, and other health professionals working with the person with Alzheimer's disease can take advantage of these resources by becoming familiar with a local chapter's activities.

Each chapter of the Alzheimer's Association offers a core of services for the family dealing with this disease: support groups, helpline, Safe Return Program, and education and information.

The national office supports the chapter network through the development of programs and materials that can be used to assist families in managing the challenges of this disease.

Support Groups

Chapters offer support groups opportunities for many special audiences: the person with early-stage Alzheimer's disease, the caregiving spouse, the teenage grandchild, or Spanish-speaking family friends.

Examples of innovative programs include:

- The Metro Denver Chapter's support group for individuals in the early-stage of Alzheimer's disease, which helps them examine issues about diagnosis, financial and legal concerns, and planning for long-term care.
- The Eastern Massachusetts Chapter, which offers support and a forum for sharing concerns that affect the teenage caregiver.
- Spanish-speaking support groups that meet through the auspices of the Los Angeles Chapter and provide educational programming in community churches through Spanish language videotape materials.

National Alzheimer's Safe Return Program

One of the most alarming and potentially life-threatening behaviors that can accompany memory impairment is wandering. In relationship to dementia, wandering has been defined as "aimless frequent ambulation." As many as 7 out of 10 people with Alzheimer's disease will wander off and get lost sometime during the course of the disease, and many do so repeatedly.

The Safe Return Program is a nationwide system designed to help identify, locate, and return to safety individuals who are memory impaired due to Alzheimer's disease or a related disorder. The program provides identification products for the person with memory impairment, a nationwide 24-hour, toll-free 800 number to contact when someone is lost or found, a national registration database of important contact information, access to 17,000 law enforcement agencies to help find the missing person, and connections to over 200 community-based Alzheimer's disease associations.

National Project Grants to Chapters

The National Association offers a variety of project grants to chapters to support their efforts in providing much-needed services to the families affected by Alzheimer's disease. Multi-year demonstration projects include the Managed Care Chapter Demonstration Project and the Alzheimer Connections Demonstration Program. The Los Angeles, Philadelphia, and Columbus, Ohio chapters, working with leading managed care providers, are examining service use by people with Alzheimer's disease, along with related outcomes and costs through the Managed Care Demonstration Project. This collaboration will lead the way in developing appropriate and effective models of care for persons with this disease in the managed care environment.

The Alzheimer Connections Demonstration Program offers chapters grants to expand their family assistance services, particularly in assessing an individual's or family's needs, developing a care plan, helping to arrange and coordinate community services, and monitoring and evaluating service delivery. Other components include public education, telephone helplines to provide emotional support, and outreach to identify afflicted individuals and caregivers needing assistance.

National Partnerships to Improve Alzheimer's Disease Care

As the Alzheimer's Association monitors the multiple services that the individual with Alzheimer's disease may need throughout the course of the disease, it strives to insure that the person will receive the appropriate care. To effectively advocate for this variety of needs, the association continually assesses and forms collabora-tive relationships with national organizations that interact with the family affected by Alzheimer's disease. One partnership is with the National Adult Day Services Association (NADSA). The focus of this cooperation is to develop standards and guidelines on respite care to encourage the support of potential payors of these services.

Assisted living options have become more prevalent for older adults who do not need the skilled care services of a nursing home, but need some assistance with daily living. However, there is a lack of a consistent definition of the care provided in these settings from state to state. To address this issue and in recognizing that up to 40% of individuals residing in these facilities have some form of dementia, the association has joined with the American Association of Retired Persons (AARP), the American Association of Homes and Services for the Aging (AAHSA), and the Association of Assisted Living Facilities of America (AALFA) to form the Assisted Living Quality Coalition. This coalition has drafted a definition of assisted living, minimal guidelines for providers, and a quality initiative for the assisted living industry.

The Alzheimer's Association commissioned the Hastings Center, a leading medical ethics institute, to identify barriers to providing hospice care to people with Alzheimer's disease. The goal of this study is to examine changes necessary to make hospice services accessible and affordable for families of patients with Alzheimer's disease.

The association supports an ongoing strategy of collaboration and cosponsorship with academic institutions, professional societies, and pharmaceutical companies for the purpose of producing consensus documents on the diagnosis and treatment of Alzheimer's disease as well as advancing techniques for managing the effects of this disease on individuals and their families.

PUBLIC AWARENESS AND EDUCATION

During the course of one year, the coast-to-coast Alzheimer's Association's network responded to calls from approximately 200,000 family members asking for direction, help, and guidance. To answer these care management and support inquiries, the association has developed an extensive catalog of more than 50 publications that is available through local chapters.

As the association has expanded its knowledge of the needs of families dealing with Alzheimer's disease on a daily basis, it has produced educational materials for the public and care professionals alike. Publications range from pamphlets to multi-media training kits and training manuals.

The Action Series pamphlets offer practical steps and tips on dealing with prominent issues, including:
• "Steps to Getting a Diagnosis: Finding Out if It's Alzheimer's Disease"
• "Steps to Enhancing Communications: Interacting with Persons with Alzheimer's Disease"
• "Steps to Planning Activities: Structuring the Day at Home"

Training kits with video and audiotapes include the "Caregiver Kit" and "An Orientation to Alzheimer's Disease."

Spanish language resources feature pictorial formats (fotonovelas), caregiver fact sheets, videotapes, and a training manual in Spanish and English and several brochures. Training manual titles include the *Multicultural Outreach Program Manual* and *Activity Programming for Persons with Dementia: A Source Book.*

Specific titles for care providers are *Terms and Tips,* a booklet of frequently used care terms, and numerous bibliographies, such as *Alternative Therapies in Alzheimer's Disease* and *Non-Alzheimer's Dementia*. *Alzheimer's Disease Research: Possible Causes . . . Potential Treatment* is a compendium of the research grants awarded by the association with brief descriptions about each study.

Since the founding of the Benjamin B. Green-Field Library and Resource Center in 1991, this premiere, privately funded facility specializing in information about Alzheimer's disease has seen a dramatic increase in use. Accessible to lay and professional publics, the collection includes patient education materials, association products, training materials, and scientific articles. New titles for reading lists and bibliographies include subjects such as behavior, aluminum, specialized dementia care, and communication. Copies are available free of charge or can be accessed on the association's Website on the Internet: http://www.alz.org.

Two professional health sciences librarians provide assistance to meet users' information needs, including basic reference services for finding statistical information, referral to other information resources within or outside of the association, and literature search and extended reference services. The preparation of literature searches is facilitated by access to over 400 online databases available through the National Library of Medicine, the OVID Search Service, and Dialogue Information services.

Bibliographical searches using local sources—the library's computerized catalog, print indexes, and periodical indexes in CD-ROM format—are provided without charge. Charges are requested for certain services. The public may use materials in the library or borrow materials via interlibrary loan through their local hospital, university, or public library. A description of the library's collection is stored in a computer database, which is readily available from anywhere in the U.S. using a computer with a modem and appropriate software.

PROFESSIONAL EDUCATION PROGRAMMING

National conference for health care professionals and paraprofessionals

Since 1992, the Alzheimer's Association has offered a national conference for health care professionals and paraprofessionals. In five years, this national forum has grown from over 1,000 to 1,500 attendees, attracting nursing home administrators; directors of nursing; physicians; social workers; administrators of home health care agencies, adult day care, and assisted living facilities; and allied health professionals. The association has premiered new products at the conference, such as *Guidelines for Dignity*, a comprehensive guide to quality care in residential settings for persons with Alzheimer's disease.

Centers for Excellence in Alzheimer Care

The new "Centers for Excellence in Alzheimer Care" training model, which is currently in development, will enhance the association's training capabilities nationwide. The National Training Center, located at the national office, will be expanded beyond its current use for in-service training classes to incorporate the education and training needs of chapters and community care professionals.

Respite Care: Strategies for the Future

In early 1996, the association invited leading respite care professionals from throughout the country to an Issues Forum, "Respite Care: Strategies for the Future," to discuss how the changing health care environment has impacted the delivery of respite care and to develop appropriate responses to identified issues.

Four issues that participants cited as central to the future development of respite services are:

1. Uneven funding
2. Difficulties in assuring quality of services—specifically recruiting, training, and retaining good staff
3. The trend to over-medicalize services
4. The need to identify appropriate outcome measures

The association continues to support the work of the Alzheimer's Disease International and is a co-sponsor of the International Symposium on Alzheimer's Disease, an educational conference that attracts the top scientists in this field.

ADVOCACY

Federal, state, and local advocacy efforts have helped to emphasize the urgency of the needs of persons with Alzheimer's disease in the legislative and regulatory arenas. Through lobbying efforts of association advocates during 1995, $4 million in federal funding was continued for community-based services for the under-served, particularly minorities and low-income citizens. Issues to be addressed are the national debate on reform of Medicare and Medicaid, nursing home quality protections, and changes in the tax code to allow deductions for the cost of long-term care.

SUMMARY

As the Alzheimer's Association stands on the threshold of a golden age of Alzheimer research, it continues to move boldly towards a future that holds great promise for creating a world without Alzheimer's disease. With the arrival of the new millennium, the association will celebrate 20 years of its accomplishments in supporting the lives of thousands of individuals and families facing the challenges of this debilitating disease. The association steadfastly stands by all who serve the person with Alzheimer's disease—to fight to help him or her retain personal dignity and to maintain existing special abilities. The Alzheimer's Association provides practical approaches to caregiving and caring approaches to service.

For a referral to a local chapter of the Alzheimer's Association or for information about educational programs and materials, call 1-800-272-3900; for the hearing impaired, use the TTD 1-312-335-8882, or contact the web page on the Internet at World Wide Web:http://www.alz.org.

BIBLIOGRAPHY

Alzheimer's Association: *Alzheimer's disease research: possible causes . . . potential treatment,* Chicago, May, 1996, The Association.

Alzheimer's Association: *Respite care: strategies for the future,* Chicago, February, 1996, The Association.

Alzheimer's Association: Alzheimer's Association Publications Catalog, Public Catalog, Chicago, 1996, The Association.

Dementia Care Units

Larry B Hudgins

We live very close together. So our prime purpose in this life is to help others. And if you can't help them, at least don't hurt them.

—Dalai Lama

Approximately 50% of long-term nursing home admissions in the U.S. are accounted for by individuals with progressive dementia. Clearly, the number of nursing home admissions, as well as the percentage of dementia residents are expected to increase as the U.S. population ages. Although there are now more than 1,000 Alzheimer Special Care Units providing care to several thousand dementia residents, there are hundreds of thousands of persons with dementia residing in the nation's general care nursing homes. Families caring for loved ones with Alzheimer's and other dementias are concerned about:
1. The appropriate indications for institutionalization
2. The type and quality of facilities available
   Families and caregivers need to know what to look for in a facility before and after placement.

DEMENTIA SPECIAL CARE UNITS (DSCU)

Dementia Special Care Units (DSCU) were developed as a result of varied groups interested in the quality of care for dementia patients. The establishment of these units represents a recognition of the special needs of dementia sufferers. DSCU benefit from the ongoing work of investigators in social work, psychology, medicine, nursing, and architecture as well as various sectors of the nursing home industry.

Dementia care units are defined as living areas that are largely self-contained and self-sufficient in terms of services, staffing, and congregate space. The unique offerings of specialized dementia care units are their ability to respond appropriately to each resident's needs and to plan innovatively according to each resident's individual situation. The items of utmost importance in accomplishing

377

this type of inclusive care are staffing, physical plant, and family-patient interaction. Such an organized treatment in carefully planned specialized dementia care units addresses the complex and ever-changing links among staff, resident, family, and the institution. The team approach to care is critical to a successful outcome in dementia care.

During the early and middle stages of Alzheimer's dementia, home is the best place for the patient to receive care. However, in most situations circumstances arise that justify strong consideration for an extended care placement. The main circumstances leading to institutionalization include:

1. The patient no longer cooperates in his own care due to marked deterioration in the activities of daily living (bathing, feeding, hygiene).
2. The patient no longer recognizes the family caregiver at home.
3. When a family caregiver and a paid caregiver jointly provide care for the patient, an interruption of the arrangements may require institutional placement.
4. The patient has become incontinent and the caregiver can no longer care for the patient at home.
5. The caregiver's health is at risk, so alternate arrangements must be considered. Caregivers may be "burned out," chronically fatigued, or "at the end of their rope."
6. Early institutional placement may be necessary if there is no family member able to fill the caregiver role. A caregiver role requires more than the will to do the job. The caregiver must have the physical strength, emotional stability, knowledge about the disease, and skill in dealing with someone who is cognitively impaired.
7. Patients with dementia may exhibit disruptive behavior, including agitation, hostility, delusions or extreme anxiety, endangering themselves and others, and hastening institutional placement.

These circumstances require extended care placement in facilities that provide a level of care sufficient to meet the patient's unique needs. The usual placement options include general care nursing homes, nursing homes that have DSCU, or dementia-specific assisted living facilities.

DISADVANTAGES OF CARING FOR PATIENTS WITH DEMENTIA IN CONVENTIONAL NURSING HOMES

The main disadvantages of caring for these patients in a custodial nursing home setting include difficulties in coping with wandering patients and intolerance of behavioral disturbances. In addition, other patients in the custodial nursing home setting may be recuperating from an acute illness or from orthopedic or other surgery, or may be receiving post-stroke rehabilitation. The probability of interference with the care of these patients would be high if wandering patients with dementia were housed within the same unit. The different care requirements for each of these groups result in such divergent goals that the staff may find it difficult to divide their attention between caring for both categories of patients at the same time.

ADVANTAGES OF DEMENTIA SPECIAL CARE UNITS

The advantages of having all the patients with dementia in one unit include the same goal orientation and expectations of the unit by staff and families. The unit staff and family caregivers are likely to have developed similar and unified coping skills to care for these patients. The separately contained dementia unit setting offers a better opportunity to develop a flexible activity schedule for the patients. With proper architectural structure, those patients inclined to wander can do so at will without requiring constant staff attention.

CONCERNS ABOUT DEMENTIA SPECIAL CARE UNITS

The concerns about having all patients with a diagnosis of dementia in one unit are threefold:
1. Morale tends to be low among staff members who must deal daily with a population of patients not expected to recover.
2. Such facilities create a closed community in which turnover is minimal and close relationships develop between family caregivers and staff.
     This situation often leads to opposition by families when the need arises to move the patient to another facility because of further deterioration of his or her condition.
3. Experience in these units has demonstrated that when the permanent staff are sick or on vacation, other staff members are reluctant to work on the unit that houses "those demented folks."

ADVANTAGES OF DEMENTIA SPECIAL CARE UNITS IN CLOSE PROXIMITY TO CONVENTIONAL CUSTODIAL NURSING HOMES

The present consensus of opinion is that it is better for specialized dementia care units to be attached to existing larger custodial nursing homes structurally but to maintain a separate identity.

The advantage of the plan is that the staff is not so isolated from general nursing home care and that the patients, once disabled to the point of requiring custodial care, can be moved easily into the custodial care unit. The family should understand this mechanism for continuity of care for their relative with dementia before admission to the dementia care unit.

This care plan arrangement alleviates some of the problems of what to do with the patient who becomes acutely ill, less mobile, and ultimately bedridden. Obviously, a team care approach is of tremendous help to the staff, family, and patient in discussing when a patient should be considered for transfer to another unit.

Should the transfer be accomplished when the patient has a noticeable decrease in ambulatory status, or should the dementia unit attempt to help the patient who requires total care and is bedridden? To settle these problems, some bargaining between the staff and the family eventually will be required. However, it should always be kept in mind that the specialized dementia unit is not designed to handle total care patients.

WHO SHOULD BE CARED FOR IN DEMENTIA SPECIAL CARE UNITS?

The ideal candidates for care in specialized dementia care units include those patients who, despite severe memory problems, are ambulatory, can feed themselves, do not need extensive medical care, are able to follow simple instructions, and can manage to perform some activities of daily living with the help of the staff.

Two decades of experience with special dementia care units has demonstrated a decrease in wandering, agitation, screaming, depression, and psychotic behavior. Other positive benefits include a decrease in (or elimination of) drugs to control behavior, weight gain, improved behavior, greater ability to sleep through the night, and reduced incontinence. Catering to the patient's needs, habits, and uniqueness rather than the dementia is the best service that the specialized dementia care unit can provide.

STAFFING ROLES

Specially trained staff are considered integral to care in DSCU. Training content for all unit personnel should address management of difficult behavior, communication skills with residents with dementia, as well as family support techniques for families of cognitively impaired residents. For staff stability and consistency, training programs for personnel in DSCU increase work skills and improve job satisfaction. Most importantly, training enables the staff to work more effectively and efficiently with patients with dementia and their families.

Staff development programs aimed at thoroughly integrated interdisciplinary team approach, improving interpersonal communication skills, emphasizing concise documentation of medical records, and fostering respect for individual rights and dignity are basic to the unit concept.

In specialized dementia care units, the staff/patient ratio is much higher than in traditional nursing homes or custodial settings. Such a situation does not necessarily mean that the patient directly requires more care but that more staff-patient interaction allows the patient to participate as fully as possible in the unit, thus helping to define his own limits and increasing his level of activity as much as practical.

> Good patient-staff interaction and communication are central features in the day-to-day management of such a unit.

Staff members invest time and energy in learning about the interests of their patients both before they come to the unit and during their stay there. This approach helps the staff to see the patients as being less dependent. Such detail in patient care may not be possible in custodial nursing home units because of time and staffing constraints.

Furthermore, in custodial care units, a tremendous amount of staff energy is required to take care of the physical needs of patients. This need is precipitated by a low staff/patient ratio and the complexity of care required for recuperating, but not yet well, patients. While in this situation, nursing home staff might know what to do for their patients but have little time or inclination to get to know them.

To suggest that the nursing home custodial care staff change their approach to patient care may be interpreted as saying that they are not doing enough or are doing their job poorly. The challenge to extended care setting nursing staff is to change from custodial care to a team approach, since no single discipline can meet the particular needs of the elderly with dementia. Communication in such a setting must be multidirectional so that most of the decision making is shared and decisions are rendered by consensus rather than by directives.

Such a model of residential living requires integrating the staff structure and understanding the needs of residents. The staff should have the ability to interact with residents according to each patient's needs and behavior in various stages of their illness. The staff should be able to determine what capacities remain in severely impaired individuals since these capacities can be used to improve the quality of life of these patients.

The attitudes of staff and facility administrators should not promote the stereotype of patients with dementia as being mentally ill and totally incapable.

> It is wrong for the staff to assume that people with dementia are no longer aware of or sensitive to their surroundings, or that they have lost all capacity to function.

Such stereotyped attitudes are noted when staff or caregivers use methods and assumptions that treat dementia as mental retardation rather than as dementia. With dementia, a person is deteriorating from a previously higher level of cognitive functioning; with mental retardation, the person did not previously have a higher level of functioning, and caregivers frequently take the role of teachers of new skills. In dementia, the teaching of new skills is generally not done.

In patients with dementia, the ability to do the task is very often intact. It is the ability of the brain to tell the body what to do or to recognize that this is the appropriate time to do it.

The differences between the two disorders may seem to be subtle, but in fact they call for very different approaches in terms of intervention, goals, and caregiver roles. Unfortunately, in many instances, the distinctions between mental retardation and dementia are not appreciated in nursing home custodial units. Therefore the remaining capacities, still intact in the person with dementia, are never recognized or utilized.

Professional people cannot serve effectively in special care units if they do not understand older people or if they have negative beliefs about them.

Specific training must be available for nurse's aides, who probably spend the most time with the patient, and their skills must be reinforced periodically.

Training in basic nursing, personal care, social needs, basic restorative services, and resident rights should be part of the continuing education of nurse's aides. Specific topics that should be included in these training sessions are an overview of dementia that explains the stages of the illness and describes the emotional and behavioral problems that may occur with this disease. Therapeutic and recreational services offered in the dementia unit should also be reviewed.

Staff members should be made aware of the importance of changing staff roles to encompass continuing periodic patient evaluation: how to assess the patient's needs, strengths, and abilities. Other important topics that must be included are mechanisms that are helpful in responding to difficult behavior problems, the importance of the physical environment of the unit, techniques used to involve families, and ways of compensating for sensory loss in old age.

▬● Staff development should also address the staff's needs.

Teaching staff caregivers how to deal with patients with dementia also helps curtail staff burnout. Adequate staff leave programs and switching staff assignments to take care of different residents at various stages of dementia illnesses help lessen the impact of personal emotional involvement by the staff. Continuing interaction with the custodial nursing home staff helps to improve dementia unit staff morale. As indicated earlier, this interaction is facilitated if the specialized dementia care unit is structurally attached to the custodial nursing home but still able to develop its own separate identity.

BEHAVIORAL ABNORMALITIES

Behavioral abnormalities are some of the more frequent and more difficult disturbances that need to be dealt with effectively in people with dementia. There are several simple mechanisms that the staff may use to help with the behavioral problems that can arise in patients in a dementia unit.

Distraction

Staff members may be able to control a patient's aberrant behavior by providing a diversion or a distraction before the patient becomes extremely agitated. They can often help the patient avoid strong reactions. Items of interest to the patient (e.g., photographs or furniture) can be incorporated into the physical environment to provide meaning and to serve as a diversion when needed. Joking and lighthearted talking sometimes help to reduce tension; however, it is important that this maneuver in no way belittles or ridicules the elderly person.

Touch

Touch is a very important method of communication with the elderly person with dementia. It may be used to focus the attention of the patient on a specific task to be accomplished and to produce a calming effect on the patient. Touch alone may be the best intervention for diffusing agitation and providing distraction during behavioral problems. Touching is one of the most beneficial therapeutic actions for combating the sensory isolation that the elderly experience. Touch can relate warmth and a genuine concern for the elderly patient with dementia that no other action can accomplish.

Explanations and Discussions

Explanations and discussions are also valuable tools in behavior adjustment, even in cognitively impaired patients. Unit staff should not assume that persons with dementia will not understand even simple explanations or instructions. Similarly, they must make an effort to give residents choices when they resist certain activities so that the patients feel that they have at least some control over their own lives.

Visual Cues

Conspicuous visual cues are used to orient the person with dementia (e.g., symbols for dining room, garden room). These cues should be simple and not arranged to overload the patient. For example, at dinner a patient may eat his dessert if no other food is on the table. Since only the dessert is placed in front of the patient along with the eating utensil, the cue is easy for him. On the other hand, placing several food items, such as appetizer, entree, and dessert in front of the patient may be overwhelming, and he may then become unable to cope (i.e., eat). Alternatively, the patient may need time to process the cues in order to act appropriately.

Avoiding Fixed Schedules

Avoiding fixed schedules and making allowances to individualize schedules for people with dementia will help to control stress and anxiety for both the patient and the staff. This approach allows the patient to follow her own lifestyle or current mood. For example, setting bath schedules, which often can be followed only if the staff uses coercion, can cause much anger and resistance on the part of residents and can result in frustration and stress for the staff. Giving the patient a choice between bathing or eating a meal may be more productive, regardless of the proximate scheduled event.

Chemical Restraints

Chemical restraints continue to be overused as a means of behavior control in custodial nursing. In general, there is too great a reliance on high-dose administration of sedatives, hypnotics, and antipsychotic drugs to achieve behavior control. Side effects associated with these particular drugs are common and are further discussed in Chapter 13.

In Dementia Special Care Units, overuse of psychoactive drugs is avoided because the staff know the patient's moods and capacities and works within these limits, learning how to bargain with the patient. When preventive mechanisms are used to deal with patients with dementia on their own terms, the need for chemical restraints should diminish.

Strategies to Help Patients with Given Tasks

The staff caregiver can use certain strategies to help the patient in a given task and simultaneously to evaluate her remaining capabilities to perform the task. The following strategies are listed from the least intrusive to the most intrusive:
1. Waiting
2. Slowing down
3. Asking if the patient wants help
4. Prompting the patient verbally or nonverbally
5. Encouraging the patient
6. Providing the patient with feedback
7. Doing all or part of the task for the patient

ARCHITECTURAL DESIGN

Another important consideration in establishing a dementia special care unit is the development and construction of the physical plant and architectural design of the building. The architectural layout should avoid the use of "institutional cues" reminiscent of the hospital setting.

Dementia care units should, as far as possible, resemble a home. In the most basic sense, specialized dementia care units should be user friendly and user protective.

In order to make patients feel comfortable, dementia units may include mirrors, pictures, and items of interest to the residents. They should provide adequate lighting and avoid shadows, glare, and loud background noise. Fenced exterior gardens may be planned as an integral part of the facility.

In general, egress control devices should be used in lieu of locked doors. For example, magnetic electrical door catches can be used to signal door openings, which alert the staff when someone is exiting from the facility. These signals can be monitored from a central station. Stress levels of the staff and the family are noted to be remarkably lower when these persons do not need to watch exit doors constantly.

Accommodations for the wandering patient with dementia require additional innovative approaches. A racetrack (circular) design has been tried in some situations so that residents can wander endlessly. Some experts believe that aimless wandering reflects a resident's desperate effort to leave an impoverished environment that provides no other stimulation for him or her. Wandering is probably important as a primal activity, but it also provides needed exercise. Although it is an energy-depleting activity, wandering is productive in the sense that it is likely to lessen the need for sedatives and hypnotics because the patient gets tired from the exercise.

The general attributes of the architectural environment should encompass the following:

1. Noninstitutionalized (homelike) image
2. Easily negotiable environment (user friendly)
3. Sensory stimulation without stress (mirrors, paintings, gardens)
4. Visitor space (affording some privacy)
5. Opportunities for meaningful wandering

Clear signs that incorporate both words and pictures should be used for concise and precise cuing to identify rest rooms, dining area, TV lounge or game areas, and walking spaces. Additional requirements to reduce environmental stressors include dampening of extraneous stimuli by using sound-absorbing material, eliminating intercoms, and "painting out" doors to storage areas. This "painting out" technique serves as a subtle camouflage; for example, a door that does not color contrast with the wall is not easily recognized. Alternatively, some units have curtains to cover doors that are exits. This simple maneuver may be a very cost-effective egress control device.

■—● Facility design should be architecturally stylized to reduce patient stress.

The goal of simulating a home environment setting should include the use of "quiet" colors. Also, the family cluster construction approach uses small, private living areas for small numbers of patients and includes a bedroom, sitting area, family area, and bath. The family area helps to provide additional privacy for visitations. Such a design respects the residents' space and allows them to keep meaningful things from the past in their living area. These living areas should be spacious enough to allow some personalization with items known to be of particular importance to the patient, such as mementos, family photographs, and furniture. The presence of personal possessions not only may help patients to maintain their identity but also may aid the staff in developing a sense of each person as an individual with a unique history. These items associated with the resident's personal history allow the staff to be creative and innovative in communication, orientation, and reminiscence.

The architectural plans of the kitchen and all other living areas should be used to create a calm and interactive environment where the demands of the physical setting are not beyond the patient's capacity to function. The staff should continually experiment with different busy activities for the residents. Residents may want to set places for the meals, wash and dry dishes, or prepare simple desserts such as cookies. Such activities provide useful recreation and therapeutic time for patients. However, some residents may choose to do such activities at odd hours of the day, and there should be enough flexibility in the program to handle such differences. These simple kitchen or dining room tasks are not done as a learning technique but as a tool for the patient to spend time in a designated task. Some assistance with kitchen tasks may be required of the unit staff, but only to assist the patient in performing the task, not do it for him.

FAMILY ROLES

Family caregivers who have invested years in caring for a loved one with dementia will certainly invest time in finding an appropriate facility for placement. What is learned by actually inspecting the facility and interviewing staff members is much more important than how the facility describes or defines itself. Interviews with family members and relatives of patients in the facility is even more revealing. The family should look for evidence that the staff and facility can provide services needed by a dementia patient. Staff training on dementia issues, a high staff to patient ratio, special environmental design of the unit, and special activity programs geared to patients with dementia are indicators that the facility is "dementia sensitive" as well as "dementia specific."

— Family participation is an integral part of dementia care.

Visitation by family members frequently helps in regard to the patient's level of activity and reinforces each patient's unique likes and dislikes to the staff. For example, one patient was reported to spend several hours folding clothes constantly before admission to the dementia care unit. Such a repetitive activity can be used effectively in the unit when there is a need to occupy the patient's attention or to divert her from a disruptive behavior. Most families prefer to remain actively involved in the caregiving process after the patient has been placed in the unit.

The staff should create an atmosphere that ensures positive family involvement. The staff must be aware of the significant burdens that the patient's family have shouldered before making the decision to institutionalize a relative with dementia. Research on caring for relatives with dementia has documented that it is a very difficult process that can have severe effects on the mental health, self-esteem, and social life of the caregiver. By the time the decision has been made to institutionalize a relative, the primary caregiver may have devoted years of his or her life to the caregiving process. Therefore the decision can be a very painful one, and it is not necessarily associated with feelings of relief. The families may continue to feel the stress of caregiving even though they are no longer responsible for the day-to-day care of the patient.

The reputation and prestige of any dementia care unit are a direct reflection of the investment made in it by family caregivers. The unit staff that pays close attention to the involvement of families will always benefit.

Resolving Complaints

One of the most important facets of good family-staff relationships is the process for resolving complaints. Family meetings are an important way of orienting and involving families at the outset. Providing the family with information in writing is important since the relatives are usually distracted and upset at the time the patient is admitted to the facility. To help keep problems from progressing to a crisis point between the facility and the family, it should be made clear initially that the family is an active participant in planning treatment.

> A family's expectations may be heightened by the guilt they feel about having sent their relative to a nursing home.

A "family buddy system" may be a good way of helping to orient new families to a unit and to adjust the family's expectations to a practical level. An excellent method of communication with the patient's family is the care planning conference. Through this conference, the family commonly feels better about having been consulted and informed. The best decisions about the resident's care can be made when staff and family are in accord and decisions are made by consensus.

In addition, introducing the family members to the staff and the key members of the team who run the unit is critical in attaining family support. Such an introduction can be done over several sessions to identify staff, their positions, and how they relate to the patient. Family-oriented educational programs offer additional benefits. These educational sessions can be used to review normal aging changes, information about Alzheimer's disease and related illnesses, emotional issues for families, communication techniques, difficult behavior, medications, depression, daily routines in the unit, and successful family visits.

One way to establish a good working relationship with the family is to ask for help in putting together a good social/medical/family history of the relative. Such a history will help the unit staff relate to and communicate with the patient in a more personal way.

The family should also be invited to become more formally involved by attending patient care conferences in which treatment plans and patient activity plans are discussed along with any particular problems that the staff is having. Such intervention planning avoids the crisis-only intervention mindset that is prevalent in custodial care settings. This type of communication among staff, family, and family caregivers optimizes the patient's functional ability to live within and up to the limits of his or her dementia. Interdisciplinary team meetings allow for direct efforts at troubleshooting and averting problems that might precipitate patient stress, family anger, and unit staff withdrawal.

Whatever the mechanism used to gain consensus in patient care, there must be a strong psychosocial component to care since the patient cannot make decisions for himself. Dementia unit care falls somewhere between medical treatment provided in custodial care nursing homes and psychiatric treatment offered in most mental health facilities. It involves an ongoing assessment that allows for continuous remodeling of approaches to patient care. The treatment team can apply whatever intervention is appropriate for the situation, affecting the patient's activities program and physical, social, and emotional environment.

Since the primary dementia disorder is progressive, the family's expectations must be adjusted to a realistic level as the goals of patient care become more existential rather than focusing on permanent gains or improvement. Through this process of ongoing reassessment and reevaluation of the patient, it is recognized that as the dementia progresses, the affected person becomes increasingly dependent on his environment to influence his actions and behavior. A major part of the patient's environment is a responsive unit staff.

THE 1992 REPORT OF THE U.S. OFFICE OF TECHNOLOGY ASSESSMENT

In 1992, the U.S. Office of Technology Assessment (OTA) released a report: *Special Care Units for people with Alzheimer's disease and other dementias: consumer education, research, regulatory and reimbursement issues.* It was requested by the Senate Special Committee on Aging and by Congresswoman Olympia J. Snowe. The principles pervading the literature on special care units, as determined by the OTA staff, were:

- *Something can be done for persons with dementia.* Treatment may improve the patient's functioning and quality of life.
- *Many factors cause excess disability in individuals with dementia.* Identifying and changing these factors may reduce disability, and improve the patient's functioning and quality of life.
- *Patients with dementia have residual strengths.* Building on these strengths will improve their functioning and quality of life.
- *The behavior of patients with dementia represents understandable feelings and needs, even if the patients are unable to express them.* Identifying and responding to these feelings and needs may reduce the incidence of behavioral symptoms. Wandering for instance may represent a variety of meaningful intentions and needs for different individuals.
- *Many aspects of the physical and social environment affect the functioning of patients with dementia.* Providing appropriate environments may improve the patients' functioning and quality of life.
- *Patients with dementia and their families constitute an integral unit.* Addressing the needs of the families and involving them in the patients' care

will benefit both the patient and the family. Families can play a positive role in the care of patients with dementia.

The characteristics of special care units, as determined by the OTA, are:

- Special care units are extremely diverse.
- Most have been established since 1983, although a few have been operational for 20 to 25 years.
- Their goals differ. For some units, the primary goal is maintaining residents' quality of life, eliminating behavioral symptoms, or meeting residents' physical needs.
- Most existing special care units were not originally constructed as special care units, and at least one fifth were neither originally constructed nor remodeled for this purpose.
- The use of specific physical design and other environmental features varies in existing special care units. Many of the physical design and other environmental features cited as important in the special care unit literature are used in only a small proportion of special care units.
- The most extensively used environmental feature is an alarm and/or locking system, found in more than three quarters of existing units.
- On average, they probably have fewer residents than nonspecialized nursing home units.
- On average, they probably have more staff per resident than nonspecialized nursing home units.
- Although the majority of existing units provide special training for the unit staff, at least one fourth of existing units do not.
- Fewer than half of existing units provide a support group for unit staff members.
- The types of activity programs provided vary greatly, but existing units are probably no more likely than nonspecialized units to provide activity programs for their residents.
- About half of existing units provide a support group for residents' families.
- They vary greatly in their admission and discharge policies. About half of all units admit residents with the intention that they will remain on the unit until they die.
- Their cost varies depending on the cost of new construction or remodeling, if any, and ongoing operating costs. On average, existing units probably cost more to operate than nonspecialized nursing home units, primarily because of the higher average staffing levels on special care units.
- Special care units generally have a higher proportion of private-pay residents than nonspecialized nursing home units, and private-pay residents are often charged more for their care in the special care unit than they would be in a nonspecialized unit.

The characteristics of special care units residents, as determined by the OTA, are:

- They are younger than other nursing home residents, and they are more likely than other nursing home residents to be male and white.
- They are more likely than other nursing home residents to have a specific diagnosis for their dementing illness.

- They are probably somewhat more cognitively impaired and somewhat less physically and functionally impaired than other nursing home residents with dementia.
- They are as likely or more likely than other nursing home residents with dementia to receive psychotropic medications.
- They are probably less likely than other nursing home residents with dementia to receive medications of all types.
- They are less likely than other nursing home residents with dementia to be physically restrained.
- They are probably somewhat more likely than other nursing home residents with dementia to participate in activity programs.
- They are more likely than other nursing home residents with dementia to fall.

BIBLIOGRAPHY

Benson DM et al: Establishment and impact of a dementia unit within the nursing home, *J Am Geriatr Soc* 35(4):319-323, 1987.

Calkins MP: *Design for dementia: planning environments for the elderly and the confused,* Owings Mills, Md, 1988, National Health Publishing.

Cohen U, Weesman G: *Holding on to home: designing environments for people with dementia,* Baltimore, 1991, Johns Hopkins University Press.

Coons DH: *Specialized dementia care units,* Baltimore, 1991, Johns Hopkins University Press.

Coons DH: Training staff to work in special care units, *Am J Alzheimer Care Res* 2(5):6-12, 1987.

Gold DT et al: Special care units: atypology of care settings for memory impaired older adults, *Gerontologist* 31(4)467-475, 1991.

Grant LA et al: Staff training and turnover in Alzheimer Special Care Units: comparison with nonspecial care units, *Geriatr Nurs* 17(6):278-282, 1996.

Hamdy RC: Nursing homes: reducing the impact of institutionalization, *J Tenn Med Assoc* 84(1):13-15, 1991.

Mace NL: *Dementia care: patient, family, community,* Baltimore, 1991, Johns Hopkins University Press.

Mace NL, Gwyther LP: *Selecting a nursing home with a dedicated dementia care unit,* Chicago, 1989, Alzheimer's Disease and Related Disorders Association.

Maslow K: Current knowledge about special care units: findings of a study by the US Office of Technology Assessment, *Alzheimer Dis Assoc Disord* 8(Suppl1):S14-240, 1994.

Matthew LP et al: What's different about a special care unit for dementia patients? A comparative study, *Am J Alzheimer Care Res* 3(2):16-23, 1988.

Pheiffer E: Institutional placement for patients with Alzheimer's disease, *Postgrad Med* 97(1):125-130, 1995.

Phillips CD: Commentary, public policy toward special dementia units, *Alzheimer Dis Assoc Disord* 8(Suppl 1):5405-5407, 1994.

Shulman MD, Mandel E: Communication training of relatives and friends of institutional elderly persons, *Gerontologist* 28(6):797-799, 1988.

Unit Six

Empiricism may serve to accumulate facts, but it will never build science. The experimenter who does not know what he is looking for will not understand what he finds.

—Claude Bernard

Future Prospects

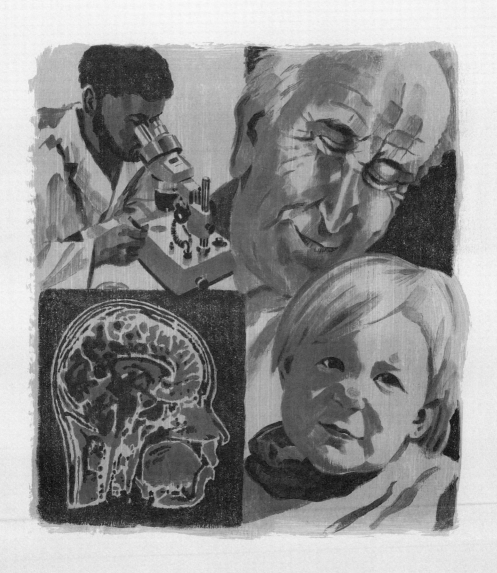

Promising Areas of Research

Robert A Kuwik
Judith A Martin

No great discovery is ever made without a bold guess.

—Isaac Newton

One cannot help but be tremendously encouraged by the explosion of knowledge that has occurred in the area of Alzheimer's disease etiology, diagnosis, and treatment in the last decade. After a long latent period during which very little movement took place, the war on Alzheimer's disease has been declared and victory is anticipated. We are now advancing on the fronts of genetics, biochemistry, molecular biology, imaging, and treatment like battalions relentlessly moving forward on a battlefield. It seems that it will be only a matter of time before we achieve a major breakthrough in halting or at least slowing the disease with a drug that is almost totally free of side effects. The decade of the 1990s has been named the "decade of the brain." It is certainly living up to its reputation. We wish to highlight some promising areas of research.

BIOMEDICAL ASPECTS

Genetics

Alzheimer's disease may have several underlying genetic causes. Three autosomal dominant genes—amyloid precursor protein (APP), presenilin I (PS I), and presenilin II (PS II)—cause an early onset (less than 65 years of age) familial form of Alzheimer's disease. Another autosomal gene called apolipoprotein E (APOE) may predispose an individual to develop the late onset (older than 65 years of age) form of Alzheimer's disease. Other as yet unmapped genes may also play roles in the causation of Alzheimer's disease and may be used in molecular testing.

Thus far no one specific clinical feature of Alzheimer's disease has been related to a particular gene. The first gene identified that causes Alzheimer's disease was the APP gene on chromosome 21, with estimates that between 4% and 20% of early onset, familial Alzheimer's disease are caused by a change in the APP gene. However, mutations within the PS I gene on chromosome 14 are a more common cause of this type of early onset, familial Alzheimer's disease, probably on the order of 50% of all such cases. Mutations in the PS II gene on chromosome 1 are a rare cause of Alzheimer's disease compared to APP and PS I. It is likely that additional Alzheimer's disease genetic loci will be found on either these three chromosomes or on other chromosomes. Most likely there will also be a focus on how and where these different gene products might interact to produce the underlying pathophysiologic defects of senile plaques and neurofibrillary tangles. Solving these types of questions should help to provide clues as to how to prevent and/or treat Alzheimer's disease either via sophisticated genetic treatments or standard biochemical and pharmaceutical means.

For the few families where a mutation can be found in APP, PS I, or PS II, the technique of mutation analysis can give an accurate assessment of whether an individual will develop Alzheimer's disease. However, the use of such genetic technology in order to do presymptomatic testing must be approached cautiously. Since there is no known effective therapeutic intervention for Alzheimer's disease yet, the negative effects of heightened worry and diminished hope may outweigh the benefits of improved awareness of Alzheimer's disease. Thus research efforts to explore the ethical implications of genetic technology will assist in the development and application of "best practice" parameters for genetic testing.

> In those families with cases of late onset Alzheimer's disease, the etiology of the illness will likely be found to be due to the admixture of genetic information and environmental factors.

The primary risk factors of advanced age and positive family history will be studied more meticulously in relation to the E4 allele of APOE on chromosome 19. Furthermore, whether and how head trauma, stroke, or female gender are related to this gene's role in the pathogenesis of late onset Alzheimer's disease will also be studied carefully in the next decade. Currently, however, APOE allelic analysis is not useful for predicting whether someone will develop Alzheimer's disease, largely because we do not comprehend the confluence of the genetic and the environmental factors. Conceivably at some future time, once the interaction between "nature" (genetics) and "nurture" (environment) is clarified, screening for APOE might allow individuals to make decisions about lifestyle changes in relation to the various risk factors, and thereby enhance prevention efforts.

Biochemistry/Physiology

Chapter 14 outlined the current application of cholinergic enhancement therapies in Alzheimer's disease. It also reviewed the potential roles of nonsteroidal antiinflammatory drugs (NSAIDs) and estrogen in the prevention and/or palliation of Alzheimer's disease. Recent reports raise the question of whether nicotine and vitamin E might have a similar positive effect in the attenuation of Alzheimer's disease. Future research is likely to deal with the judicious combination of these various therapeutic/preventive agents. For example, the use of a cholinesterase inhibitor like tacrine (Cognex) or donezepil (Aricept) could be linked to the use of an NSAID like ibuprofen (Motrin, Advil) to determine if there is an additive benefit. Alternatively, donezepil or tacrine could be used along with estrogen compounds in a cohort of females. END 713, metrifonate, selegiline, and vitamin E are other important compounds that will need to be carefully examined clinically, either alone or in combination with one another. Indeed, the recently published results of one such prototypical study involving 341 patients appeared to indicate that high doses of vitamin E or standard antiparkinson doses of selegiline can delay certain consequences of dementia. Such encouraging reports on palliative therapy will foster even more clinical trials in the near future. In addition, more complex pharmaceuticals like nerve growth factor, ganglioside(s), and the neuroimmuno-philins will be subject to careful clinical investigation in order to determine if alone, or in combinations, they may hold the solution to the puzzle of Alzheimer's disease.

In the future, family physicians, internists, geriatricians, neurologists, and psychiatrists will become more adept in neuropharmacology in an effort to minimize or to eliminate the destructive symptoms of Alzheimer's disease. Complex polypharmacy may be potentially as fruitful for Alzheimer's disease as combination therapy has been for Parkinson's disease, hypertension, and other serious chronic diseases of our population.

Radiography

The ongoing refinement and application of structural brain imaging techniques like computerized axial tomography (CAT) and magnetic resonance imaging (MRI) will enhance diagnostic capability with respect to Alzheimer's disease. Functional brain imaging procedures like single photon emission computerized tomography (SPECT) and positron emission tomography (PET) are going to be improved so that diagnostic ability will be much better, and therapeutic effectiveness can be monitored in a more immediate and responsive manner by visualizing changes in brain physiology as active therapies are applied. Of course the best basic scientists and engineers continue to work to develop new and even better devices and techniques for brain imaging.

PSYCHOSOCIAL ASPECTS

Executive Functioning/Activities of Daily Living

During the next decade it will be essential to apply scientific observation to the activities that are crucial in daily functioning in our society. Handling one's finances and driving are but two of the main areas for potential study. The development of a national model of how to objectify and standardize criteria for financial competency will constitute one major clinical challenge. Carefully controlled studies that coordinate the legal and psychiatric aspects of this area of competency are needed. Collaboration between the families of patients, local Alzheimer's disease chapters, and professional caregivers, including attorneys, in a team-oriented framework should produce "best practice" guidelines that should elevate the standard of care provided to Alzheimer's disease patients.

Another area that would benefit from the systematic application of research principles is that of driving safety and competency. Clinicians presently have no universally accepted method of assessing driving competency. Programs meant to perform this task are surprisingly scarce and research on driving ability is in its infancy. A promising development has been the introduction of virtual reality devices. Currently these are primarily used to entertain, but have great potential for clinical use. There is a genuine need for a shared database on this issue so that caregivers (family and professionals) can work to implement a course of remediation to upgrade residual skills or to enforce driving cessation. Once again the development of a "best practice" paradigm would enhance the successful education of Alzheimer's disease patients, caregivers, as well as appropriate local and state agencies. Such protocols to educate and counsel patients and responsible family members would help to overcome the difficult challenge of restricting mobility in a culture like ours, where independence and autonomy are highly valued.

Site of Care/Placement

Systematic research comparing home, day, and institutional care settings is ongoing. A holistic model that focuses on the needs of the individual patient with Alzheimer's disease, as well as the optimal circumstances for specific types of caregivers, will be delineated in the future. Outcomes research of this nature would ideally speed the evolution of treatment planning algorithms that would allow professionals and caregivers to time and sequence interventions in a more ideal manner, e.g., when to try day care enrichment programs, how and when to initiate nursing home placement.

Studies comparing different environmental designs, as well as the effect of variable staffing patterns, may allow us to determine how to best approach wandering and other problematic behaviors that involve psychomotor agitation. For example, research protocols evaluating color schemes, room layout, and other elements of unit design may lead to more naturalistic solutions to complex behavioral problems. Other research could address how lighting patterns and changes in the intensity and duration of light exposure affect "sundowning," a major management dilemma in many institutional settings.

Yet another fruitful area of study might include active testing of the "use it or lose it" approach to the residual cognitive skills of Alzheimer's disease patients. Adding a rich milieu of options like gardening, exposure to pet animals, and other vigorous psychosocial interventions to standard individual and group aspects of care like physical exercise, reality orientation, and occupational therapies might well allow us to document the benefits of such vigorous efforts. Tangible proof of the outcome of more intensive therapies will be needed to establish a rationale for investing in such therapies instead of simply warehousing the elderly Alzheimer's disease patient. Such a diligent effort will be increasingly essential in a managed health care environment where payers (private or governmental) are demanding the results of outcomes research before agreeing to reimburse for treatment(s).

Caregiver Stress

The benefits of support groups, as well as formal therapy groups, for the family and collateral caregivers seem to be apparent, at least at an intuitive level. However, the best way(s) to implement the educative and counseling elements of such groups are not completely clear. The optimal scheduling of initial and follow-up sessions so as to effectively reinforce training efforts has to be determined. The goals of delivering effective high quality and financially responsible care can be attained by implementing the "best practice" approach described earlier. How to time episodes of respite care so as to minimize the psychosocial trauma to both patient and caregiver could also be addressed by utilizing the systematic methods of basic and social sciences.

SUMMARY

The prospects for continued, steady improvement in the diagnosis and treatment of Alzheimer's disease will hinge on the energy and effort devoted to all types of research. This relentless pursuit of excellence is a hallmark of American medicine and has led to tremendous advances in the care of heart disease, cancer, HIV/AIDS, and other chronic ailments. The groundswell of interest in Alzheimer's disease may lead to one dazzling breakthrough discovery that will constitute the solution to Alzheimer's disease. It is more likely that an incremental series of advances will give us a sequence of clues that allow us to solve the riddle. In either scenario, the coordinated efforts of caregivers, professionals, as well as public and private entities, will be of crucial importance.

BIBLIOGRAPHY

Adler G, Rottunda SJ, Dysken MW: The driver with dementia, *Am J Geriat Psychiatry* 4(2):110-120, 1996.

Aisen PS, Davis KL: Inflammatory mechanisms in Alzheimer's disease: implication for therapy, *Am J Psychiatry* 151(8):1105-1113, 1994.

Bachman DL, Wolf PA, Linn R et al: Prevalence of dementia and probable senile dementia of the Alzheimer type in the Framingham Study, *Neurology* 42:115-119, 1992.

Evans DA, Funkenstein HH, Albert MS et al: Prevalence of Alzheimer disease in a community population of older persons: higher than previously reported, *JAMA* 262:2551-2556, 1989.

Hall GR, Gerdner L, Zwygart-Stauffacher M et al: Principles of nonpharmaco-logical management: caring for people with Alzheimer's disease using a conceptual model, *Psychiatr Ann* 25(7):432-440, 1995.

Hutton M, Busfield F, Wragg M et al: Complete analysis of the presenilin I gene in early onset Alzheimer disease, *Neuroport,* 7:801-805, 1996.

Katzman, Kawas: The epidemiology of dementia and Alzheimer disease. In Terry R, Katzman R, Bick K, editors: *Alzheimer disease,* New York, 1994, Raven Press, 105-122.

Kumar V, editor: Management of Alzheimer disease, *Psychiatr Ann* 26(5):261-288, 1996.

Lendon C, Ashall F, Goate A: Exploring the etiology of Alzheimer disease using molecular genetics, *JAMA* 277:825-832, 1997.

Payami H, Grimslid M, Oken B et al: A prospective study of cognitive health in the elderly (Oregon Brain Aging Study): effects of family history and apolipoprotein E genotype, *Am J Hum Genet* 60:948-956, 1997.

Payami H, Zareparsi S, Montee KR et al: Gender difference in apolipoprotein E associated risk for familial Alzheimer disease: a possible clue to the higher incidence of Alzheimer's disease in women, *Am J Hum Genet* 58:803-811, 1996.

Rao VS, Cupples A, Van Duijn CM: Evidence for major gene inheritance of Alzheimer disease in families of patients with and without apolipoprotein E epsilon 4, *Am J Hum Gen* 59:664-675, 1996.

Reyes-Ortiz CA, Modigh A: Promoting successful aging of the brain, *Clin Geriatr* 5(3):120-128, 1997.

Sano M, Ernesto C, Thomas RG et al: A controlled trial of selegiline, alpha-tocopherol, or both as treatment for Alzheimer's disease, *N Engl J Med* 336(17):1216-1222, 1997.

Schneider LS: New therapeutic approaches to Alzheimer disease, *J Clin Psychiatry* 57(Suppl 14):30-35, 1996.

Schneider LS, Olin JT, Pawcuczyk S: A double-blind crossover pilot study of L-deprenyl (Selegiline) combined with cholinesterase inhibitor in Alzheimer disease, *Am J Psychiatry* 150(2):321-323, 1993.

Snowdon DA, Greiner LH, Mortimer JA et al: Brain infarction and the clinical expression of Alzheimer disease—the nun study, *JAMA* 277(10):813-817, 1997.

Stern Y, Tang M, Albert M et al: Predicting time to nursing home care and death in individuals with Alzheimer disease, *JAMA* 277(10):806-812, 1997.

Strittmatter WJ, Saunders AM, Schmichel D et al: Apolipoprotein E: high avidity binding to beta-amyloid and increased frequency of type 4 allele in late onset familial Alzheimer disease, *Proc Natl Acad Sci USA* 90:1977-1981, 1993.

Sussman N: Facing our limitations: the accidental dilemma of drug augmentation (editorial), *Prim Psychiatry* 4(3)7, 1997.

Some Useful Addresses and Phone Numbers

Administration on Aging
330 Independence Ave, SW
Washington, DC 20201
Tel.: 202-619-1006

Agency for Health Care Policy and Research
US Department of Health and Human Services
2101 East Jefferson St., Suite 501
Rockville, MD 20852

Alliance for Aging Research
2021 K St. NW, Suite 305
Washington, DC 20006
Tel.: 202-293-2856
    800-639-2421

Alliance of Information and Referral Systems
P.O. Box 31668
Seattle, WA 98103
Tel.: 206-632-2477

Alzheimer's Association
919 N Michigan Ave, Suite 100
Chicago, IL, 60601
Tel.: 800-272-3900
    312-335-8700

Alzheimer's Disease Education and Referral Center National Institute of Aging
P.O. Box 8250
Silver Spring, MD 20907
Tel.: 800-438-4380
    301-495-3311

Alzheimer's Disease AHCPR Publications Clearinghouse
P.O. Box 8547
Silver Spring, MD 20907
Tel.: 800-358-9295

Alzheimer's Family Care
Parke-Davis
12051 Indian Creek Court
Beltsville, MD 20705
Tel.: 800-600-1600

American Academy of Family Physicians
8880 Ward Parkway
Kansas City, MO 64114
Tel.: 800-944-0000

American Association for Geriatric Psychiatry
7910 Woodmont, Suite 1350
Bethesda, MD 20814
Tel.: 301-654-7850

American Association of Homes and Services for the Aging
901 E St. NW, Suite 500
Washington DC, 20004
Tel.: 202-783-2242

American Association of Retired Persons (AARP)
601 E St. NW
Washington, DC 20049
Tel.: 202-434-2277
     800-424-3410

AARP Pharmacy Price Quote Center (Open 24 hours a day)
Tel.: 800-456-2226

American Bar Association Commission on Legal Problems of the Elderly
740 Fifteenth Street, NW
Washington, DC 20005
Tel.: 202-662-8690

American Federation for Aging Research
1414 Avenue of the Americas, 18th Floor
New York, NY 10019
Tel.: 212-752-2327

American Geriatrics Society
770 Lexington Ave., Suite 300
New York, NY 10021
Tel.: 212-308-1414

American Health Assistance Foundation
15825 Shady Grove Rd., Suite 140
Rockville, MD 20850
Tel.: 301-948-3244
    800-437-2423

American Health Care Association
1201 L St NW
Washington, DC 20005
Tel.: 202-842-4444

American Society on Aging
833 Market St., Suite 511
San Francisco, CA 94103
Tel.: 415-974-9600

Children of Aging Parents
1609 Woodbourne Road, Suite 302-A
Levittown, PA 19057
Tel.: 215-945-6900

Consortium to Establish a Registry for Alzheimer's Disease (CERAD)
Durham, NC
Tel.: 919-286-6405
    919-286-6406

Eldercare Locator
Washington, DC
Tel.: 800-677-1116

Family Caregiver Alliance
425 Bush St., Suite 500
San Francisco, CA 94108
Tel.: 415-434-3388
    800-445-8106

Family Service America
11700 W Lake Park Dr.
Milwaukee, WI 53224
Tel.: 414-359-1040

Food and Drug Administration
Information and Outreach Staff
HFE-88, Room 16-63
5600 Fishers Lane
Rockville, MD 29857
(301) 443-3170

Foundation for Hospice and Homecare
513 C St. NE
Washington, DC 20002
Tel.: 202-547-6586

French Foundation for Alzheimer Research
11620 Wilshire Blvd., Suite 820
Los Angeles, CA 90025
Tel.: 800-477-2243

Gerontological Society of America
1275 K St. NW, Suite 350
Washington, DC 20005
Tel.: 202-842-1275

Gray Panthers
2025 Pennsylvania Ave. NW, Suite 821
Washington, DC 20006
Tel.: 202-466-3132
      800-280-5362

Insurance Consumer Helpline
Washington, DC
Tel.: 800-942-4242

Medicare Hotline
Baltimore, MD
Tel.: 800-638-6833

National Alliance for the Mentally Ill
2101 Wilson Boulevard, Suite 302
Arlington, VA 22201
Tel.: 800-950-6264

National Association for Continence
P.O. Box 8310
Spartanburg, SC 29305
Tel.: 864-579-7900
      800-252-3337 (800-BLADDER)

National Association for Home Care
228 7th St. SE
Washington, DC 20003
Tel.: 202-547-7424

National Association of Professional Geriatric Care Managers
1604 North Country Club Rd
Tucson, AZ 85716
Tel.: 612-881-8008

National Association of Social Workers
750 1st St. NE
Washington, DC 20002
Tel.: 202-408-8600

National Citizens Coalition for Nursing Home Reform
1424 16th St. NW, Suite 202
Washington, DC 20036
Tel.: 202-332-2275

National Council on Aging
409 3rd St. SW, Suite 200
Washington, DC 20024
Tel.: 202-479-1200
       800-424-9046

National Foundation for Depressive Illness
P.O. Box 2257
New York, NY 10116
Tel.: 800-239-1265

National Hospice Organization
1901 N Moore St., Suite 901
Arlington, VA 22209
Tel.: 703-243-5900
       800-658-8898

National Institute on Adult Day Care
600 Maryland Avenue, SW, West Wing 100
Washington, DC 20024
Tel.: 202-479-1200

National Institute on Aging
Public Information Office
Federal Building, Room 6C12
Bethesda, MD 20892
Tel.: 301-496-1752

National Institute of Mental Health
Public Inquiries and Publications, Room 7C-02
5600 Fishers Lane
Rockville, MD 20857
Tel.: 301-443-4513

National Mental Health Association
1021 Prince St.
Alexandria, VA 22314
Tel.: 703-684-7722

National Parkinson's Foundation
East Coast: Miami, FL
Tel.: 800-327-4545
West Coast: Encino, CA
Tel.: 800-522-8855

National Stroke Association
96 Inverness Drive East, Suite 1
Englewood, CO 80112
Tel.: 303-649-9299
    800-787-6537 (800-STROKES)

Older Women's League
666 11th St. NW, Suite 700
Washington, DC 20001
Tel.: 202-783-6686

Social Security Information
Office of Public Inquiries
6401 Security Boulevard
Baltimore, MD 21235
Tel.: 410-965-7700
    800-772-1213

TriAD Disease Management Program
Pfizer Inc. and Eisai Inc.
Tel.: 888-874-2343

US Department of Veterans Affairs
810 Vermont Ave. NW
Washington, DC 20420
Tel.: 202-418-4343
    800-827-1000

ALZHEIMER'S DISEASE CENTERS PROGRAM DIRECTORY

The National Institute on Aging currently funds 29 Alzheimer's Disease Centers (ADCs) at major medical institutions across the nation. Researchers at these centers are working to translate research advances into improved care and diagnosis for Alzheimer's patients while, at the same time, focusing on the program's long-term goal—finding ways to cure and possibly prevent Alzheimer's disease.

Areas of investigation range from basic mechanisms of Alzheimer's disease to managing the symptoms and helping cope with the effects of the disease. Center staff conduct basic, clinical, and behavioral research.

Each of the 29 centers has its own unique areas of emphasis. One of the program's major benefits is the opportunity for collaborative studies that draw upon the expertise of scientists from many different disciplines.

Centers also have significant responsibilities related to information transfer and the training of scientists and health care providers new to Alzheimer's disease research. A common goal of the ADCs is to enhance research by providing a network for sharing new ideas as well as research results.

Currently, 27 ADC-affiliated satellite facilities offer diagnostic and treatment services and collect research data in underserved, rural, and minority communities.

For patients and families affected by Alzheimer's disease, many ADCs offer:
- Diagnosis and medical management (costs may vary—many centers accept Medicare, Medicaid, and private insurance)
- Information about the disease and services and resources
- Opportunities for volunteers to participate in drug trials and other clinical research projects (and support groups and other special programs for volunteers and their families)

For more information, you may contact any of the centers on the following list. While the name, address, and telephone number given are for the center director, you may ask for information about any of the activities described above and about offices and satellite clinics at other locations throughout the country.

For E-mail addresses of the directors of ADCs with Web Sites, see the Alzheimer's Disease Education and Referral (ADEAR) Center's Web Site at: http://www.alzheimers.org/adear/adcdir.html

ALABAMA

University of Alabama at Birmingham
Lindy E. Harrell, M.D., Ph.D.
Professor
Department of Neurology
University of Alabama at Birmingham
1720 7th Avenue South
Sparks Center 454
Birmingham, AL 35294-0017
Director's Tel: 205-934-3847
Director's Fax: 205-975-7365
Information: 205-934-9775

CALIFORNIA

University of California, Davis
William J. Jagust, M.D.
Director
University of California, Davis
Alzheimer's Disease Center
Alta Bates Medical Center
2001 Dwight Way
Berkeley, CA 94704
Director's E-mail: wjjagust@lbl.gov
Director's Tel: 510-204-4530
Director's Fax: 510-204-4524

University of California, Los Angeles
Jeffrey L. Cummings, M.D.
Professor
Department of Neurology and Psychiatry
University of California, Los Angeles
710 Westwood Plaza
Los Angeles, CA 90095-1769
Director's Tel: 310-206-5238
Director's Fax: 310-206-5287

University of California, San Diego
Leon Thal, M.D.
Chairman
Department of Neuroscience (0624)
University of California, San Diego School of Medicine
9500 Gilman Drive
La Jolla, CA 92093-0624
Director's E-mail: lthal@ucsd.edu
Director's Tel: 619-534-4606
Director's Fax: 619-534-2985
Information: 619-622-5800

University of Southern California
Caleb E. Finch, Ph.D. and Carl Cotman, Ph.D.
Co-Directors
Division of Neurogerontology
Ethel Percy Andrus Gerontology Center
University Park, MC-0191
University of Southern California
3715 McClintock Avenue
Los Angeles, CA 90089-0191
University of California at Irvine's Web Site: http://www.alz.uci.edu/

Dr. Finch's Tel: 213-740-1758
Dr. Finch's Fax: 213-740-0853
Dr. Cotman's Tel: 714-824-5847
Dr. Cotman's Fax: 714-824-2071
Information: 213-740-7777

GEORGIA

Emory University/VA Medical Center
Suzanne S. Mirra, M.D.
Professor
Department of Pathology and Laboratory Medicine
Emory University School of Medicine
VA Medical Center (151)
1670 Clairmont Road
Decatur, GA 30033
ADC's E-mail: emoryadc@emory.edu
Web Site: http://www.emory.edu/WHSC/MED/ADC
Director's Tel: 404-728-7714
Director's Fax: 404-728-7771

ILLINOIS

Northwestern University
Marsel Mesulam, M.D.
Director
Cognitive Neurology and Alzheimer's Disease Center
Northwestern University Medical School
320 East Superior Street, Searle 11-450
Chicago, IL 60611
Director's E-mail: mmesulam@nwu.edu
Web Site: http://www.brain.nwu.edu
Director's Tel: 312-908-9339
Director's Fax: 312-908-8789

Rush-Presbyterian-St. Luke's Medical Center
Denis A. Evans, M.D.
Professor of Medicine
Rush Alzheimer's Disease Center
Rush-Presbyterian-St. Luke's Medical Center
1645 West Jackson Boulevard, Suite 675
Chicago, IL 60612
ADCs E-mail: radc@neuro.rpslmc.edu
Web Site: http://www.rpslmc.edu/Med/RADC/

Director's Tel: 312-942-3350
Director's Fax: 312-942-2861
Information: 312-942-4463

INDIANA

Indiana University
Bernardino Ghetti, M.D.
Professor of Pathology, Psychiatry, and Medical and Molecular Genetics
Department of Pathology, MS-A142
Indiana Alzheimer's Disease Center
Indiana University School of Medicine
635 Barnhill Drive
Indianapolis, IN 46202-5120
Director's E-mail: bghetti@indyvax.iupui.edu
Web Site: http://medgen.iupui.edu/research/alzheimer/
Director's Tel: 317-274-1590
Director's Fax: 317-274-4882
Information: 317-278-2030

KANSAS

University of Kansas
Charles DeCarli, M.D.
Director
Department of Neurology
University of Kansas Medical Center
3901 Rainbow Boulevard
Kansas City, KS 66160-7314
Web Site: http://www.kumc.edu/instruction/medicine/neurology/resAD.html
Director's Tel: 913-588-6979
Director's Fax: 913-588-6965

KENTUCKY

University of Kentucky
William R. Markesbery, M.D.
Director
Sanders-Brown Research Center on Aging
University of Kentucky
101 Sanders-Brown Building
800 South Lime
Lexington, KY 40536-0230

Director's E-mail: wmarkesbery@aging.coa.uky.edu
Web Site: http://www.coa.uky.edu/
Director's Tel: 606-323-6040
Director's Fax: 606-323-2866

MARYLAND

The Johns Hopkins Medical Institutions
Donald L. Price, M.D.
Professor of Pathology, Neurology, and Neuroscience
The Johns Hopkins University School of Medicine
558 Ross Research Building
720 Rutland Avenue
Baltimore, MD 21205-2196
ADCs E-mail: adrc@welchlink.welch.jhu.edu
Director's Tel: 410-955-5632
Director's Fax: 410-955-9777

MASSACHUSETTS

Boston University
Neil William Kowall, M.D.
Boston University
Alzheimer's Disease Center
Geriatric Research, Education, and Clinical Center (182B)
Bedford VA Medical Center
200 Springs Road
Bedford, MA 01730
Director's E-mail: nkowall@bu.edu
Web Site: http://med-www.bu.edu/alzheimer/home.html
Director's Tel: 617-687-2632
Director's Fax: 617-687-3515
Information: 617-687-2916

Harvard Medical School/Massachusetts General Hospital
John H. Growdon, M.D.
Department of Neurology
Massachusetts Alzheimer's Disease Research Center
Massachusetts General Hospital
WAC 830
15 Parkman Street
Boston, MA 02114
Director's E-mail: growdon@helix.mgh.harvard.edu
Web Site: http://dem0nmac.mgh.harvard.edu/postings/Alzheimer.html

Director's Tel: 617-726 1728
Director's Fax: 617-726-4101

MICHIGAN

University of Michigan
Sid Gilman, M.D.
Professor and Chair
Department of Neurology
Michigan Alzheimer's Disease Research Center
University of Michigan
1914 Taubman Street
Ann Arbor, MI 48109-0316
Director's E-mail: sgilman@umich.med
Web Site: http://www.med.umich.edu/madrc/MADRC.html
Director's Tel: 313-936-9070
Director's Fax: 313-936-8763
Information: 313-764-2190

MINNESOTA

Mayo Clinic
Ronald Petersen, M.D., Ph.D.
Professor
Department of Neurology
Mayo Clinic
200 First Street SW
Rochester, MN 55905
Director's E-mail: peter8mayo.edu
Director's Tel: 507-284-4006
Director's Fax: 507-266-4752
Information: 507-284-1324

MISSOURI

Washington University
Leonard Berg, M.D.
Alzheimer's Disease Research Center
Washington University Medical Center
4488 Forest Park Avenue
St. Louis, MO 63108-2293
ADRCs E-mail: adrc@neuro.ewstl.edu
Web Site: http://www.biostat.wustl.edu/adrc/

Director's Tel: 314-286-2881
Director's Fax: 314-286-2763
Information: 314-286-2881

NEW YORK

Columbia University
Michael L. Shelanski, M.D., Ph.D.
Director
Alzheimer's Disease Research Center
Columbia University
Department of Pathology
630 West 168th Street
New York, NY 10032
Director's E-mail: mls7@columbia.edu
Director's Tel: 212-305-3300
Director's Fax: 212-305-5498
Information: 212-305-6553

Mount Sinai School of Medicine/Bronx VA Medical Center
Kenneth L. Davis, M.D.
Professor and Chairman
Department of Psychiatry
Mount Sinai School of Medicine
Mount Sinai Medical Center
1 Gustave L. Levy Place, Box #1230
New York, NY 10029-6574
Director's Tel: 212-824-7008
Director's Fax: 212-860-3945
Information: 212-241-8329
Fax: 212-996-0987

New York University
Steven H. Ferris, Ph.D.
Aging and Dementia Research Center
Department of Psychiatry (THN314)
New York University Medical Center
550 First Avenue
New York, NY 10016
Director's Tel: 212-263-5703
Director's Fax: 212-263-6991
Information: 212-263-5700

University of Rochester
Paul D. Coleman, Ph.D.

Director
Alzheimer's Disease Center
Department of Neurobiology and Anatomy, Box 603
University of Rochester Medical Center
601 Elmwood Avenue
Rochester, NY 14642
Director's E-mail: coleman@medinfo.rochester.edu
Director's Tel: 716-275-2581
Director's Fax: 716-273-1132
Information: 716-275-2581

NORTH CAROLINA

Duke University
Allen D. Roses, M.D.
Director
Joseph and Kathleen Bryan Alzheimer's Disease Research Center
2200 Main Street, Suite A-230
Durham, NC 27705
ADRC's E-mail: psansing@acpub.duke.edu
Director's Tel: 919-286-3228
Director's Fax: 919-286-3406
Information: 919-286-3228
Clinic: 919-286-7299

OHIO

Case Western Reserve University
Peter J. Whitehouse, M.D., Ph.D.
Director
Alzheimer's Disease Research Center
University Hospitals of Cleveland
11100 Euclid Avenue
Cleveland, OH 44106
Web Site: http://www.cwru.edu/orgs/adsc/intro.html
Director's Tel: 216-844-7360
Director's Fax: 216-844-7239

OREGON

Oregon Health Sciences University
Jeffrey A. Kaye, M.D.
Director

Oregon Alzheimer's Disease Center (L226)
Oregon Health Sciences University
3181 SW Sam Jackson Park Road
Portland, OR 97201-3098
Director's E-mail: kaye@ohsu.edu
Director's Tel: 503-494-6976
Director's Fax: 503-494-7499
Information: 503-494-6976

PENNSYLVANIA

University of Pennsylvania
John Q. Trojanowski, M.D., Ph.D.
Professor
Pathology and Laboratory Medicine
University of Pennsylvania School of Medicine
Room A009, Basement Maloney/HUP
36th and Spruce Streets
Philadelphia, PA 19104-4283
Director's E-mail: trojanow@mail.med.upenn.edu
Director's Tel: 215-662-6399
Director's Fax: 215-349-5909
Information: 215-662-6921

University of Pittsburgh
Steven DeKosky, M.D.
Director
Alzheimer's Disease Research Center
University of Pittsburgh Medical Center
Montefiore University Hospital, 4 West
200 Lothrop Street
Pittsburgh, PA 15213
Director's E-mail: dekosky@vms.cls.pitt.edu
Director's Tel: 412-624-6889
Director's Fax: 412-624-7814
Information: 412-692-2700

TEXAS

Baylor College of Medicine
Stanley H. Appel, M.D.
Director
Alzheimer's Disease Research Center
Department of Neurology

Baylor College of Medicine
6501 Fannin, NB302
Houston, TX 77030-3498
Director's E-mail: lappel@bcm.tmc.edu
Web Site: http://www.bcm.tmc.edu/neurol/struct/adrc/adrcl.html
Director's Tel: 713-798-6660
Director's Fax: 713-798-8573
Information: 713-798-6660

University of Texas, Southwestern Medical Center
Roger N. Rosenberg, M.D.
Director
Alzheimer's Disease Research Center
Zale Distinguished Chair and Professor of Neurology and Physiology
University of Texas
Southwestern Medical Center at Dallas
5323 Harry Hines Boulevard
Dallas, TX 75235-9036
Director's Tel: 214-648-3239
Director's Fax: 214-648-6824
Information: 214-648-3198

WASHINGTON

University of Washington
George A. Martin, M.D.
Director
Alzheimer's Disease Research Center
Department of Pathology
Box 357470, HSB K-543
University of Washington
1959 NE Pacific Avenue
Seattle, WA 98195-7470
Director's E-mail: gmmartin@u.washington.edu
Director's Tel: 206-543-5088
Director's Fax: 206-685-8356
Information: 206-543-6761

Additional References

Appendix B

The following is a list of references that may be of interest to some of our readers who may wish to acquire a more in-depth knowledge of the subject.

CLINICAL MANIFESTATIONS

Armstrong RA, Syed AB: Alzheimer's disease and the eye, *Ophthalmic Physiol Opt* 16 Suppl 1: S2-8, March 1996.

Brooks JO III: A comment on age at onset as a subtype of Alzheimer disease, *Alzheimer Dis Assoc Disord* 9 Suppl 1: S28-9, 1995.

Brooks JO III, Yesavage JA: Identification of fast and slow decliners in Alzheimer disease: a different approach, *Alzheimer Dis Assoc Disord* 9 Suppl 1: S19-25, 1995.

Esiri MM: The basis for behavioural disturbances in dementia [editorial], *J Neurol Neurosurg Psychiatry* 61(2): 127-30, August 1996.

Herskovits E: Struggling over subjectivity: debates about the "self" and Alzheimer's disease, *Med Anthropol Q* 9(2): 146-64, June 1995.

Lyketsos CG, Corazzini K, Steele C: Mania in Alzheimer's disease, *J Neuropsychiatry Clin Neurosci* 7(3): 350-2, Summer 1995.

Migliorelli R, Teson A, Sabe L et al: Anosognosia in Alzheimer's disease: a study of associated factors, *J Neuropsychiatry Clin Neurosci* 7(3): 338-44, Summer 1995.

Prince MJ: Predicting the onset of Alzheimer's disease using Bayes' theorem, *Am J Epidemiol* 143(3): 301-8, February 1, 1996.

Randolph C, Tierney MC, Chase TN: Implicit memory in Alzheimer's disease, *J Clin Exp Neuropsychol* 17(3): 343-51, May 1995.

Raskind MA, Carta A, Bravi D: Is early-onset Alzheimer disease a distinct subgroup within the Alzheimer disease population? *Alzheimer Dis Assoc Disord* 9 Suppl 1: S2-6, 1995.

Ripich DN, Petrill SA, Whitehouse PJ et al: Gender differences in language of AD patients: a longitudinal study, *Neurology* 45(2): 299-302, February 1995.

Sandson TA, Sperling RA, Price BH: Alzheimer's disease: an update, *Compr Ther* 21(9): 480-5, September 1995.

Stern Y, Jacobs DM: Preliminary findings from the predictors study: utility of clinical signs for predicting disease course, *Alzheimer Dis Assoc Disord* 9 Suppl 1: S14-8, 1995.

Talwalker S, Overall JE, Srirama MK et al: Cardinal features of cognitive dysfunction in Alzheimer's disease: a factor-analytic study of the Alzheimer's Disease Assessment Scale, *J Geriatr Psychiatry Neurol* 9(1): 39-46, January 1996.

Terry RD: Biologic differences between early- and late- onset Alzheimer disease, *Alzheimer Dis Assoc Disord* 9 Suppl 1: S26-7, 1995.

Trick GL, Trick LR, Morris P et al: Visual field loss in senile dementia of the Alzheimer's type, *Neurology* 45(1): 68-74, January 1995.

DIAGNOSIS

Forstl H, Hentschel F, Sattel H et al: Age-associated memory impairment and early Alzheimer's disease. Only time will tell the difference, *Arneimittelforschung* 45(3A): 394-7, March 1995.

George AE, Holodny A, Golomb et al: The differential diagnosis of Alzheimer's disease. Cerebral atrophy versus normal pressure hydrocephalus, *Neuroimaging Clin N Am* 5(1): 19-31, February, 1995.

Hansen LA, Crain BJ: Making the diagnosis of mixed and non-Alzheimer's dementias, *Arch Pathol Lab Med* 119(11): 1023-31, November 1995.

Herholz K: FDG PET and differential diagnosis of dementia, *Alzheimer Dis Assoc Disord* 9(1): 6-16, Spring 1995.

Hock C, Villringer K, Muller-Spahn F et al: Near infrared spectroscopy in the diagnosis of Alzheimer's disease, *Ann N Y Acad Sci* 777: 22-9, January 17, 1996.

Jagust WJ: Functional imaging patterns in Alzheimer's disease. Relationships to neurobiology, *Ann N Y Acad Sci* 777: 30-6, January 17, 1996.

Jagust WJ, Johnson KA, Holman BL: SPECT perfusion imaging in the diagnosis of dementia, *J Neuroimaging* 5 Suppl 1: S45-52, July 1995.

Klatka LA, Schiffer RB, Powers JM et al: Incorrect diagnosis of Alzheimer's disease. A clinicopathologic study, *Arch Neurol* 53(1): 35-42, January 1996.

Kolanowski A: Everyday functioning in Alzheimer's disease: contribution of neuropsychological testing [see comments], *Clin Nurse Spec* 10(1): 11-7, 56; quiz 18-9, January 1996.

McClure RJ, Kanfer JN, Panchalingam K et al: Magnetic resonance spectroscopy and its application to aging and Alzheimer's disease, *Neuroimaging Clin N Am* 5(1): 69-86, February 1995.

National Institute of Aging/Alzheimer's Association Working Group: Apolipoprotein E genotyping in Alzheimer's disease, *Lancet* 347(9008): 1091-5, April 20, 1996.

Newberg AB, Alavi A, Payer F: Single photon emission computed tomography in Alzheimer's disease and related disorders, *Neuroimaging Clin N Am* 5(1): 103-23, February 1995.

Ott BR, Noto RB, Fogel BS: Apathy and loss of insight in Alzheimer's disease: a SPECT imaging study, *J Neuropsychiatry Clin Neurosci* 8(1): 41-6, Winter 1996.

Rosiers G, Hodges JR, Berrios G: The neuropsychological differentiation of patients with very mild Alzheimer's disease and/or major depression, *J Am Geriatr Soc* 43(11): 1256-63, November 1995.

Rossor MN, Kennedy AM, Frackowiak RS: Clinical and neuroimaging features of familial Alzheimer disease, *Ann N Y Scad Sci* 777: 49-56, January 17, 1996.

Sandson TA, Price BH: Diagnostic testing and dementia, *Neurol Clin* 14(1): 45-59, February 1996; *Eur J Radiol*, 21(3): 183-7, February 1996.

Schellenberg GD: Progress in Alzheimer's disease genetics, *Curr Opin Neurol* 8(4): 262-7, August 1995.

Smith CD: Quantitative computed tomography and magnetic resonance imaging in aging and Alzheimer's disease. A review, *J Neuroimaging* 6(1): 44-53, January 1996.

Soininen H, Helkala EL, Kuikka J et al: Regional cerebral blood flow measured by 99mTc-HMPAO SPECT differs in subgroups of Alzheimer's disease, *J Neural Transm Park Dis Dement Sect* 9(2-3): 95-109, 1995.

Standish TI, Molloy DW, Bedard M et al: Strang-DImproved reliability of the Standardized Alzheimer's Disease Assessment Scale (SADAS) compared with Alzheimer's Disease Assessment Scale (ADAS), *J Am Geriatr Soc* 44(6): 712-6, June 1996.

Starkstein SE, Vazquez S, Merello M et al: A SPECT study of parkinsonism in Alzheimer's disease, *J Neuropsychiatry Clin Neurosci* 7(3): 308-13, Summer 1995.

Stoppe G, Staedt J, Kogler A et al: 99mTc-HMPAO-SPECT in the diagnosis of senile dementia of Alzheimer's type—a study under clinical routine conditions, *J Neural Transm Gen Sect* 99(1-3): 195-211, 1995.

Talbot PR, Testa HJ: The value of SPECT imaging in dementia, *Nucl Med Commun* 16(6): 425-37, June 1995.

EPIDEMIOLOGY

Corrada M, Brookmeyer R, Kawas C: Sources of variability in prevalence rates of Alzheimer's disease, *Int J Epidemiol* 24(5): 1000-5, October 1995.

Keefover RW: The clinical epidemiology of Alzheimer's disease, *Neurol Clin* 14(2): 337-51, May 1996.

van Duijn CM: Epidemiology of the dementias: recent developments and new approaches, *J Neurol Neurosurg Psychiatry* 60(5): 478-88, May 1996.

ETIOLOGY

Harman D: A hypothesis on the pathogenesis of Alzheimer's disease, *Ann N Y Acad Sci* 786: 152-68, June 15, 1996.

Harvey RJ, Rossor MN: Does early-onset Alzheimer disease constitute a distinct subtype? The contribution of molecular genetics, *Alzheimer Dis Assoc Disord* 9 Suppl 1: S7-13, 1995.

Hull M, Strauss S, Berger M et al: Inflammatory mechanisms in Alzheimer's disease, *Eur Arch Psychiatry Clin Neurosci* 246(3): 124-8, 1996.

Ii K: The role of beta-amyloid in the development of Alzheimer's disease, *Drugs Aging* 7(2): 97-109, August 1995.

Mera SL: Alzheimer's disease: genetics or environment? *Br J Biomed Sci* 53(2): 91-2, June 1996.

Mortel KF, Meyer JS: Lack of postmenopausal estrogen replacement therapy and the risk of dementia, *J Neuropsychiatry Clin Neurosci* 7(3): 334-7, Summer 1995.

Oken RJ, McGeer PL: Schizophrenia, Alzheimer's disease, and anti-inflammatory agents, *Schizophr Bull* 22(1): 1-4, 1996.

Pericak Vance MA, Haines JL: Genetic susceptibility to Alzheimer's disease, *Trends Genet* 11(12): 504-8, December 1995.

Riggs JE: The "protective" influence of cigarette smoking on Alzheimer's and Parkinson's diseases. Quagmire or opportunity for neuroepidemiology? *Neurol Clin* 14(2): 353-8, May 1996.

Rogers J: Inflammation as a pathogenic mechanism in Alzheimer's disease, *Arzneimittelforschung* 45(3A): 439-42, March 1995.

Roses AD: Apolipoprotein E alleles as risk factors in Alzheimer's disease, *Annu Rev Med* 47: 387-400, 1996.

Rossor MN: Catastrophe, chaos and Alzheimer's disease. The F E Williams Lecture, *J R Coll Physicians Lond* 29(5): 412-8, September-October, 1995.

Savory J, Exle C, Forbes WF et al: Can the controversy of the role of aluminum in Alzheimer's disease be resolved? What are the suggested approaches to this controversy and methodological issues to be considered? *J Toxicol Environ Health* 48(6): 615-35, August 30, 1996.

Smith MA, Perry G: Free radical damage, iron, and Alzheimer's disease, *J Neurol Sci* 134 Suppl: 92-4, December 1995.

St George Hyslop P: Genetic determinants of Alzheimer disease, *Prog Clin Biol Res* 393: 139-45, 1995.

Yankner BA: New clues to Alzheimer's disease: unraveling the roles of amyloid and tau [comment], *Nat Med* 2(8): 850-2, August 1996.

MANAGEMENT

Bedard M, Molloy DW, Standish T et al: Clinical trials in cognitively impaired older adults: home versus clinic assessments, *J Am Geriatr Soc* 43(10): 1127-30, October 1995.

Brennan PF, Moore SM, Smyth KA: The effects of a special computer network on caregivers of persons with Alzheimer's disease, *Nurs Res* 44(3): 166-72, May-June 1995.

Clipp EC, Moore MJ: Caregiver time use: an outcome measure in clinical trial research on Alzheimer's disease, *Clin Pharmacol Ther* 58(2): 228-36, August 1995.

Cohen GD: Management of Alzheimer's disease, *Adv Intern Med* 40: 31-67, 1995.

Devanand DP, Levy SR: Neuroleptic treatment of agitation and psychosis in dementia, *J Geriatr Psychiatry Neurol* 8 Suppl 1: S18-27, October 1995.

Golden R: Dementia and Alzheimer's disease. Indications, diagnosis, and treatment [see comments] *Minn Med* 78(1): 25-9, January 1995.

Griffith CH III, Wilson JF, Emmett KR et al: Knowledge and experience with Alzheimer's disease. Relationship to resuscitation preference, *Arch Fam Med* 4(9): 780-4, September 1995.

Hewawasam L: Floor patterns limit wandering of people with Alzheimer's, *Nurs Times* 92(22): 41-4, May 29-June 4, 1996.

Hollister L, Gruber N: Drug treatment of Alzheimer's disease. Effects on caregiver burden and patient quality of life, *Drugs Aging* 8(1): 47-55, January 1996.

Kirby M, Lawlor BA: Biologic markers and neurochemical correlates of agitation and psychosis in dementia, *J Geriatr Psychiatry Neurol* 8 Suppl 1: S2-7, October 1995.

Knesper JD: The depressions of Alzheimer's disease: sorting, pharmacotherapy, and clinical advice, *J Geriatr Psychiatry Neurol* 8 Suppl 1: S40-51, October 1995.

Lemke MR: Effect of carbamazepine on agitation in Alzheimer's inpatients refractory to neuroleptics, *J Clin Psychiatry* 56(8): 354-7, August 1995.

Marchello V, Boczko F, Shelkey M: Progressive dementia: strategies to manage new problem behaviors, *Geriatrics* 50(3): 40-3; quiz 44-5, March 1995.

Mendez MF: Dementia and guns [see comments], *J Am Geriatr Soc* 44(4): 409-10, April 1996.

Pheiffer E: Institutional placement for patients with Alzheimer's disease. How to help families with a difficult decision, *Postgrad Med* 97(1): 125-6, 129-32, January 1995.

Procter AW: Psychopharmacology of Alzheimer's disease, *Br J Hosp Med* 55(4): 191-4, February 21-March 5, 1996.

Quayhagen MP, Quayhagen M: Discovering life quality in coping with dementia, *West J Nurs Res* 18(2): 120-35, April 1996.

Sambandham M, Schirm V: Music as a nursing intervention for residents with Alzheimer's disease in long-term care, *Geriatr Nurs* 16(2): 79-83, March-April 1995.

Sloane PD, Lindeman DA, Phillips C et al: Evaluating Alzheimer's special care units: reviewing the evidence and identifying potential sources of study bias, *Gerontologist* 35(1): 103-11, February 1995.

Snyder M, Egan EC, Burns KR: Interventions for decreasing agitation behaviors in persons with dementia, *J Gerontol Nurs* 21(7): 34-40, July 1995.

OTHER DEMENTIAS

Beck J: Neuropsychiatric manifestations of diffuse Lewy body disease, *J Geriatr Psychiatry Neurol* 8(3): 189-96, July 1995.

Bowler JV, Hachinski V: Vascular cognitive impairment: a new approach to vascular dementia, *Baillieres Clin Neurol* 4(2): 357-76, August 1995.

Butters N, Delis DC, Lucas JA: Clinical assessment of memory disorders in amnesia and dementia, *Annu Rev Psychol* 46: 493-523, 1995.

Cummings JL: Lewy body diseases with dementia: pathophysiology and treatment, *Brain Cogn* 28(3): 266-80, August 1995.

Filley CM: Neuropsychiatric features of Lewy body disease, *Brain Cogn* 28(3): 229-39, August 1995.

Kalra S, Bergeron C, Lang AE: Lewy body disease and dementia. A review, *Arch Intern Med* 156(5): 487-93, March 11, 1996.

Katzman R, Galasko D, Saitoh T et al: Genetic evidence that the Lewy body variant is indeed a phenotypic variant of Alzheimer's disease, *Brain Cogn* 28(3): 259-65, August 1995.

PATHOLOGY

Braak H, Braak E: Staging of Alzheimer's disease-related neurofibrillary changes, *Neurobiol Aging* 16(3): 271-8; discussion 278-84, May-June 1995.

Haass C: The molecular significance of amyloid beta-peptide for Alzheimer's disease, *Eur Arch Psychiatry Clin Neurosci* 246(3): 118-23, 1996.

Octave JN: The amyloid peptide and its precursor in Alzheimer's disease, *Rev Neurosci* 6(4): 287-316, October-December, 1995.

TREATMENT

Baldinger SL, Shroeder DJ: Nicotine therapy in patients with Alzheimer's disease, *Ann Pharmacother* 29(3): 314-5, March 1995.

Brietner JC: The role of anti-inflammatory drugs in the prevention and treatment of Alzheimer's disease, *Annu Rev Med* 47: 401-11, 1996.

Corey-Bloom J, Galasko D: Adjunctive therapy in patients with Alzheimer's disease. A practical approach, *Drugs Aging* 7(2): 79-87, August 1995.

Domingo JL: Adverse effects of potential agents for the treatment of Alzheimer's disease: a review, *Adverse Drug React Toxicol Rev* 14(2): 101-15, Summer 1995.

Eagger SA, Harvey RJ: Clinical heterogeneity: responders to cholinergic therapy, *Alzheimer Dis Assoc Disord* 9 Suppl 2: 37-42, 1995.

Fakouhi TD, Jhee SS, Sramek JJ et al: Evaluation of cycloserine in the treatment of Alzheimer's disease, *J Geriatr Psychiatry Neurol* 8(4): 226-30, October 1995.

Filley CM: Alzheimer's disease: it's irreversible but not untreatable, *Geriatrics* 50(7): 18-23, July 1995.

Frolich L, Riederer P: Free radical mechanisms in dementia of Alzheimer type and the potential for antioxidative treatment, *Arzneimittelforschung* 45(3A): 443-6, March 1995.

Harvey R, Rosseror M: Treatments for Alzheimer's disease, *Practitioner* 239(1552): 440-3, July 1995.

Hock FJ: Therapeutic approaches for memory impairments, *Behav Brain Res* 66(1-2): 143-50, January 23, 1995.

Huff FJ: Preliminary evaluation of besipirdine for the treatment of Alzheimer's disease. Besipirdine Study Group, *Ann N Y Acad Sci* 777: 410-4, January 17, 1996.

Jinnah HA, Friedmann T: Gene therapy and the brain, *Br Med Bull* 51(1): 138-48, January 1995.

Kanowski S, Herrmann WM, Stephan K et al: Proof of efficacy of the ginkgo biloba special extract EGb 761 in outpatients suffering from mild to moderate primary degenerative dementia of the Alzheimer type or multi-infarct dementia, *Pharmacopsychiatry* 29(2): 47-56, March 1996.

Lyketsos CG, Corazzini K, Steele CD et al: Guidelines for the use of tacrine in Alzheimer's disease: clinical application and effectiveness. Johns Hopkins Dementia Research Clinic, *J Neuropsychiatry Clin Neurosci* 8(1): 67-73, Winter 1996.

Marin DB, Bierer LM, Lawlor BA et al: L-deprenyl and physostigmine for the treatment of Alzheimer's disease, *Psychiatry Res* 58(3): 181-9, October 16, 1995.

Martin JB: Gene therapy and pharmacological treatment of inherited neurological disorders, *Trends Biotechnol* 13(1): 28-35, January 1995.

McCarten JR, Kovera C, Maddox MK et al: Triazolam in Alzheimer's disease: pilot study on sleep and memory effects, *Pharmacol Biochem Behav* 52(2): 447-52, October 1995.

McGeer PL, McGeer EG: Anti-inflammatory drugs in the fight against Alzheimer's disease, *Ann N Y Acad Sci* 777: 213-20, January 17, 1996.

Messier C, Gagnon M: Glucose regulation and cognitive functions: relation to Alzheimer's disease and diabetes, *Behav Brain Res* 75(1-2): 1-11, February 1996.

Mimori Y, Katsuoka H, Nakamura S: Thiamine therapy in Alzheimer's disease, *Metab Brain Dis* 11(1): 89-94, March 1996.

Mohr E, Knott V, Sampson M et al: Cognitive and quantified electroencephalographic correlates of cycloserine treatment in Alzheimer's disease, *Clin Neuropharmacol* 18(1): 28-38, February 1995.

Paganini Hill A: Oestrogen replacement therapy and Alzheimer's disease, *Br J Obstet Gynaecol* 103 Suppl 13: 80-6, May 1996.

Parnetti L: Clinical pharmacokinetics of drugs for Alzheimer's disease, *Clin Pharmacokinet* 29(2): 110-29, August 1995.

Parnetti L, Ambrosoli L, Abate G et al: Posatirelin for the treatment of late-onset Alzheimer's disease: a double-blind multicentre study vs citicoline and ascorbic acid, *Acta Neurol Scand* 92(2): 135-40, August 1995.

Patel SV: Pharmacotherapy of cognitive impairment in Alzheimer's disease: a review, *J Geriatr Psychiatry Neurol* 8(2): 81-95, April 1995.

Rother M, Kittner B, Rudolphi K et al: HWA 285 (propentofylline)—a new compound for the treatment of both vascular dementia and dementia of the Alzheimer type, *Ann N Y Acad Sci* 777: 404-9, January 17, 1996.

Schneider LS, Farlow MR, Henderson VW et al: Effects of estrogen replacement therapy on response to tacrine in patients with Alzheimer's disease, *Neurology* 46(6): 1580-4, June 1996.

Schwartz BL, Hashtroudi S, Herting RL et al: Id-Cycloserine enhances implicit memory in Alzheimer patients, *Neurology* 46(2): 420-4, February 1996.

Soares JC, Gershon S: THA—historical aspects, a review of pharmacological properties and therapeutic effects, *Dementia* 6(4): 225-34, July-August 1995.

Sramek JJ, Anand R, Wardle TS et al: Safety/tolerability trial of SDZ ENA 713 in patients with probable Alzheimer's disease, *Life Sci* 58(15): 1201-7, 1996.

Sramek JJ, Hurley DJ, Wardle TS et al: The safety and tolerance of xanomeline tartrate in patients with Alzheimer's disease, *J Clin Pharmacol* 35(8): 800-6, August 1995.

Whitehouse PJ, Voci J: Therapeutic trials in Alzheimer's disease, *Curr Opin Neurol* 8(4): 275-8, August 1995.

Wilcock GK, Harrold PL: Treating Alzheimer's disease, *QJM* 88(9): 673-6, September 1995.

Wilson AL, Langley LK, Monley J et al: Nicotine patches in Alzheimer's disease: pilot study on learning, memory, and safety, *Pharmacol Biochem Behav* 51(2-3): 509-14, June-July 1995.

Wood DM, Ford JM, Roberts CJ: Variability in the plasma protein binding of velnacrine (1-hydroxy tacrine hydrochloride). A potential agent for Alzheimer's disease, *Eur J Clin Pharmacol* 50(1-2): 115-9, 1996.

Zemlan FP, Keys M, Richter RW et al: Double-blind placebo-controlled study of velnacrine in Alzheimer's disease, *Life Sci* 58(21): 1823-32, 1996.

Glossary

abscess Accumulation of pus caused by infection.

abstracting ability Ability to shift voluntarily from one aspect of a situation to another. A characteristic of Alzheimer's disease and other psychiatric disorders is the inability to shift readily from the concrete to the abstract and back again as demanded by circumstances.

abulia Loss or impairment of the ability to perform voluntary actions or to make decisions.

acetylcholine Neurotransmitter that is deficient in patients with Alzheimer's disease.

agnosia Inability to recognize various objects. Although agnosia often is present in the early stages of Alzheimer's disease, it may be so subtle and slight that it goes unnoticed. In the early stages of Alzheimer's disease, this condition can be recognized only through detailed psychological tests.

akathisia Syndrome characterized by an inability to remain in the sitting position because of motor restlessness and a feeling of muscular quivering.

akinesia Absence or loss of the power of voluntary motion.

amitriptyline (Elavil) Tricylic antidepressant commonly given at bedtime. It has both sedative and anticholinergic side effects.

amnesia Memory impairment.

amyloid deposition Deposit of an abnormal protein (amyloid) in the brain of a patient with Alzheimer's disease.

analgesics Medications used to relieve pain; painkillers.

angina See **anginal pain.**

anginal pain Chest pain experienced by a patient with coronary artery disease. Typically the pain occurs during exercise and is relieved by rest or appropriate medication. If such measures do not relieve the pain within a few minutes, the patient may have developed a myocardial infarction.

anhedonia   Loss of pleasure in things that normally interest the individual.

anomia   Difficulty in finding the correct word for an object. For example, the patient may recognize a pencil and may know what it is used for but may be unable to think of the word "pencil." Often the patient uses a sentence to describe a particular word. For instance, instead of "pencil," the patient may say "the thing you use to write with," or instead of "key," he may say "the thing used to open a door." Anomia is one of the first manifestations of Alzheimer's disease. Usually the patient initially has difficulty naming objects that he does not deal with in everyday life.

anosognosia   Failure to recognize a disease or deficit.

antacids   Drugs given to reduce the acidity of the contents of the stomach.

antibiotics   Group of drugs used to combat infection. For severe infections, antibiotics usually are administered intravenously. In most other cases, they are administered orally.

anticholinergic side effects   Side effects produced by medication that inhibit the parasympathetic branch of the autonomic nervous system (e.g., dry mouth, blurred vision, urinary retention). Medications with anticholinergic side effects include antihistamines, neuroleptic drugs, and antidepressants. These drugs sometimes are combined with antacids.

antihistamines   Drugs taken for allergies and the common cold. Most antihistamines induce a certain degree of drowsiness and may cause sedation. They often are included in sleeping medications bought over the counter.

apathy   Condition in which the patient shows little or no emotion.

aphasia   Impairment in the speech process. *Receptive aphasia* is an inability to comprehend what one hears. *Expressive aphasia* is an inability to express oneself, even though the question has been heard and understood. The two types of aphasia can be differentiated by asking the patient to execute a certain command, such as closing the eyes, sticking out the tongue, or raising the left arm. If the patient hears and understands what is being said, he will execute the command. If he cannot hear or cannot comprehend what he hears (receptive aphasia), he will be unable to comply. When these commands are given, it is important not to mimic the gesture that the patient is expected to perform. For instance, while asking the patient to raise his arm, the examiner must refrain from raising an arm.

apnea   Cessation of breathing. *Sleep apnea* is the cessation of breathing while sleeping, which characteristically occurs in grossly overweight and obese individuals. With apnea, insufficient oxygen reaches the brain, and the individual may wake up distressed.

apolipoprotein E (APOE)   Type of protein that is attached to a fat molecule, which transports cholesterol in the bloodstream. According to the genes inherited, 3 different forms of apolipoprotein E can be present: E2, E3, or E4. Whereas E2 appears to protect the person from developing Alzheimer's disease, E4 appears to predispose to it.

apraxia   Inability to carry out purposeful movements and actions despite intact motor and sensory systems. Apraxia usually is present early in Alzheimer's disease, but it may be confined to actions that the patient does not routinely perform during daily activities. For example, the patient may not be able to tie a bow tie but may still be able to tie a regular tie. This situation is often attributed to a lack of practice. In the early stages, apraxia may be more apparent when the patient faces several choices. He may have no difficulty putting his shirt on, but when faced with a variety of shirts, ties, underwear, trousers, and coats, he may become confused as to which one to pick first. As the disease progresses, apraxia comes to affect even daily activities, and the patient no longer can dress, feed, or wash himself, even though he has no paralysis.

Aricept   Name of a medication (donezepil) approved for the treatment of Alzheimer's disease. The usual dose is 5 to 10 mg once a day, preferably in the evening, to be taken with or without food. It is meant to have few side effects and no toxic effect on the liver. Monitoring of liver functions by regular blood tests is not necessary.

arteriosclerosis   Condition in which the inner lining of the arteries is coated with cholesterol, triglycerides, and other fatty substances. This deposition, which often also invades other layers of an artery, causes the arteries to become rigid and their lumens to narrow. This change diminishes the amount of blood that flows through these arteries and the amount that reaches the various organs supplied by them. If arteriosclerosis affects the arteries that carry blood to the brain, the blood supply to the brain is reduced and the patient is at increased risk of developing a stroke.

aspiration pneumonia   Pneumonia caused by inhaling gastric contents or food into the lungs.

asthma   Disease in which the trachea and the bronchi (airways) become constricted, reducing the amount of air that reaches the lungs. Asthma characteristically occurs in attacks, with the patient experiencing sudden breathlessness and an inability to breathe comfortably. In many instances asthma reflects an allergic reaction to a number of substances that may contain pollen. Asthmatic attacks also are often precipitated by smoking.

ataxia   Inability to coordinate voluntary actions.

atrophy   Wasting of tissues, organs, or the entire body. One of the characteristic features of Alzheimer's disease is the wasting away of the brain, which becomes much smaller than that of an individual of the same age and sex who does not have the disease.

atypical antipsychotics   New drugs used to treat delusional and/or hallucinating patients. They have few extrapyramidal side effects and include: clozaril (clozapine), riperdal (resiperidone) and zyprexa (olanzepine).

audiometric testing   Use of an electrical instrument to measure hearing acuity.

autoanalysis   See **biochemical screening**.

autonomic nervous system   Part of the nervous system that is not under voluntary control. The autonomic nervous system has two main subdivisions: parasympathetic and sympathetic. On the whole, the parasympathetic system takes over while a person is relaxing or sleeping, whereas the sympathetic system is active predominantly when an individual is in an excited state.

benzodiazepines   Class of drugs used to treat anxiety and insomnia. The group includes flurazepam (Dalmane), chlordiazepoxide (Librium), diazepam (Valium), and alprazolam (Xanax). Some patients become addicted to these drugs, and abrupt withdrawal may lead to seizures.

b.i.d.   (Latin: *bis in die*) Abbreviation designating that a medication is to be administered twice daily.

biochemical screening   Series of laboratory tests for measuring the concentration of various blood substances. The screening often is done on automated equipment and sometimes is referred to as autoanalysis or sequential multi-channel autoanalysis (SMA).

bipolar disorder   Mood disorder comprising episodes of both mania and depression; formerly called "manic depressive illness." Patients with bipolar disorder may appear either manic or depressed.

bradyphrenia   Slowing of information processing.

bulimia   Episodic eating binges or excessive intake of food or fluid, generally beyond voluntary control. Although often a condition of young women, it is also seen in patients with Alzheimer's disease.

cachexia   Severe weight loss associated with dehydration.

calculi   (singular, *calculus*) Crystals or very small stones present in the urinary tract system. If a stone is present in the kidneys or ureters, the patient will have very severe flank pain radiating to the groin and will pass blood in the urine. If the stone is located in the urinary bladder, the patient may feel a constant urge to empty the bladder, but only a few drops of urine are passed at a time. A bladder stone also is often associated with pain or scalding. When calculi are present in the bladder, they increase the excitability of the bladder and may be responsible for bouts of urinary incontinence.

cardiac reserve capacity   Heart's ability to increase its output to meet the body's increased demand during exercise.

cataract   Condition in which the lens of the eye becomes opaque. It is frequently seen in old age and is one of the most common causes of impaired visual acuity in older people. In some instances cataracts are caused by specific diseases, such as diabetes mellitus or hyperparathyroidism, but most often the cause is unknown. Patients with cataracts often see better in dim light because the pupils are dilated and a larger portion of the lens is exposed (in bright light, the pupils are constricted and only a small part of the lens is exposed). Cataract surgery is the treatment of choice.

cerebrovascular accident   See **stroke.**

chlorpromazine (Thorazine)   Neuroleptic agent that belongs to the class of drugs known as phenothiazines. It causes extrapyramidal side effects, sedation, and orthostatic hypotension.

cholesterol   Fatty substance present in the bloodstream that is essential for the adequate functioning of a number of body cells. However, if the concentration rises above a certain level, cholesterol tends to be precipitated along the inner lining of the arteries, giving rise to arteriosclerosis. This situation, in time, is associated with an increased risk of developing coronary heart disease, stroke and peripheral vascular insufficiency.

cholinergic   Relating to nerve cells that use acetylcholine as their neurotransmitter.

cholinesterase   Group of enzymes capable of breaking down acetylcholine.

chromosomes   Microscopic rod-shaped structures that contain genes and are found in every living cell. The genes transmit the characteristics inherited from the parent cell to the next generation. It has been postulated that Alzheimer's disease may involve some defect in chromosome 21, the same chromosome that is defective in Down syndrome. Most patients with Down syndrome who survive the third decade of life develop the manifestations of Alzheimer's disease. Other chromosomes that have been implicated with Alzheimer's disease include 1, 14, and 19.

circadian rhythm   See **sleep/wake cycle.**

circumstantial (tangential) thinking   Disturbance in thinking characterized by an excessive amount of detail that is irrelevant.

Cognex   Name of a medication (tacrine) approved for the treatment of Alzheimer's disease. It has to be given 4 times a day. Its main side effect is that it is toxic to the liver. This necessitates that it be started in a low dose that is gradually increased. The usual starting dose is 10 mg 4 times a day. The maximum dose is 40 mg 4 times a day. It also often causes adverse gastrointestinal effects.

cognitive functions   Operations of the mind by which an individual becomes aware of objects of thought or perception. Includes all aspects of perceiving, thinking, and remembering.

computed tomography (CT) scan   Special radiological test in which a very large number of x-ray films are taken simultaneously from different angles. The various films are put together by a computer to produce a detailed view of the brain. In advanced stages of Alzheimer's disease, the CT scan often reveals that the brain has atrophied and that the ventricles of the brain are dilated. In early stages of the disease, however, the CT scan is essentially within normal limits. Although there has been a great deal of controversy over whether a CT scan should be done routinely in patients suspected of having Alzheimer's disease, the current consensus is that such an investigation is necessary. It must be emphasized, however, that such an investigation is not necessary to confirm the diagnosis of Alzheimer's disease but to exclude other conditions that may mimic Alzheimer's disease, such as a brain tumor, brain hemorrhage, or stroke. A CT scan may be done with or without contrast medium. The former technique usually is preferred so that the various parts of the brain can be clearly visualized. The main problem with performing a CT scan is that the patient must lie still on the table, which is sometimes difficult for patients who have advanced Alzheimer's disease.

congestive cardiac failure   Condition in which the heart cannot maintain an adequate output. The common manifestations of heart failure include swelling of the legs (particularly worse toward the end of the day) and breathlessness on exertion. One of the first signs is awakening several times a night to pass a large amount of urine. In the early stages the patient tends to wake up in the middle of the night short of breath. This breathlessness usually is relieved when the patient sits up. In the later stages the patient cannot lie flat in bed and must be in a semisitting position supported by two, three, or four pillows.

coronary heart disease   Condition in which the lumina (inside diameter) of the arteries supplying blood to the heart are narrowed by deposition of cholesterol along their inner linings. Patients with coronary heart disease may have anginal pain or a myocardial infarct.

cortex   Outer layer of the brain. Alzheimer's disease affects the cortex: the number of brain cells (neurons) is reduced, and certain typical microscopic findings are noted, including neurofibrillary tangles and plaques.

cross-sectional study   Study done at one point in time on several people of different ages. Many such studies have been done in an attempt to examine the aging process, but it now is generally thought that those studies can be misleading because it is inaccurate to compare generation with generation and to attribute changes to the aging process when, in fact, most changes could be the result of alterations in economic, cultural, and social circumstances. Currently, longitudinal studies are preferred because they do follow-up studies on a group of individuals as they age. The main drawback of longitudinal studies is the long period before results become apparent, often exceeding 20 to 30 years. Two major longitudinal studies in progress are the Framingham study and the Baltimore study.

decubitus ulcer (plural, *decubiti*)   Ulcer that develops when a patient is bedridden for prolonged periods. The usual sites for these ulcers are the sacral region, the heels, and, in rare cases, the shoulder blades and the back of the head. To prevent decubiti, foam mattresses or special beds should be used and the patient should be turned regularly while in bed.

delirium   Acute medical condition manifested by disorientation, confusion, and fluctuating levels of consciousness. Unlike Alzheimer's disease, delirium has an acute onset and is associated with semiconsciousness or an impaired state of consciousness. It usually is caused by a reversible condition.

delusions   False beliefs firmly held despite obvious evidence to the contrary. These beliefs are not accepted by other members of the person's culture. Some examples are delusions of being controlled, delusions of grandeur (an exaggerated idea of one's own importance or identity), and delusions of persecution.

dementia   Irreversible mental deterioration caused by a medical condition.

diabetes mellitus   Disease in which the body's utilization of glucose (sugar) is reduced, resulting in an increase in the blood glucose level. Patients with diabetes mellitus often may experience acute confusion if the blood glucose level reaches a high level or if the condition is treated, if the blood glucose level is inadvertently reduced to a very low value.

diaphragm   Muscle that separates the chest from the abdominal cavity. The diaphragm plays an important role in breathing. By contracting and relaxing, it pulls on the chest wall, increases tile volume of the chest, and facilitates the drawing of air into the lungs.

diazepam (Valium)   Benzodiazepine used to treat anxiety and muscle spasms. It is long acting and particularly liable to accumulate in the bodies of elderly patients, and therefore has a long duration of action.

digitalis   Drug often used to treat heart failure, especially when the heart rate is irregular and rapid.

digoxin   See **digitalis.**

diuretics   Drugs that increase the volume of urine produced. All diuretics increase the amount of sodium and water in the urine, and most also increase the amount of potassium lost in the urine. This effect may be particularly serious if the patient is simultaneously taking digitalis. The incidence of digitalis toxicity is increased if the patient has a low blood potassium level. Some diuretics also increase the amount of calcium lost in the urine.

diurnal pattern   See **sleep/wake cycle.**

donezepil   See **Aricept.**

double-blind studies   Research method used to evaluate the efficacy of a drug in which neither the patient nor the physician knows whether the patient is receiving the agent being tested or a placebo.

dysarthria   Difficulty in articulating words.

dysphagia   Difficulty with swallowing.

dysphasia   Mild form of aphasia.

dysuria   Pain or a burning sensation while passing urine. Dysuria often denotes an infection in the bladder.

echolalia   Tendency to repeat a question asked or a word of a question without being able to answer the question.

electrocardiogram (ECG)   Graphic record of the heart's electrical activity. ECGs usually are obtained to detect insufficient blood supply to the heart or cardiac irregularities.

electroencephalogram (EEG)   Graphic record of the brain's electrical activity. In patients with Alzheimer's disease, the EEG shows that most brain waves are of smaller magnitude than those of normal individuals; generalized slowing may also be observed. Currently, an EEG is not necessary in the routine diagnostic workup of a patient suspected of having Alzheimer's disease.

electrolyte   Chemical substance in the blood. Examples include sodium, potassium, calcium, and magnesium. Electrolyte levels can be reduced or elevated by various diseases or medications.

embolism   Development of an embolus.

embolus   Clot or other blockage brought to a blood vessel from another part of the body.

endocrine disease   Disease of the endocrine or hormonal glands, including the thyroid, parathyroid, pituitary, adrenal glands, and gonads.

estrogens   Hormones secreted by the ovaries. Estrogen secretion tends to decrease drastically during menopause; this sudden reduction may be responsible for a number of signs and symptoms, including atrophic vaginitis.

etiology   Study of the causes of a particular disease.

excoriation Breaking down of the skin's surface; a condition associated with irritation. Excoriation often occurs when urine is left in contact with the skin.

extrapyramidal side effects Variety of signs and symptoms that includes muscular rigidity, tremors, drooling, shuffling gait, restlessness, peculiar involuntary posture, and motor inertia. Neuroleptic drugs are particularly liable to cause these side effects.

fibroblast Connective tissue cell capable of forming collagen.

flurazepam (Dalmane) Hypnotic medication that tends to remain in the body for a long period, particularly in elderly patients. This situation may lead to drowsiness and unsteadiness the morning after the drug is taken.

gag reflex Retching or gagging caused by contact of a foreign body with the mucous membrane of the space between the inside of the mouth and the pharynx.

genes Microscopic structures located on the chromosomes that transmit specific characteristics from generation to generation. Current studies in Alzheimer's disease are focusing on identifying one or more particular genes that may be defective. This approach would allow identification and accurate diagnosis of individuals with the disease and possible "repair" of the defective gene through genetic engineering. (See also **chromosomes.**)

genetic markers Substances produced by abnormal genes. They can be found in individuals possessing these abnormal genes but not in people with normal genes.

genetic pattern Organization and structure of various genes. It is possible to identify abnormal genes in a number of diseases and to diagnose these diseases by finding the abnormal gene and abnormal genetic pattern.

geropsychology Psychology of old age.

glaucoma Condition in which the fluid in the eye is under increased pressure. Glaucoma is a serious condition since, if allowed to persist, the pressure may interfere with the blood supply of the optic nerve and lead to blindness. A characteristic feature of glaucoma is the halos a patient often sees around objects; headaches also are common. Glaucoma can be managed relatively easily by administering eye drops regularly. Surgery also is sometimes used to treat this condition. In late stages, before vision is completely lost, the patient may have tunnel vision.

granulovacuolar degeneration Microscopic finding describing degenerative changes in the brain cells.

gray matter Structures in the brain that appear gray when the brain is cut. These include the outer layer of the cortex and a few structures in the center of the brain known as the basal ganglia. The gray matter contains most of the neurons.

gyri (singular, *gyrus*) Convolutions on the surface of the brain. In Alzheimer's disease the gyri tend to become narrower and less convoluted.

hallucinations Apparent subjective sensory perception of sight, sound, or smell with no basis in external reality.

haloperidol (Haldol) Neuroleptic drug that is one of the butyrophenones. A powerful medication that produces severe extrapyramidal side effects, haloperidol should be given only for delusions, hallucinations, or bizarre behavior.

Heimlich maneuver   Emergency procedure designed to clear an airway obstructed by a foreign object, usually food.

hematoma   Collection of blood within an organ tissue or space resulting from trauma to a blood vessel.

Hippocrates   Greek physician who lived on the island of Cos in the fifth century BC and is generally considered to be the Father of Medicine.

histopathology   Study of diseased tissue through microscopic examination.

human immunodeficiency virus (HIV) test   Test performed to detect the virus responsible for acquired immunodeficiency syndrome (AIDS).

Huntington's disease   Genetic neurological disorder, usually appearing in midlife, characterized by involuntary movements and eventually dementia.

hyperinnervation   Excessive nerve stimulation.

hyperthyroidism   Disease in which the thyroid gland is overactive. Patients with hyperthyroidism tend to be overactive and to feel as if they have an enormous amount of energy. They also commonly lose weight and prefer cold weather.

hypnotics   Drugs that are given to induce sleep. Since drugs are metabolized more slowly as an individual ages, the effect of hypnotics may be prolonged in an older individual, causing increased sleepiness. Also, older people may be more sensitive to these drugs.

hypothermia   Condition resulting when the body temperature falls to 35° C or less (compared to the normal temperature of approximately 37° C).

hypothyroidism   Disease in which the thyroid gland does not produce sufficient thyroxin. Patients with hypothyroidism tend to tire easily, to become constipated, to sleep most of the time, and to be oversensitive to cold (preferring very warm environments).

illusion   Misperception of a real external stimulus, for example, a shadow on the wall caused by the moon and a tree outside is perceived as a stranger entering the room.

imipramine (Tofranil)   Drug used to treat depression; it is one of the tricyclic antidepressants. Imipramine is particularly prone to causing anticholinergic side effects.

indwelling Foley catheter   Tube introduced through the urethra into the urinary bladder. A balloon at the end of the tube is inflated to keep the catheter in position. This type of catheter should be used only as a last resort in the treatment of urinary incontinence. Its use is associated with a number of side effects, most importantly urinary tract infections, which often spread from the bladder to the kidneys.

insight   Person's ability to be aware of her problems. In the early stages of Alzheimer's disease, the patient usually has insight into her impaired mental functions, particularly poor memory. As time passes and the patient's condition deteriorates, this insight is gradually lost and the patient may not realize that she has a poor memory. Lack of insight is particularly useful in differentiating Alzheimer's disease from depression, which sometimes can give rise to apparently impaired mental functions, a condition referred to as pseudodementia. In all but the early stage of Alzheimer's disease, the patient has no insight into her poor memory, whereas with depression the patient usually has this insight and often tends to exaggerate this memory problem. A depressed patient commonly will state that her memory is poor and thus she cannot remember what day of the week it is or cannot recall recent events. A patient with Alzheimer's disease, on the other hand, will maintain that her memory is quite good and readily confabulate, that is, give wrong answers about recent events or incorrectly identify the day of the week.

intramuscular   Within a muscle. Denotes the route of administration of medication by injection into a muscle. The usual sites for intramuscular injection are the buttocks, thighs, and occasionally the shoulders.

intravenous   Within a vein. Denotes the route of administration of medication or fluids into a vein.

intravenous line   Slender tube that is inserted into a vein and kept in position to allow regular administration of medication or fluids.

ischemic attack   Condition resulting from an interference with blood flow.

Kegel exercises   Set of exercises designed to strengthen the pelvic floor and perineal muscles to control stress incontinence. These exercises mainly consist of constricting the external urinary sphincter and some of the perineal and pelvic muscles. The easiest way of knowing when these muscles contract is to attempt to interrupt the flow of urine while micturating. To be effective, Kegel exercises must be repeated as often as possible.

kyphoscoliosis   Condition in which the curvature of the thoracic vertebrae (upper part of back) is increased and is associated with a sideways deformity of the spine. This condition often is the result of osteoporosis.

kyphosis   Condition involving excessive curvature of the thoracic vertebrae. It often results from osteoporosis because the increased fragility of the vertebrae causes them to become wedge shaped, thus exaggerating the normal curvature of the thoracic spine.

lacuna   Small space or cavity.

laxative   Drug taken to increase the bowel motions and to prevent constipation.

lewy bodies   Small, round structures first identified in parts of the brain in the basal ganglia of patients with Parkinson's disease. They are also often seen throughout the brains of patients with Alzheimer's disease. A separate type of dementia, diffuse Lewy body dementia (DLBD), has also been described. The main differentiating clinical features from Alzheimer's disease include hallucinations, paranoid ideations, and repeated falls.

lipofuscin   Pigment that accumulates in the nerve cells as a person ages. It also collects in muscle, heart, and liver cells. The significance of this pigment is not fully understood.

lithium   Lithium carbonate is a salt used in the treatment of acute mania and as a maintenance medication to help reduce the duration, intensity, and frequency of recurrent episodes of bipolar disorder.

logoclonia   Repetition of the first syllable of a word that has just been heard.

lumbar puncture   Test that involves introducing a needle through the back between two lumbar vertebrae to obtain a sample of the fluid that surrounds the spinal cord (cerebrospinal fluid). Until recently, a lumbar puncture was part of the routine diagnostic workup of patients suspected of having Alzheimer's disease, but it currently is not done routinely in these patients. It is reserved for the diagnosis of infections, tumors, multiple sclerosis, and other conditions affecting the spinal cord or brain.

magnetic resonance imaging (MRI)   Specialized radiological test that allows a clear view of various body organs. When MRI is done on the head, the brain can be clearly visualized. This imaging method is sometimes used in the diagnostic workup of patients suspected of having Alzheimer's disease. It is more sensitive than the CT scan and can detect abnormalities too small to be detected by it.

metabolic diseases   Diseases that interfere with the body's metabolism. The concentration of various substances in the blood is maintained within a very narrow range of normality by a number of factors. For instance, glucose is controlled by the amount of insulin produced by the pancreas (in addition to a number of other factors). In metabolic diseases the concentration of these various substances is altered.

mood disorders   Group of disorders characterized by prominent and persistent disturbances in mood (depression or mania). The disorders usually are episodic but may be chronic.

morbidity   State of being diseased.

mucosal smear   Test in which a few cells from the lining of the vagina (mucosa) are smeared on a glass slide and examined microscopically to determine whether enough estrogens (female hormones) are circulating in the blood. By examining these mucosal cells, it is possible to tell whether a patient has atrophic vaginitis.

multiinfarct dementia   Condition in which the dementia is caused by repeated small strokes. Often these strokes do not give rise to any paralysis or other neurological deficit. However, as time goes by and more strokes are produced, the number of brain cells gradually diminishes and the patient may slowly manifest a dementing illness. It is important to differentiate multiinfarct dementia from Alzheimer's disease since the incidence of repeated strokes can be reduced and thus the progress of multiinfarct dementia sometimes can be stopped, leading to stabilization of the patient's condition. With Alzheimer's disease, progression of the disorder is usually relentless.

muscarinic   Having a muscarine-like action, i.e., producing parasympathetic stimulation, such as cardiac slowing, vasodilation, salivation, lacrimation, bronchoconstriction, and gastrointestinal stimulation.

mutism   Condition in which the patient does not communicate verbally.

myocardial infarction   Condition that results when the blood flow through one of the coronary arteries that carried blood to the heart is completely stopped. This usually happens when a blood clot develops in one of the coronary arteries, accompanied by complicating arteriosclerosis. The condition usually is manifested by severe central chest pain that is not relieved by either rest or sublingual nitroglycerine. The patient is apprehensive, is usually sweating, and has a sense of impending death.

nasogastric tube   Tube that is passed through the nasal cavity into the stomach. It usually is used to feed patients who have difficulty swallowing or who cannot feed themselves.

neoplasm   Cancerous growth.

neurofibrillary tangles   Aggregations of neurofilaments and neurotubules in neurons, which are noted through microscopy. Neurofibrillary tangles are commonly seen in normal aged brains but usually are few in number. In Alzheimer's disease, however, these tangles are widespread throughout the cortex and are quite dense.

neurofilament   Slender filament present in neurons. Neurofilaments are thought to be involved in intracellular transport of metabolites.

neuroleptics   Drugs used to treat psychotic symptoms. They include phenothiazines (e.g., Thorazine, Mellaril, Stelazine), butyrophenones (e.g., Haldol), and thioxanthenes (e.g., Navane [thiothixene]).

neuromelanin   Pigment within the nerve cells.

neuron   Nerve cell.

neuropathy   Condition resulting from the degeneration of nerve fibers.

neurotransmitters   Chemical substances that conduct electrical impulses from one cell to another and thus enable an electrical impulse to proceed. The main neurotransmitters that are deficient in Alzheimer's disease are acetylcholine, somatostatin, and, to a lesser extent, serotonin and dopamine.

nonsteroidal antiinflammatory compounds   Medications given to patients with arthritis and other painful conditions. These drugs reduce inflammation and relieve pain. Common examples are aspirin and ibuprofen.

nootropics   Class of chemical compounds that help to correct the decline in learning and behavior in patients with dementia by increasing metabolic activity within the neurons.

o.d.   (Latin: *omni die*) Abbreviation designating that a medication be administered once a day.

oropharynx   Anatomical term referring to the back of the mouth and upper part of the pharynx.

osteoarthritis   Disease affecting the joints—particularly the hands, knees, and hips—that causes pain and stiffness. Characteristically the pain is much worse after exercise and tends to be relieved somewhat by rest. With osteoarthritis the cartilage that lines the bones becomes less efficient at protecting the bones and preventing them from rubbing against each other in the joint. The cartilage gradually becomes frayed, and loose bits of cartilage may become dislodged in the joint. The exact cause of osteoarthritis is not known, although currently it is thought to be mainly a degenerative disease. It usually is treated with analgesics or nonsteroidal antiinflammatory drugs.

paralalia   Any speech defect, especially in the production of a vocal sound different from the one desired.

paranoid disorders   Also called delusional disorders, these mental conditions involve a persistent delusion of persecution or jealousy. Schizophrenia, mood disorders, and organic mental disorders have been excluded as causes in these cases.

paraphasia   Sometimes referred to as paraphrasia. A form of speech in which the individual substitutes one word for another or describes an object for which he has forgotten the name. For example, when presented with a key and asked to name it, the person states "something that opens a door."

parasympathetic nervous system Division of the autonomic nervous system.

paresis Weakness resulting in a neurological disorder, such as a stroke.

Parkinson's disease Disease characterized by muscle stiffness and tremors. It is also known as "shaking palsy" or "shaking paralysis." The muscles are not weakened, but the tremors interfere with the patient's daily activities. Parkinson's disease is caused by damage to certain parts of the brain (substantia nigra). Some patients with Parkinson's disease develop dementia, a condition often referred to as a subcortical dementia because the affected area of the brain lies below the cortex. The main biochemical abnormality in Parkinson's disease is a deficiency of the neurotransmitter dopamine. Many drugs can be used to treat Parkinson's disease.

pathognomonic Characteristic of a disease.

peripheral vascular insufficiency Disease in which the lumina (inside diameter) of the arteries that carry blood to the legs are considerably reduced. As a result the patient may develop intermittent pain in the leg muscles during exercise, but this pain usually is relieved by rest.

phosphorylation Addition of phosphate to an organic compound.

physostigmine Chemical substance that decreases the breakdown of acetylcholine in the synapse.

pica Craving and eating of unusual foods or other substances. Pica is seen in a variety of medical conditions, including Alzheimer's disease. Common examples include eating of paint, paper, or excessive amounts of ice.

placebo Inactive substance identical in appearance with the material being tested in experimental research.

plaque See **senile plaque.**

positron emission tomography (PET) Highly specialized test that reflects the metabolic activity of the brain. Currently it is not routinely available.

pressure areas Regions of the body that are under pressure when an individual lies down, including the sacral region, heels, shoulder blades, and back of the head. Patients who are immobile or bedridden for prolonged periods develop a decubitus ulcer.

pressure sore See **decubitus ulcer.**

progesterone Hormone secreted by the ovaries. Secretion of this hormone tends to decrease dramatically during menopause.

prognosis Forecast of what is likely to happen when an individual contracts a particular disease. In the case of Alzheimer's disease, the prognosis currently is poor because there is no effective cure and the disease is known to have a slow, progressive course. In general, the younger the individual when the disease manifests itself, the worse the prognosis.

prolapse Displacement of an organ or part of an organ. Uterine prolapse denotes the displacement and descent of the uterus into the vagina. Bladder prolapse denotes the protrusion of the bladder into the vaginal wall. Both conditions are associated with urinary incontinence secondary to the altered architecture and relationship of the urinary bladder, uterus, and vagina.

promazine (Sparine) Neuroleptic drug that is one of the phenothiazines. Promazine is no longer widely used because of its sedative side effects.

prostatic hypertrophy Enlargement of the prostate gland, which is present in men at the junction of the bladder and the urethra. An enlarged prostate may compress the urethra and obstruct the flow of urine. When the pressure of urine in the bladder exceeds that of the sphincter, incontinence results; this type of incontinence is called overflow incontinence. Other signs of prostatic hypertrophy include difficulty in starting the flow of urine and a weak stream.

proteolysis Protein breakdown.

proton magnetic resonance See **magnetic resonance imaging.**

pruritus Itching.

pseudodementia Condition in which the patient shows impaired mental functions and signs and symptoms of dementia but in which the underlying diagnosis is not dementia but depression.

psychoactive drugs Drugs that affect the mind or behavior, such as antidepressant, anxiolytic, and neuroleptic medications.

psychological testing Series of tests performed by psychologists to assess a patient's mental functions.

psychosis Form of mental illness in which the patient suffers from delusions, hallucinations, and/or bizarre behavior.

psychotropic drugs Drugs that exert an effect on the mind and modify mental activity. (See also **psychoactive drugs.**)

q.i.d. (Latin: *quater in die*) Abbreviation designating that a medication be given four times a day.

respiratory reserve capacity Ability of the respiratory system to increase its work to meet the body's increased demands during exercise.

rigidity, muscle rigidity Condition in which the muscles become rigid and thus movement becomes difficult. Muscle rigidity often is seen in patients with Parkinson's disease and in the late stages of Alzheimer's disease. In the latter condition, the excessive rigidity causes the body to assume a generalized flexed position while the patient is lying in bed.

sacral plexus Agglomeration of nerve fibers from the autonomic nervous system that is present in the sacral area. This part of the autonomic nervous system partly controls micturition.

schizophrenia Severe chronic mental disorder characterized by extreme difficulty in thinking and associated with delusions and hallucinations.

sedatives Medications used to calm a patient. These agents are particularly useful when a patient is agitated, irritable, and violent. Sedatives should not be used routinely in patients with Alzheimer's disease since a major side effect is drowsiness, which may, in turn, worsen the patient's confusion.

senile macular degeneration Degenerative condition of the retina that occurs in old age and causes diminished visual acuity and eventually blindness. Currently there is no satisfactory treatment for this condition.

senile plaque Microscopic finding that describes a small mass between the neurons of the brain. Senile plaques are found in many older people, but they tend to be more numerous in patients with Alzheimer's disease. The center of the plaque is made of amyloid.

sensorium   Term used to describe orientation to time, place, and person. Sometimes it also includes an assessment of short-term memory.

sensory information   Information sent to the brain by one of the five senses (sight, hearing, touch, smell, and taste). For instance, when a person sees a pencil, the shape and appearance of the object are transmitted through the eye to the brain, where they are interpreted as a pencil. Similarly, when the ears detect a sound, this information is transmitted to the brain, where it is interpreted and the individual becomes aware of the meaning of the sound. In the late stages of Alzheimer's disease, the patient may not be able to recognize common objects or the people he lives with, such as his spouse, children, or fellow residents in a nursing home.

septicemia   Condition in which an infection spreads to involve the blood. As a result of septicemia, bacteria or other infective organisms circulate in the bloodstream and may reach any organ.

serotonin   Neurotransmitter present in the brain. The concentration of serotonin usually is reduced in patients with Alzheimer's disease.

sleep apnea   See **apnea.**

sleep/wake cycle   Twenty-four-hour cycle during which individuals tend to sleep at night and remain awake during the day. This cycle often is referred to as the "circadian rhythm" or "diurnal rhythm." Although the sleep/wake cycle generally is regulated by a number of hormonal glands, which secrete various hormones at different concentrations at different times of the day. These glands seem to be regulated by an internal clock. Even when people are deprived of sunlight and timekeeping devices, they tend to retain a circadian sleep/wake cycle. Patients with Alzheimer's disease often have a disturbed sleep/wake cycle and tend to be awake and agitated at night and sleepy during the day. They commonly become particularly confused early in the evening, a phenomenon sometimes called the "sundown syndrome." The altered sleep/wake cycle is particularly stressful for caregivers and has been found to be the least tolerated symptom of Alzheimer's disease.

SMA 6, 18, or 29   See **biochemical screening.**

social judgment   Ability to determine behaviors and actions that are appropriate to any given social situation.

somatic complaints   Body symptoms such as headache, backache, and dizziness. These complaints may be caused by physical or emotional disorders.

somatization   Conversion of feelings (usually anxiety and depression) into physical symptoms.

SPECT   Single Photon Emission Computed Tomography. Technique to measure blood flow through various parts of the brain.

stroke   Condition in which part of the brain is deprived of blood. It often occurs as a complication of arteriosclerosis. The three most common causes of strokes are thrombosis, embolism, and hemorrhage. In older patients thrombosis is the most common cause and hemorrhage the least common.

subcortical dementia   Dementia caused by abnormalities in the areas of the brain that lie below the cortex. In Alzheimer's disease the cortex and certain other areas below it are grossly affected. In subcortical dementia the cortex is generally spared, but the structures below it are largely affected. A common example of subcortical dementia is that seen in some patients with Parkinson's disease.

subdural Space below the dura mater, which is a membrane lining the outside of the brain and spinal cord.

sulci (singular, *sulcus*) Fissures seen on the outer surface of the brain. In Alzheimer's disease, sulci tend to become shallow.

sundown syndrome Condition characterized by a period of severe confusion, occasionally associated with agitation, irritability, and sometimes violence, that typically occurs toward the end of the day. The cause of this syndrome is not well understood but probably is related to the concentrations of various hormones in the blood. It has also been suggested that this syndrome may stem from the reduced natural light at the end of the day, which may precipitate a confused state in the patient.

sympathetic nervous system Division of the autonomic nervous system.

synapse See **synaptic cleft.**

synaptic cleft Space between two nerve cells. The electrical impulses generated in one nerve cell can pass across the synaptic cleft (synapse) by the release of chemical compounds known as neurotransmitters, which, in effect, transmit the electrical impulses from one nerve cell to the other.

tardive dyskinesia Involuntary movements, generally of the lips, tongue, or jaw but sometimes of other parts of the body, that occur 5 to 10 years after neuroleptic drugs have been taken.

tau A protein normally present in the nerve fibers and seen in the neurofibrillary tangles of patients with Alzheimer's disease. This protein is meant to stabilize the structure of the neurofibril. Several forms of the tau protein exist. When their chemical structure is altered by excessive phosphorylation they may lead to the formation of neurofibrillary tangles. Tau protein binds less to APOE4 than APOE2 or APOE3, which also may lead to nerve cell damage and the formation of neurofibrillary tangles and amyloid plaques.

thioridazine (Mellaril) Neuroleptic drug that is one of the phenotiazines. Although it causes fewer extrapyramidal side effects than haloperidol, thioridazine produces far more sedation and orthostatic hypotension.

thrombosis Development of a thrombus.

thrombus Blood clot that forms inside a blood vessel. A thrombus often is precipitated by arteriosclerosis.

thyroid Gland situated in the neck that secretes thyroid hormone. If the secretion of thyroid hormone is excessive or insufficient, the patient may show a confusional state. Either imbalance worsens the degree of mental impairment seen in patients with Alzheimer's disease.

t.i.d. (Latin: *ter in die*) Abbreviation designating that a particular medication is to be administered three times a day.

tranquilizers Drugs intended to calm an individual without causing undue sedation. These drugs are better avoided or used sparingly in patients with Alzheimer's disease because they tend to cause some drowsiness. Since elderly individuals cannot eliminate most drugs through their urine (or bile) as quickly and efficiently as younger people can, repeated use of a tranquilizer or other drug may cause the medication to accumulate in the body and lead to drowsiness and even sedation.

triglycerides   Fatty substances present in the blood that are essential for the proper functioning of many cells. As with cholesterol, if the concentration of triglycerides is excessive, arteriosclerosis may develop.

tropic functions   Nourishing functions.

urethral stricture   Constriction in the urethra that can lead to obstruction of the flow of urine and overflow incontinence.

urinary sphincters   Two sphincters located on the urethra. One is close to the junction of the urethra and the urinary bladder (internal urinary sphincter), and the other is closer to the surface of the body (external urinary sphincter). The external urinary sphincter can be contracted at will, and its main use is to postpone micturition for a short time. Normally, urine is prevented from leaving the urinary bladder by the constant contraction of the internal urinary sphincter, which is controlled by the autonomic nervous system. The sympathetic division of this system causes the internal urinary sphincter to constrict, preventing the passage of urine. The parasympathetic component causes the internal sphincter to relax, encouraging voiding.

urinary stasis   Presence of urine in the bladder after voiding (also called residual urine). This condition which frequently is seen in men with prostatic hypertrophy, often invites infection.

urodynamic tests   Series of tests that evaluate the relationship between the bladder, the urethra, and abdominal pressure to determine the cause of urinary incontinence.

venous return   Blood returning from various parts of the body to the heart.

visual spatial skills   Skills that enable individuals to integrate incoming information so that they can orient themselves geographically and find their way. A common manifestation of this impairment is a tendency to become lost.

vital signs   Pulse, temperature, blood pressure, and respiratory rate.

white matter   Structure of the brain below the cortex that appears white when the brain is dissected. White matter is mainly made up of nerve fibers that connect the neurons in the gray matter to other parts of the brain or the body.

Index

A

Abnormal involuntary movement scale, 175-176
Absorbent products, 217
Accident prevention. *See* Safety/accident prevention
Acetylcholine, 18, 184
Acetylcholine precursors, 184
Acetylcholine releasers, 185
Acetyl-L-carnitine, 192
Activities of daily living. *See* Daily care
Activity. *See also* Treatment programs
  importance of, 148
Adult day care, 357
  respite, 356
Adult foster homes, 361
Advance directives, 288, 297-298
  durable power of attorney for health care, 297, 307-311
  living will, 297-298, 311-312
Ageism, 329
Aggressive behavior, 157-158
  drugs and, 178
  restraints and, 238
Agitated behavior, 157
  bathing and, 248
  restraints and, 238
Agnosia, 78
AIDS, 100
  dementia due to, 125-128
Alcohol, 114
  in differential diagnosis, 90, 97-98
Alcohol-induced dementia, 133-134
Alpha-glycerylphosphorylcholine, 121
Alzheimer's Association, 87, 365
  advocacy by, 375
  mission of, 368
  national partnerships to improve Alzheimer's disease care, 372-373
  national project grants to chapters, 372
  organization of, 367-368
  origins of, 367
  patient and family services, 371-373
  professional education programming, 374-375
  public awareness and education, 373-374
  Reagan institute initiative, 371
  research activities of, 368-371
  safe return program, 372
  support groups, 371
  Zenith Awards, 370
Alzheimer's disease
  clinical manifestations, 3
  diagnosis for, 3-4
  discovery of, 55-56
  economic implications of, 2
  etiology of, 3
  false positive for, 31-32

Alzheimer's disease—cont'd
  historical perspective of, 53-58
  incidence of, 57-58
  information on, 344-346
  vs. multiinfarct dementia, 30-31
  prevalence of, 1-2
  risk factors and potential protective factors, 69
  sequence of disruption and most distinguishing cognitive features, 30, 31
Alzheimer's Disease Education and Referral Centers, 343
Alzheimer, Alois, 54-56
Amitriptyline, 178, 179
Amygdala, 23
Amyloid, 61-62
Angiotension converting enzyme inhibitors, 192
Anomia, 77
Antidepressants, 178-181
  considerations for, 178
Antioxidant drug therapy, 188
Antipsychotic drugs, 19, 172-177
  side effects for, 177
Anxiety, meaning of, 261
Anxiolytics, 177-178
Apathy, 164-165
Aphasia, 78
Apraxia, 78-79
Area Agency on Aging, 354-355
Aricept, 4, 186-187
Arrhythmias, 107-108
Arteriosclerosis, 100
Aspirin, 120
Assessment
  terminal care and, 276-278
  in treatment program, 269
Assisted living, 360

B

Basal ganglia, 22-23
Basal nucleus of Meynert, 15, 16
  Alzheimer's disease and, 16, 18-19
Bathing, 246-248
  causes for difficulty in, 246
  frequency of, 247
  hair care, 247-248
  handling agitation, 248
  routines for, 246-247
  safety and, 230, 247
  terminal care and, 277
  useful strategies for, 248
Beck Depression Inventory, 33
Bedpans, 216-217
Behavior, difficult, 80-81
  aggression and combativeness, 157-158
  agitation and restlessness, 157
  analysis of, 261

441

Behavior—cont'd
    basic intervention techniques for, 153-154
    catastrophic reactions, 158-159
    communication and, 150-151
    in dementia care units, 382-383
    depression and apathy, 164-165
    eating difficulties, 169
    environment and, 151
    inappropriate sexual behavior, 161-164
    insurmountable task and, 150
    management strategies, 154-155
    meaning of, 260-261
    paranoid thinking, 164
    problem-solving behavior management
        defining desired change, 152
        defining problem, 151-152
        evaluation of plan, 153
        plan of action, 152-153
    repetitive behaviors, 168-169
    sleep disturbances, 165-168
    validation as means of communication and
            problem solving, 155-157
        centering, 155
        eye contact, 156
        imagining opposite, 156
        music, 157
        non-threatening words, 155-156
        polarity, 156
        reminiscing, 156
        rephrasing, 156
        touching, 156
    vocalization/screaming, 159-160
Benign forgetfulness, 75-76
Benzisoxazole, 174
Benzodiazepines, 19, 177-178
Bethanechol, 187
Binswanger's disease, 118-119
Bladder training/retraining programs, 223
Blessed Dementia Scale, 93
Blood
    altered quality of blood to brain, 108-109
    sudden decrease of supply to brain, 107-
        108
Boundary homes, 361
Bowel function. See also Incontinence, fecal
    fecal impaction, 254
    laxatives, 252-254
    maintaining, 251
    natural stimulants, 251-252
    terminal care and, 284
    useful strategies for, 252
Bradycardia, 108
Brain. See also Central nervous system
    basal ganglia, 22-23
    blood supply to
        altered quality of, 108-109
        sudden decrease in, 107-108
    dysexecutive syndrome, 22
    executive function of, 22
    functions of, 13-15
    gray matter, 16-17

Brain   cont'd
    hemispheres of, 11-12
        integration of, 15
        specialization of, 14-15
    hippocampus, 23-24
    imaging techniques for, 41-47
    integration and specialization of higher corti-
        cal functions, 24-25
    integration of brain functions, 20-22
    levels of functioning, 20
    limbic system, 23-24
    lobes of, 12-14
    nerve cells, 15-20
    space-occupying lesions in skull, 106-107
    stages of Alzheimer's disease and changes in
        function, 25
    stroke, 105-106
    structure of, 11-12
    subdural hematoma, 106
Bristol Activities of Daily Living Scale, 269
Buflomedil, 121
Bupropion, 179-181
Burnout, 322
    administrative support, 325-326
    institutional setting, 322-323
    job satisfaction, 323
    preventive measures, 324
    staff development, 324
    stress and personality, 323
    support groups, 326
    time-out, 325
    workload, 325
Buspirone, 177
Butyrophenone, 173

C
Calcium channel blockers, 191-192
Caregivers
    as "hidden victims", 2
    education for, 341-348
    family
        caregiver reactions, 318
        caregiver training, 320
        coping skills, 319
        emotional burden, 317
        male family caregivers, 318
        nursing home placement, 320-321
        pastoral counseling, 321
        physical burden, 317
        respite care, 319
        sickness in caregivers, 318
        support groups, 319-320
    interpersonal relationships between caregivers
            and patients, 143-144
    professional, stress in, 321-326
    psychological reactions of, in ethical issues,
        295-296
    reaction to treatment programs, 274
    stress and, 316-326
    support groups for, 348-352
Cars, driving and safety, 227-228

Catastrophic reactions, 158-159
Catheter devices, 219-222
    external, 220-222
    internal, 219-220
Centering, 155
Centers for Excellence in Alzheimer Care, 374
Central nervous system, 11-12
Chemical restraints, 383
Chest infections, 110-111
Chloroprppiophenones, 179
Chlorpromazine, 19, 127, 172
Chlorprothixene, 173
Choice in Dying, 298
Cholinergic agonists, 187
Cholinesterase inhibitors, 185-187
Chromosome 1, mutation, 64
Chromosomes 14, mutation, 64
Chromosome 19, mutation, 64-65
Chromosomes 21, mutation, 64
Chronic care, definition of, 276
Cicero, 52
Clinical presentation of Alzheimer's disease,
        74-85
    behavioral problems, 80-81
    impaired visuospatial skills and apraxia,
        78-79
    inability to acquire and process, 76-77
    insidious onset, 81
    language difficulties, 77-78
    memory impairment, 74-76
    personality changes, 77, 80
    physical deterioration, 81
    poor judgment, 79
    self-neglect, 79-80
    stages of, 81-85
Clonazepam, 177
Clozapine, 172, 174, 177
Clozaril, 174
Cognex, 185-186
Combativeness, 157-158
Commode chairs, 215-216
Communication
    establishing good communication with
        patient, 145-146
    inability to, and incontinence, 205
    validation as means of
        centering, 155
        eye contact, 156
        imagining opposite, 156
        music, 157
        non-threatening words, 155-156
        polarity, 156
        reminiscing, 156
        rephrasing, 156
        touching, 156
Computed tomography, 41-42
Consortium to Establish a Registry for Alzhei-
        mer's Disease, battery for assessment,
        27, 29
Constipation. See Bowel function
Cortical atrophy, 19-20

Court-appointed guardians, 314-315
Crafts, 265, 266
Creating excess disability, 346-347
Creutzfeldt-Jakob disease, 130-131
Cytosine diphosphocholine, 121

D

Daily care
    bathing, 246-248
    dressing, 248-250
    ears, 255
    nail care, 254
    nutrition/eating, 255-257
    oral care and hygiene, 244-246
    shaving, 255
    task breakdown, 244
    in terminal care, 277-280
    toileting, 250-254
Day care program. See Treatment programs
Declarative memory, 24
Delusions, 101
Dementia
    alcohol-induced, 133-134
    Creutzfeldt-Jakob disease, 130-131
    depression in, 171
    diffuse Lewy body disease, 123-125
    HIV disease, 125-128
    historical perspective of, 51-53
    Huntington's disease, 132
    hypothyroidism, 133
    Lacunas, 118
    neuropsychological assessment of, 27-37
    Normal Pressure Hydrocephalus, 129-130
    Parkinson's disease, 121-123
    Pick's disease, 128-129
    presenile vs. senile dementia, 56-57
    Progressive Supranuclear Palsy, 131-132
    subdural hematoma, 132-133
    vascular, 117-121
Dementia care units, 377-387
    advantages of, 379
        in close proximity to conventional custodial
            nursing homes, 379
    architectural design, 384-385
    behavioral abnormalities, 382-383
    concerns about, 379
    definition of, 377-378
    establishment of, 377
    family roles in, 385-387
    1992 report of U. S. Office of technology as-
        sessment on, 387-389
    patients for, 380
    resolving complaints, 386-387
    staffing roles, 380-382
Dementia Severity Rating Scale, 94-96
Denture care, 245-246
Depression, 90, 99, 144, 164-165
    brain imaging and, 43
    case study of, 35
    dementia and, 36, 171
    drugs and, 178-181
    memory and, 35, 36

Desipramine, 10, 179
Detrusor instability, 202
Dextroamphetamine, 179
Diabetes mellitus, 99
Diagnosis, clinical, 3-4
  criteria for, 88-89
  differential diagnosis, 90-100
  importance of early diagnosis, 4
  laboratory tests, 102
  medical history in, 88-90
Diagnosis, disclosure of, 302
Diapers, adult, 218-219
Dibenzodiazepine, 174
Dibenzoxazepine, 173
Differential diagnosis
  alcohol in, 90
  arteriosclerosis, 100
  drugs in, 90, 97-98
  emotional disorders, 99
  eyes and ears in, 98-99
  infection, 100
  mental status examination, 100-102
  metabolic, endocrine diseases and nutritional
    deficiency, 99
  neurological disorders, 99-100
  tumors and trauma, 100
Diffuse Lewy body disease, 123-125
  management of, 124-125
Diphenylbutylpiperidine, 174
Discomfort, aggravation of Alzheimer's disease,
  113
Distraction, as management of difficult behavior,
  154
Diversion, as management of difficult behavior,
  154
Domiciliary homes, 361
Donepezil, 186-187
Dopamine, 19, 188
Dopaminergic therapy, 188
Doxepin, 178, 179
Dressing, 248-250
  ease of, 249
  organization, 249
  terminal care and, 279-280
  unusual patterns of, 249-250
  useful strategies for, 250
Driving safety, 396
Drug holidays, 172
Drugs. See also names of specific drugs
  aggravation of Alzheimer's disease, 113-114
  antidepressants, 178-181
  antipsychotic, 19
  antipsychotics, 172-177
  anxiolytics, 177-178
  fecal incontinence and, 209
  general considerations, 181
  hypnotics, 177-178
  incontinence and, 203, 205-207
  increased vulnerability to, with age and Alz-
    heimer's, 19
  physiological changes in aging and, 171-172

Drugs—cont'd
  psychoactive, 19
  safety/accident prevention, 233-234
  sleep disturbances and, 166, 167
  stimulants, 19
Drug therapy, 183-193
  acetyl-L-carnitine, 192
  angiotension converting enzyme inhibitors,
    192
  calcium channel blockers, 191-192
  cholinergic strategies
    acetylcholine precursors, 184
    acetylcholine releasers, 185
    cholinergic agonists, 187
    cholinesterase inhibitors, 185-187
    other agents, 187
  development of, 193
  dopaminergic and antioxidant strategies, 188
  estrogen, 192-193
  gangliosides, 190
  hydergine, 183-184
  introduction to, 183
  neurothrophic factors, 190
  NMDA receptor strategies, 188-189
  nonsteroidal antiinflammatory drugs, 191
  nootropics, 189-190
Dup 996, 185
Durable power of attorney for health care, 6,
  297, 307-311
  living will and, 312
Dysexecutive syndrome, 22

E

Ears
  daily care of, 255
  in differential diagnosis, 98-99
Eating, 160, 255-257
  problems with, 256-257
Echolalia, 78
Education caregiver
  Alzheimer's Association and, 373-375
  anticipatory guidance, 345-346
  baseline information, 344
  day-to-day management, 348
  formal teaching, 342-343
  informal teaching, 341-342
  information on Alzheimer's disease, 344-346
  objectives for, 342
  over involvement, 347
  preparing caregivers for emotional reactions,
    346
  prevention of excess disability, 346-347
  role reversal, 348
  written material for, 343
Elder abuse, 328-336
  abuser profile, 331-332
  ageism, 329
  definition of, 330-331
  diagnosis of abuse, 332-334
  geriatric abuse intervention team, 334-336
  incidence of, 329-330

Elder abuse—cont'd
  physical indicators of abuse, 334
  recognition of abuse, 331
  relationship to caregiver stress, 328
  victim profile, 332
Electrical safety, 229-230
Emotional disorders, in differential diagnosis, 99
Emotional factors in neuropsychological assess-
    ment, 36-37
ENA-713, 187
Endorphins, 19
Enkephalins, 19
Environment
  maintaining supportive, 147
  manipulation of, and behavioral management,
    154
  safety and, 237-238
  sudden change in, and aggravation of Alzhei-
    mer's disease, 113
Ergoloid mesylates, 183-184
Estates, 312-313
Estrogen, 67-68, 192-193
Ethical issues, 5-6
  advance directives, 297-298
  broad concerns for, 304
  care at end of life, 297
  disclosure of diagnosis, 302
  genetics and, 5-6
  limited familial autonomy, 297
  management of medical problems, 302-303
  obligation to give equitable treatment, 301-
    302
  obligation to preserve life and prevent suffer-
    ing, 298-299
  obligation to respect caregiving unit, 303
  obligation to support, 296
  paternalism and, 288, 296
  physician-assisted suicide and active euthana-
    sia, 299-301
  principles governing care, 294-295
  psychological reactions of caregivers, 295-296
  refusing treatment, 296
  restraints, 297
  right to decide, 296
  right to die, 299
  substituted judgment, 297
  terminal care and, 288-289
Etiology/pathogenesis, 60-71
  abnormalities of tissues other than brain, 68
  amyloids in, 61-62
  free radicals, 70
  genetics and, 63-65
  head trauma, 68-70
  infection, 70
  inflammatory process, 62-63
  inorganic compounds, 70-72
  Lewy bodies, 66
  neuritic plaques, amyloid and genetics, 61
  neurofibrillary tangles, 65
  neurotransmitters, neurotrophic factors and
    estrogen, 66-68
  thyroid disease, 70

Euthanasia, 299-301
  negative, 299
  positive, 299
Exercise
  importance of, 148
  in treatment program, 263
External catheters, 220-222
Eye contact, as communication, 156
Eyes, in differential diagnosis, 99

F
Falls, safety and accident prevention, 231-232
False positive for Alzheimer's disease, 31-32
Family. See also Caregivers, family
  role in dementia care units, 385-387
Fecal impaction, 208-209, 254. See also Bowel
    function
Final Exit (Humphrey), 299
Finger Oscillation Test, 33
Fire hazards, 229-230
Fluoxamine, 180
Fluoxetine, 179, 180
Fluphenazine, 172, 173
Fluphenazine decanoate, 177
Foley catheters, 220
Free radicals, 70
Frontal lobe, 12, 13
Fuld profile, 31-33
Functional imaging of brain, 43-45
Functional incontinence, 203-204
  characteristics of, 204
  drug-induced, 205-206
  inability to locate toilet, 204-205

G
Gangliosides, 190
Genetics, 5-6, 63-65
  ethical issues and, 5-6
  research on, 393-394
Geriatric abuse intervention team, 334-336
Geriatrics, 54
Glutamate, 188
Glycine agonists, 189
Greeks, dementia and, 51-52

H
Hachinski Ischemic Scale, 97
Hair care, 247-248
Haldol, 19, 173
Hallucinations, 101
  due to diffuse Lewy body disease, 123
Haloperidol, 127, 173
Haloperidol decanoate, 177
Halstead-Reitan Neuropsychological Test
    Battery, 33
Head trauma, 68-70
Hearing
  differential diagnosis, 98-99
  impaired, and aggravation of Alzheimer's
    disease, 112-113
Heart rate, 107-108

Hepatic functions, impaired, 110
"Hidden victims" of Alzheimer's disease, 2
Hippocampus, 23-24
　memory and, 24
Hippocrates, 52
Histamine, 114
Historical perspective of Alzheimer's dementia
　Alois Alzheimer, 54-56
　Alzheimer's disease research, 58-59
　early history of, 51-53
　first patient with Alzheimer's disease, 55-56
　patient care reform movement and origins of
　　contemporary view of, 53-58
　presenile vs. senile dementia, 56-57
HIV disease, dementia due to, 125-128
Holindone, 174
Home health aides, 359
Home health care, 358-360
Homes for the aged, 361
Horace, 52
Hospice care, 357-358
Housing alternatives, 360-362
Humphrey, Derek, 299
Huntington's disease, 132
Hydergine, 183-184
Hydrocephalus, 99-100
Hyperthermia, 231
Hypnotics, 177-178
Hypoglycemia, 109
Hypothalamus, 23
Hypothermia, 230
Hypothyroidism, 133
Hypoxemia, 108-109

I

Imaging techniques for brain, 41-47
Imaging the opposite, as communication, 156
Imipramine, 19, 178, 179
Immobility, 286-287
Incontinence, fecal. *See also* Bowel function
　clinical evaluation, 210
　common causes of, 208-210
　fecal impaction, 208-209
　gastrointestinal conditions, 210
　medications and, 209
　neurogenic factors in, 209
Incontinence, urinary
　clinical examination, 208
　curtailed patient mobility, 204
　discussing, 200
　functional incontinence, 203-204
　　drug-induced, 205-206
　inability to communicate and, 205
　inability to locate toilet, 204-205
　information for physicians on, 206-207
　laboratory investigations, 208
　as main reason for institutionalization, 200
　management of
　　absorbent and protective products, 217-218
　　access to facilities, 222
　　adult diapers, 218-219

Incontinence—cont'd
　management of—cont'd
　　behavioral techniques for, 222-223
　　catheter devices, 219-222
　　commode chairs, 215-216
　　fluid and dietary management, 223-224
　　habit training, 223
　　key points in, 224
　　prompted voiding, 223
　　protective underpads, 218
　　scheduled toiletry, 222-223
　　shields and guards, 218
　　skin care, 224-225
　　special considerations for Alzheimer's dis-
　　　ease, 214
　　strategies to reduce, 216
　　urinals and bedpans, 216-217
　patient factors affecting
　　flexibility, 215
　　manual dexterity, 214-215
　　mobility, 214
　physical restraints and, 205
　reluctance to admit, 199-200
　stress, 201
　urge incontinence, 202
Indole derivative, 174
Infection
　aggravation of Alzheimer's disease, 110-111
　in differential diagnosis, 100
In-home services, 358-360
Instrumental Activities of Daily Living, 30
Intellectual functioning, in mental status exami-
　nation, 101
Internal catheters, 219-220
Irritability, meaning of, 261

J

Judgment, poor, 79

K

Kegel exercises, 201
Kevorkian, Jack, 299
Kraepelin, Emil, 54-56

L

Laboratory tests, 102
Lacunar dementia, 118
Language difficulties, 30, 77-78
　agnosia, 78
　anomia, 77
　aphasia, 78
Laxatives, 252-254
　bulk-forming, 253
　lubricants, 254
　natural stimulants, 251-252
　osmotic, 253
　stimulant, 253-254
　surfactant, 253
Left hemisphere
　integration of, 15
　specialization of, 14

Legal issues, 306-315
    choosing lawyer for, 308
    court-appointed guardians, 314-315
    durable, 307
    living wills, 311-312
    powers of attorney, 307-311
    trusts, 313-314
    wills and estates, 312-313
Lewy bodies, 66
Life care facilities, 360-361
Light room, 166
Limbic system, 23-24
Lithium, 180
Liver, impaired function and aggravation of Alz-
        heimer's disease, 110
Living will, 297-298, 311-312
Logoconia, 78
Long-term care insurance, 364-365
Loop diuretic drugs, 205-206
Loxapine, 173
Loxitane, 173
Luria, A. R., 20-21

M

Magnetic Resonance Imaging, 42-43
Management
    general principles of, 143-148
    goals for, 4-5
Manual dexterity, urinary incontinence and,
        214-215
Maprotiline, 179
Mashed potato syndrome, 97
Mattis Dementia Rating Scale, 30
Meals on Wheels, 355-356
Medical history in clinical diagnosis, 88-90
Medicare hospital insurance (Part A), 363
Medicare supplementary medical insurance (part
        B), 363
Medication. See also Drugs; specific names of
        medication
    review of, 5
    safety/accident prevention, 233-234
    sleep disturbances and, 166, 167
Mellaril, 173
Memory
    declarative, 24
    depression and, 35, 36
    working, 24
Memory aids, 168
Memory impairment, 30, 31
    Alzheimer's disease vs. benign forgetfulness,
        75-76
    as clinical symptom of Alzheimer's disease,
        74-76
    late stages of, 76
Mental status examination, 91, 100-102
    intellectual functioning, 101
    mood, 101
    sensorium, 101
    thinking processes, 101
Mesoridazine, 173

Methylphenidate, 127, 179
Metrifonate, 187
Microtubules, 65-66
Mini-Mental State Examination, 29, 33, 269
    instructions for administration, 91-92
Minnesota Multiphasic Personality Inven-
        tory, 36
Mirtazapine, 179
Moban, 174
Mobility
    assisting patients with difficulty walking, 271-
        272
    incontinence and, 204
    urinary incontinence and, 214
Modified Blessed Dementia Scale, 29-30
Monoamine oxidase inhibitors, 179
Mood, in mental status examination, 101
Multiinfarct dementia, 29, 99, 100, 119
    vs. Alzheimer's disease, 30-31
    case study of, 35
Music, as communication, 157
Myocardial infarction, 107, 109

N

Nail care, 254
National Alzheimer's Safe Return Program, 372
National Institute of Neurological and Commu-
        nicative Disorders and Strokes, 87
Navane, 173
Needs
    patient's, 260
    security, 260
Nefazodone, 179, 181
Neocortex. See also Brain
    characteristics of, 12
    hemispheres of, 12
    lobes of, 12-14
    map of, 12
Nerve cells, 15-20
Nerve growth factor, 190
Neuritic plaque, 61
Neurofibrillary tangles
    discovery of, 55-56
    etiology of, Alzheimer's disease, 65
Neuroleptic, 124, 127
Neurons, 15-20
    cell body of, 15, 17, 18
    function of, 17-20
    gray matter, 16-17
    importance of, 15-16
    senile plaques, 16
    sudden reduction in number of, 105-107
    white matter, 17
Neuropsychological assessment of dementia,
        27-37
    brief cognitive screening tests for, 29-30
    case studies of, 34-36
    clinical differentiation, 30-36
    clinical evaluation procedures, 28-30
    cultural and racial considerations, 28
    emotional factors in, 36-37
    goals of, 27-28

Neurotransmitters, 67, 184
  drugs effects on, 19
  neurons and, 18-20
Neurotrophic factors, etiology of Alzheimer's
    and, 66-68
Nimodipine, 121, 192
Nissl, Franz, 54-55
NMDA receptor strategies, 188-189
  AMPA receptor strategies, 189
  glycine agonists, 189
  NMDA agonists, 188-189
  NMDA receptor antagonists, 189
Nonsteroidal antiinflammatory drugs, 191
Non-threatening words, 155-156
Nootropics, 189-190
Noradrenaline, 19
Normal Pressure Hydrocephalus, 129-130
Nortriptyline, 179
Nurses, in home, 359-360
Nursing homes. See also Dementia care units
  advantage of dementia care units in close
      proximity to conventional, 379
  disadvantages of, 378
  financing, 362
  placement in, 320-321
Nutrition/eating, 255-257
  problems with, 256-257
  terminal care and, 284-286
Nutrition programs, 355-356

O

Occipital lobe, 12, 14
Olanzepine
Olanzepine, 172, 177
Oral care and hygiene, 244-246
  edentulous patients, 245
  patients with dentures, 245-246
  patients with natural teeth, 245
  terminal care and, 279
Orap, 174
Over involvement, caregiver's education and,
    347

P

Pain, aggravation of Alzheimer's disease, 113
Palliative care, definition of, 276
Paralalia, 78
Paranoid thinking, 164
Parietal lobe, 12, 13
Parkinson's disease, 58-59, 100
  dementia due to
    management of, 122-123
    risk factors for, 122
Paroxetine, 180
Paternalism, 288
  ethical issues and, 288, 296
Patients
  activity and exercise, 148
  establishing good communication, 145-146
  interpersonal relationships between caregivers
      and patients, 143-144

Patients—cont'd
  maintaining consistency and routine, 147-148
  maintaining supportive environment, 147
  need for individuality, 144-145
  reaction to treatment program, 272-274
  treating the person, 143-144
Patient Self-Determination Act, 298
Permitil, 173
Perphenazine, 172, 173
Personal care homes, 361
Personality changes, 77, 80
Perusini, Gaetano, 56
Phenelzine, 179
Phenothiazine, 173
Phenylpiperazine, 179
Physical environment
  for dementia care unit, 384-385
  for treatment program, 262-263
Physical restraints. See Restraints
Physician-assisted suicide, 299-301
Physostigmine, sustained-release, 187
Pica, 233
Pick's disease, 128-129
Pimozide, 172, 174
Pinel, Philippe, 53
Pituitary gland, 23
Pneumonia, 100
Poisoning, 232-233
Polarity, as communication, 156
Positioning, 280-282
Positron Emission Tomography, 43-44
Power of attorney, ethical issues and, 6
Presenile dementia, vs. senile dementia, 56-57
Pressure ulcers
  environmental factors, 283-284
  positioning and, 280-282
  skin protection, 282-283
  support surfaces, 283
Problem-solving method of behavior manage-
    ment, 151-153
  defining desired change, 152
  defining problem, 151-152
  evaluation of plan, 153
  plan of action, 152-153
Progressive Supranuclear Palsy, 131-132
Prolixin, 173
Propentoxifilline, 120-121
Protective underpads, 218
Psychoactive drugs, 19

Q

Qualified Medicare beneficiary, 363-364

R

Reagan Institute Initiative, 371
Reality Orientation Therapy (ROT), 267
Redirection, 154
Reminiscing, as communication, 156
Renal functions, impaired function and aggrava-
    tion of Alzheimer's disease, 109-110
Repetitious behaviors, 168-169

Rephrasing, as communication, 156
Research, 58-59
    Alzheimer's Association and, 368-371
    biochemistry/physiology, 394-395
    caregiver stress, 397
    executive functioning/activities of daily living,
        395-396
    genetics, 393-394
    radiography, 395
    Reagan Institute Initiative, 371
    site of care/placement, 396-397
    targeted research grants, 370
    Zenith awards, 370
Respite care, 319
    adult day care, 356-357
    Alzheimer's Association and, 375
Restlessness, 157
    meaning of, 261
Restraints, 114, 158
    aggravation of Alzheimer's disease, 114
    alternatives to, 239
    chemical, 383
    ethical issues and, 297
    incontinence and, 205
    safety and accident prevention, 238-241
    sundowning and, 166
    use of, 238-241
Retirement villages, 360
Rey Auditory Verbal Learning Test, 33
Right hemisphere
    integration of, 15
    specialization of, 14-15
Risk factors, 69
Risperdal, 174
Risperidone, 172, 174, 177
Rorschach, 36
Roswell, Gilbert, 303
Routine, maintaining consistency, 147-148

S

Safe Return Program, 372
Safety/accident prevention, 227-241
    bathing, 247
    becoming lost, 228-229
    considerations in later disease stages, 237-241
    driving car, 227-228, 396
    environmental safety, 237-238
    falls, 231-232
    fire and electrical safety, 229-230
    guns, 237
    heat and cold injuries, 230-231
    medication, 233-234
    poisoning and pica, 232-233
    poor judgment and gullibility, 229
    restraints, 238-241
    wandering, 234-237
Screaming, 159-160
Second victims of Alzheimer's disease, 347
Security, patient's need for, 260
Selegiline hydrochloride, 19

Self Help Alzheimer's Caregivers Training and
        Information (SHACTI), 365-366
Self-neglect, 79-80
Senile dementia
    early history of, 51-53
Senile plaques, 16
    discovery of, 55-56
Senior citizen apartments and condominiums,
        360
Senior citizen centers, 365
Senior Companion Program, 358-359
Sensorium, in mental status examination, 101
Sensory-Perceptual Examination, 33
Serentil, 173
Serotonin, 19
Serotonin Reuptake Inhibitors, 179, 180
    drugs interacting with, 180
Sertraline, 179, 180
Setting limits, 154-155
Sexual behavior
    considerations in patients with Alzheimer's
        disease, 161-162
    elderly and, 161
    inappropriate, 161
        context of, 162
        meaning of, 162
        management of, 163-164
Shaving care, 255
    terminal care and, 279
Shear, 282
Sheltered housing, 360
Single photon emission computer tomography,
        43, 44-46
Skin care
    bathing and, 247
    pressure ulcers
        environmental factors, 283-284
        positioning and, 280-282
        skin protection, 282-283
        support surfaces, 283
    for terminal care and, 280
    urinary incontinence and, 224-225
Sleep deprivation, aggravation of Alzheimer's
        disease, 114
Sleep disturbances, 165-168
    management of, 166-168
    medication and, 166, 167
    sundowning, 166
Social Security, 364
Social services, 354-365
    area agency on aging, 354-355
    case management services, 363
    financing nursing home care, 362
    home health care and in-home services, 358-
        360
    hospice care, 357-358
    housing alternatives, 360-362
    insurance and medical benefits, 363-364
    nutrition programs, 355-356
    respite care, adult day care, 356-357
    transportation services, 362

Spastic bladder, 202
Staff
  in Dementia care units, 380-382
  for treatment program, 264
Stages of Alzheimer's disease, 3, 82, 84-85
  brain function and, 25
  stage 1, 82-83
  stages 2, 82-84
Stelazine, 173
Stimulant drugs, 19, 179-180
Stress
  elder abuse and, 328
  family caregivers, 316-321
    caregiver reactions, 318
    caregiver training, 320
    coping skills, 319
    emotional burden, 317
    male family caregivers, 318
    nursing home placement, 320-321
    over involvement, 347
    pastoral counseling, 321
    physical burden, 317
    respite care, 319
    sickness in caregivers, 318
    support groups, 319-320
  professional caregivers, 321-326
    administrative support, 325-326
    institutional setting, 322-323
    job satisfaction, 323
    personality and, 323
    preventive measures, 324
    staff development, 324
    support groups, 326
    time-out, 325
    workload, 325
Stress incontinence, 201
  characteristics of, 201
Stroke, 100
  aggravating Alzheimer's disease, 105-106
  post-stroke dementia, 119
  risk of, 120
Subacute bacterial endocarditis, 111
Subdural hematoma, 106, 132-133
Suicide, 164-165
Sundowning, 166-168
Support groups, 319-320, 348-352
  Alzheimer's Association and, 371
  benefits of, 349-350
  negative aspects of, 350-352
  for professional caregivers, 326

T
Tachycardia, 108
Tacrine, 185-186
Tacrine hydrochloride, 4
Taractan, 173
Task breakdown, 154, 244
Taste, communication and, 146
Tau protein, 65
Temporal lobe, 12, 14

Terminal care, 276-289
  assessment in, 276-278
  comfort needs, 287-288
  daily care and management of advanced, 277
  definition of, 276
  elimination, 284
  environmental factors, 283-284
  ethical considerations, 288-289
  hospice care, 357-358
  immobility, 286-287
  nutrition and, 284-286
  personal hygiene needs, 277-280
  positioning, 280-282
  skin protection, 282-283
  sleep and rest, 287
  support surfaces, 283
Tetracyclines, 179
Therapy programs, 357
Thienobenzodiazepine, 174
Thinking process, in mental status examination,
    101
Thioridazine, 172, 173
Thiothixene, 172, 173
Thioxanthenes, 173
36-Hour Day, The (Mace & Rabins), 331
Thorazine, 19, 173
Thyroid disease, 70
Toileting, 250-254
  maintaining bowel function, 251
Touch, 382
  as communication, 156
  communication and, 146
Trail Making Test, 33
Transportation services, 362
Trazodone, 179
Treatment programs
  activities
    crafts and work-oriented activities, 265,
      266
    grooming activities, 264
    individual tasks, 266
    physical exercise, 264
    reality orientation therapy, 267
    sample, 265-266
    socialization, 264, 266
    special activities, 267
  caregiver's reaction to, 274
  meaning of aberrant behavior, 260-261
  patient needs, 260
  patient reactions to, 272-274
  patient strengths, 261-262
  program design
    physical environment, 262-263
    staffing, 264
  selection of activities
    assessment scales, 269
    assistance with mobility, 270-271
    functional evaluation, 267-269
    provision of guidance, 270-271
    scheduling, 269-270
Triazolopyridine, 179

Tricyclic antidepressants, 19, 179
Trifluoperazine, 173
Trilafon, 173
Trusts, 313-314

U

Uninhibited bladder, 202
Unstable bladder, 202
Urge incontinence, 202
  characteristics of, 202
Urinals, 216-217
Urinary tract infection, 100
  terminal care and, 284
Urine. *See* incontinence, urinary

V

Valium, 19
Vascular dementia, 117-121
  Binswanger's disease, 118-119
  dementia stage, 120-121
  lacunar, 118
  multiinfarct dementia, 119
  patients with risk factors for vascular, 119-
    120
  post-stroke dementia, 119
  predementia stage, 120
  treatment and prevention, 119
Velnacrine, 187

Venlafaxine, 179, 181
Veterans Affairs Benefits, 364
Vision
  differential diagnosis, 99
  impaired, and aggravation of Alzheimer's dis-
    ease, 112
Visual agnosia, 22
Visuospatial skills, impaired, 78-79
Vocalization, 159-160

W

Walking, assisting patients with difficulty, 271-
    272
Wandering, 384
  becoming lost and safety, 228-229
  I.D. bracelets, 234
  safety/accident prevention, 233-237
Warfarin, 120
Wechsler Adult Intelligence Scale, 31, 33
Wechsler, David, 25
Wechsler Memory Scale Russell Revision, 33
Wills, 312-313
Working memory, 24

Z

Zenith Awards, 370
Zidovudine, 127
Zyprexa, 174